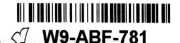
Robert E. C. Wildman, PhD, RD

The Nutritionist
Food, Nutrition,
and Optimal Health

Pre-publication
REVIEWS,
COMMENTARIES,
EVALUATIONS . . .

"*The Nutritionist: Food, Nutrition, and Optimal Health* is refreshing in its approach to the subject. The organization of this text is clear and logical, particularly tables and figures which are self-explanatory without constant reference to the text. A salient defining aspect of this text which separates it from other introductory texts in nutrition is the organization of each chapter. In this book, rather than having the usual academic subheadings as topics, the subheadings are articulated as questions. For instance, the chemical nature of carbohydrates is discussed under the subheading 'Where do carbohydrates come from?'

The manner in which the text is written is user friendly and largely devoid of technical jargon. The major nutrients are discussed in terms of need and how they optimize health and prevent certain diseases. Applications to physical activity, pregnancy, and weight control issues, for example, are discussed from a consumer perspective. The content is accurate and up-to-date. Academicians will find this useful as a text for an introductory nutrition class and nonacademicians will find it useful in their home libraries. The reader of this book will discover significant information for personal use on how to lead a healthy lifestyle."

Denis M. Medeiros, PhD, RD
Professor and Head,
Department of Human Nutrition,
Kansas State University, Manhattan

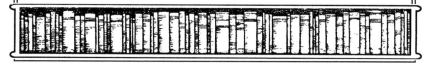

More pre-publication
REVIEWS, COMMENTARIES, EVALUATIONS . . .

"Nutrition is perhaps one of the most confusing topics for students, health professionals, and the general public. A large part of the confusion stems from the fact that nutrition is a relatively `young' field of study and, as such, new information is being generated every day. In *The Nutritionist*, Dr. Wildman has taken a complex topic and distilled it down to its most fundamental elements—the result being a highly useful and easy-to-understand overview of nutrition from theory, to science, to practice. *The Nutritionist* uses a friendly question and answer format to focus the reader on the primary elements necessary for understanding first the basic concepts of general nutrition and then the subtler nuances of nutrition and health. Using this format, *The Nutritionist* provides value for nonscience majors with an interest in nutrition as well as for science majors looking for practical nutrition knowledge."

Shawn M. Talbott, PhD
Senior Scientist,
Pharmacology and Clinical Affairs,
Pharmanex, LLC,
Provo, UT

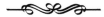

"This book will certainly be of interest and use to the general public as well as an introductory course in nutrition with no prerequisites. The book covers the basics and later uses and integrates this information to discuss topics such as exercise nutrition, lifespan nutrition, and nutrition and disease. It covers not only material on nutrition for our well-being but also nutrition to enhance the quality of our lives. The text is amply complemented with easily understood tables and figures. Dr. Wildman writes in a snappy, yet authoritative, style. He gives us much food for thought."

Ira Wolinsky, PhD
Professor of Nutrition,
University of Houston, TX

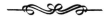

"This book would be a very good text for use in an introduction to nutrition course, and an excellent text for a general education requirements (nonmajor) class in nutrition. The text will also be very helpful for professionals engaged in the fitness and wellness areas (for example, personal trainers). It also would be very digestible for the layperson wanting to learn more about nutrition and how it affects the human body.

The question/answer style of the text makes it easy to read and engages the reader. The introductory chapters do a nice job of laying the groundwork for later discussions. In general, it is a very nice read for understanding the 'nuts and bolts' of human nutrition while still including more technical information. It also presents nutrition information relative to the lifespan, which will reach a broader audience."

Barry Miller, PhD
Assistant Director, Recreation;
Assistant Professor, Department
of Health and Exercise Science,
University of Delaware,
Newark

More pre-publication
REVIEWS, COMMENTARIES, EVALUATIONS . . .

"Dr. Wildman has truly compiled a one-stop primer into the basic chemistry, biology, and physiology related to human nutrition. He has presented a most excellent and painless description of human nutrition along with an outstanding complement of figures and tables to further aid in one's understanding. In fact, the title of this book is most appropriate, since Dr. Wildman presents the information as answers to commonly asked questions. He has demonstrated the admirable quality of synthesizing difficult material and concepts into straightforward and comprehensive explanations. After presenting a general, but thorough, overview of the science of nutrition, he demonstrates the application of these concepts in exercise and sport, the life cycle, and in disease states. His description of nutritional factors and their role in cardiovascular disease and cancer are particularly pertinent in a society where these disease states are leading causes of death. Along the way, he addresses popular nutritional myths and misconceptions with scientific evidence and sound nutritional advice.

In reality, this text allows anyone from the student to the enthusiast to learn the basics of nutrition without years of schooling. In Dr. Wildman's text, the science of nutrition is packaged for ready consumption. This book should be mandatory reading for every basic nutrition course and for every dietary program. An excellent reflection of his scientific understanding and his teaching capabilities."

Arny A. Ferrando, PhD
Associate Professor, Surgery, Metabolism,
Shriners Hospital for Children,
Galveston, TX

"I wish I could persuade everyone who wants to learn about nutrition to read this book instead of picking up one of the many popular books published every year that are full of gimmicks, hype, and self-promotion. In one comprehensive text, Dr. Robert Wildman presents modern nutrition science in a user-friendly package suitable for those with a personal interest and beyond. The major strength of this book is the deft use of examples and analogies to both entertain and educate readers while maintaining an easy-to-read and personalized writing style. In fact, reading this book feels like having a one-on-one conversation with the author.

Readers, you will learn about nutrition as it truly is, a science residing at the interface between biology, chemistry, and medicine. Best of all, a background in science isn't required as *The Nutritionist* does a splendid job of explaining any relevant science that comes up in the reading. You will find tools in this book that will empower you to make important decisions regarding optimal health and disease prevention. If you want to learn more about nutrition and health, then this book is for you."

Thunder Jalili, PhD
Director of Nutrition Science,
Division of Foods and Nutrition,
University of Utah

The Nutritionist
*Food, Nutrition,
and Optimal Health*

THE HAWORTH PRESS
Nutrition, Exercise, Sports, and Health
Robert E. C. Wildman, PhD, RD, LD
Senior Editor

The Nutritionist: Food, Nutrition, and Optimal Health by Robert Wildman

A Guide to Understanding Dietary Supplements: Magic Bullets or Modern Snake Oil? by Shawn M. Talbott

Fragments: Coping with Attention Deficit Disorder by Amy Stein

The Nutritionist
Food, Nutrition, and Optimal Health

Robert E. C. Wildman, PhD, RD

The Haworth Press®
New York • London • Oxford

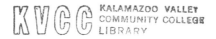

© 2002 by The Haworth Press, Inc. All rights reserved. No part of this work may be reproduced or utilized in any form or by any means, electronic or mechanical, including photocopying, microfilm, and recording, or by any information storage and retrieval system, without permission in writing from the publisher. Printed in the United States of America.

The Haworth Press, Inc., 10 Alice Street, Binghamton, NY 13904-1580.

Cover design by Jennifer M. Gaska.

Library of Congress Cataloging-in-Publication Data

Wildman, Robert E. C., 1964-
  The nutritionist : food, nutrition, and optimal health / Robert Wildman.
    p. cm.
  Includes bibliographical references and index.
  ISBN 0-7890-1478-5 (alk. paper) — ISBN 0-7890-1479-3 (alk. paper)
  1. Nutrition. I. Title.

QP141 .W487 2002
613.2—dc21

2001051469

CONTENTS

ABOUT THE AUTHOR

Robert Wildman, PhD, RD, is Associate Professor in the Nutrition Program at the University of Louisiana at Lafayette. He has published numerous research articles and is co-author of *Advanced Human Nutrition* and *Sport & Fitness Nutrition* and editor of *The Handbook of Nutraceuticals and Functional Foods*. His forthcoming books include *Dr. Wildman's Sport, Fitness, and Nutrition* and *The DNA Diet*. Dr. Wildman is co-editor of the *Journal of Nutraceuticals, Functional & Medical Foods*. His current research efforts involve cardiovascular and exercise performance aspects of nutrition. He provides seminars throughout the world. For more information on the author, please visit <www.ucs.Louisiana.edu/~rew5073> and <www.Dr.Wildman.com> or <www.athletefactory.net>.

Preface

The seeming simplicity of our daily activities is greatly contrasted by the complexity of our true nature—quite a paradox, no doubt. We appear simple in that, on the outside, the goals of our body may appear few. We internalize food, water, and oxygen, while at the same time ridding ourselves of carbon dioxide and other waste materials. These operations support reproduction, growth, maintenance, and defense. Yet on the inside our body seems very complex, as various organs participate in a tremendous number of complicated processes intended to meet the simple goals previously mentioned.

Nutrition is just one part of the paradoxical relationship mentioned. The objective of nutrition is simple: to supply our body with all of the necessary nutrients, and in appropriate quantities, to promote optimal health and function. However, in practice, nutrition is far from that simple. Too many nutrients, controversial nutrients, and different conditions such as growth, pregnancy, and exercise are involved to allow nutrition to be a simple topic.

Although we have long appreciated food, it has only been in more recent years that we have really begun to understand the finer relationship between food and our body. Most nutrients have been identified only within the past century or so, and right now nutrition is one of the most prevalent areas of scientific research. However, our understanding of nutrition is by no means complete. It continues to evolve in conjunction with the most current nutrition research. Discoveries in nutrition occur seemingly on a weekly basis.

Just a few decades ago the *basic four* food groups were pretty much all the nutrition information known by the average American. Today, nutrition deeply penetrates many aspects of our lives including preventative and treatment medicine, philosophy, exercise training, and weight management. Diet has been linked to cardiovascular health, cancer, bowel function, moods, and brain activity, along with many other health domains. Humans no longer eat merely to satisfy hunger. Nutrition has become a matter of great curiosity and/or concern for most of us today.

A few problems have developed along with this most recent illumination of nutrition. One such problem is that we may have generated too much knowledge too fast. Even though we, as humans, have been eating throughout our existence, the importance of proper nutrition seems to have been thrust upon us suddenly. We did not have time to first wade into the waters of nutrition science, slowly increasing our depth. The reality is that we may be in over our heads, barely treading water to keep up with the latest recommendations. Sometimes, all we can do is try our best to follow the latest nutrition recommendations without really having the background or accessibility to proper resources to truly understand the reasons behind the recommendations.

Although nutrition has become a very complex subject, many authors still try to present it in an oversimplified manner. Perhaps they believe that people are not interested in the scientific details and merely wish to be told what to do. This book attempts to break that pattern. We will spend time laying a foundation with some of the basic concepts of science and the body in hope that this effort will make nutrition a simpler subject.

I believe that deep down a scientist lurks within each of us. Every day we ponder the effects of certain actions before performing them. This is the so-called *cause and effect* relationship, the very basis of scientific experimentation. Furthermore, since most of us give at least some thought to the foods we eat, humans are all a special breed of scientist. We are nutrition scientists! A nutrition scientist is one who ponders the relationship between food components and the body. One does not have to work in a laboratory to be a nutrition scientist. All one needs is simple curiosity and the dedication of his or her time to pursue a greater understanding of nutrition. This book is written in a question and answer format to satisfy the reader's curiosity.

Fundamental questions regarding nutrition and our body will be posed and then answered based upon the most current research. If your educational background includes a solid foundation of biology and chemistry you may wish to skip the first few chapters. However, if your science background is weak or far in the past, you may find the first few chapters of service. So, here we go. Good luck and good science!

Acknowledgments

The author wishes to acknowledge the following people for their knowing or unknowing participation in the development of this book: my family, the Hamiltons, all of the Beems, the faculty of the College of Applied Life Sciences at the University of Louisiana, my mentors, Dr. Denis Medeiros and Dr. Bruce Rengers, and the background sounds of dada, Pink Floyd, Neil Young, Alice in Chains, GD, and Metallica.

The author would also like to acknowledge the following facilities and people for their assistance in the development of *The Nutritionist*. Research assistants: Carol Haas, Melissa Guillory, Jody Williams, Jennifer Gautreaux, Denise Darjean, Gena LeMaire, Dolly Zeringue, Dani Marsh, Jennifer Zimmerman, Sara Myers, Christine Lister, and Charity Humphrey. Exercise photo models: Mark Doyle, Noelle LeJeune, Ashley Martin, and Barrett Richard. Facilities: Red Lerille's Health and Racquet Club, Lafayette, Louisiana, and the Exercise Laboratory of the Department of Kinesiology at the University of Louisiana at Lafayette.

Chapter 1

The Very Basics of Humans
and the World We Inhabit

OUR MOST BASIC OBJECTIVES

We humans are just one of millions of different species inhabiting this planet. Like our planetmates we must abide by the basic objectives of life. These are to

1. function independently or self-operate,
2. defend ourselves (externally and internally),
3. nourish ourselves, and
4. reproduce, which is without question the ultimate objective.

Yet we humans enjoy a relatively massive brain and intellectual capability. This quality allows us to try to understand ourselves and in accordance how to nourish ourselves.

What is nutrition?

We will start out as simple as possible. The shortest definition for nutrition is the science pertaining to the factors involved in nourishing our body. Nutrition hinges upon the special relationship between our body and the environment that we inhabit. It is this environment that dictates our nourishment needs as well as provides the substances that will do the nourishing. These nourishing substances are called *nutrients,* which are chemicals that are used by our body for energy or other human processes.

From the moment of conception to the waning hours of advanced age, we find ourselves in a continuum to nourish our body. Nourishment supports body businesses such as growth, movement, immunity, injury and disease recovery, and, of course, the ultimate business at hand for all life-forms, reproduction. All that we are, ever were, or are going to be is actually borrowed from the environment that we inhabit. This unique state of indebtedness is primarily attributed to our nutrition intake.

We must be grateful to the earth's crust for lending us minerals that strengthen our bones and teeth and allow us to be electrical. We must also pay homage to plants for the carbohydrate forms that power our operations and for the amino acids that make the protein in our muscle.

All too often we do not truly appreciate the relevance of nutrition to our basic being. But again, please keep in mind that nearly everything we are and are able to do is either a direct or indirect reflection of our past and current nutrition intake. No matter how oversimplified nutrition may seem in television commercials and on cereal boxes, it is without a doubt one of the most complex and interesting sciences out there.

How do we begin to understand nutrition?

Certainly any great building must be constructed upon a solid foundation. So let us go ahead and commit ourselves to building our own scientific foundation for nutrition as well. Before we try to learn how to nourish our body we should have a better understanding of what needs to be nourished. Our body is the product of nature and being so it must adhere to the basic laws of nature. In fact, the science of nutrition is really an offspring science, with chemistry and biology being the proud parents. Therefore, understanding the whats, whys, and hows of nutrition will be a lot easier once a few basic areas of chemistry and biology are appreciated. Following are some basic principles of chemistry and biology and a description of their relevance to nutrition and the body.

ATOMS AND MOLECULES MAKE THE HUMAN, NOT CLOTHES

What is the most basic composition of our body?

Let's say that we had access to fancy laboratory equipment capable of determining the most fundamental composition of an object. If we used this equipment to assess a person it would spit out data on our most basic level of composition, *elements*. Elements are substances that cannot be broken down into other substances. Scientists have determined that there are 100 or so of these elements in nature. Some of the more recognizable elements include carbon, oxygen, hydrogen, nitrogen, iron, zinc, copper, chromium, calcium, nickel, silver, aluminum, helium, gold, sodium, potassium, and chlorine. All of the elements known to exist can be found on the Periodic Table of Elements, which we have all come across at one point or another in our schooling. A Periodic Table of Elements is included as Appendix A in case you feel the need for another peek. Now, imagine, if you will, that everything that you can think of is merely a skillful combination of these same elements. This includes cars, boats, buildings, clouds, oceans, trees, and of course our body. In fact, our body employs about twenty-seven of the elements (see Table 1.1 and Appendix A).

The great Carl Sagan in his personal exploration of the cosmos believed that we are made up of the stuff of stars. He was alluding that our body is made up of many of the very same elements that make up planets and other celestial bodies in the universe. We humans as well as other life-forms on our planet have simply borrowed these ele-

TABLE 1.1. Elements of Our Body

Major Elements	% of Body Weight	Minor Elements	% of Body Weight
Oxygen (O)	63.0	Iron (Fe)	< 0.1
Carbon (C)	18.0	Selenium (Se)	< 0.1
Hydrogen (H)	9.0	Copper (Cu)	< 0.1
Nitrogen (N)	3.0	Cobalt (Co)	< 0.1
Calcium (Ca)	1.5	Fluorine (F)	< 0.1
Phosphorus (P)	1.0	Iodine (I)	< 0.1
Potassium (K)	0.4	Molybdenum (Mo)	< 0.1
Sulfur (S)	0.3	Manganese (Mn)	< 0.1
Sodium (Na)	0.2	Vanadium (V)	< 0.1
Chlorine (Cl)	0.2	Chromium (Cr)	< 0.1
Magnesium (Mg)	0.1	Boron (B)	< 0.1
		Zinc (Zn)	< 0.1
		Aluminum (Al)	< 0.1
		Tin (Sn)	< 0.1
		Silicon (Si)	< 0.1
		Arsenic (As)	< 0.1

ments. Interestingly, four of these elements, namely oxygen, carbon, hydrogen, and nitrogen, make up greater than 90 percent of our body weight. Since the majority of these elements are found in our body as part of substances such as water, proteins, carbohydrates, fats, and nucleic acids (DNA and RNA), it only makes sense that these substances must be the major chemicals of our body. For example, a lean, young adult male's body weight may be approximately 62 percent water, 16 percent protein, 16 percent fat, and < 1 percent carbohydrate. Most of his remaining weight (about 5 percent) would be attributed to minerals. We will spend a lot more time talking about the finer details of body composition in later chapters.

What is the relationship between elements and atoms?

Atoms are the building blocks of everything that exists. From the clothes on your back to the car you drive to the food you eat—everything is comprised of atoms. Each individual atom belongs to only one element. This is to say that even though there are an incomprehensible number of atoms on this planet and the universe making up everything we know and are yet to know, all of these atoms belong to only one of 100 or so elements (see Appendix A). This is similar to each one of the billions of people living on this planet being native to only one of a hundred or so countries.

In a world where size is judged relative to the size of humans, the size of the atom is indeed miniscule. It has been said that if we could line up a million atoms end to end they would barely cover the distance across the period that follows this sentence. However, they do indeed exist even though you cannot see them with the naked eye.

All atoms have a similar blueprint to the image displayed in Figure 1.1. There are three principal particles called *neutrons, protons,* and *electrons.* Because they are smaller than the atom that they come together to form, they are often called *subatomic* particles. Two of these particles (protons and neutrons) are found in the tightly packed center region of the atom, referred to as the *nucleus,* which literally means "the center." Protons bear a positive charge (+). Meanwhile, neutrons do not bear any charge at all and are thus deemed neutral. Revolving around the nucleus of the atom at the speed of light is the third type of subatomic particle, the electron. Electrons bear a negative charge (−). By design, there are the same number of electrons revolving around

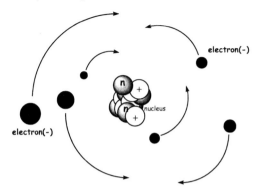

FIGURE 1.1. This is a carbon atom. Protons (white [+]) and neutrons (shaded [n]) are in the nucleus. Electrons (black [–]) orbit the nucleus at the speed of light.

the nucleus as there are protons within the nucleus. This balances the *net charge* of the atom.

We classify an atom as belonging to a specific element based on the number of protons it has. In fact, the Periodic Table organizes the elements in order of increasing proton number. Hydrogen atoms have only one proton; helium atoms have two protons; carbon six; calcium twenty; and so forth. Again, the general design of an atom is to have an equal number of electrons as protons, thereby "balancing" the electrical charge, creating a neutral atom. Meanwhile, the number of neutrons can vary for a given atom.

It is the electrons that generally dictate how atoms will behave in relation to one another. Electrons are the interacting portion or "business portion" of an atom and will be involved in many nutrition aspects to follow.

Is it possible for certain atoms to become charged?

Atoms of certain elements do possess the ability to lose or gain electrons. Since electrons bear a negative charge, this results in the development of a net electrical charge on that atom. It is a matter of simple algebra. If an atom gives up an electron, it will develop a single positive charge (1^+). This is shown in Figure 1.2. If an atom concedes two electrons it will develop a double positive charge (2^+). On the contrary, if an atom gains an electron, it develops a single negative

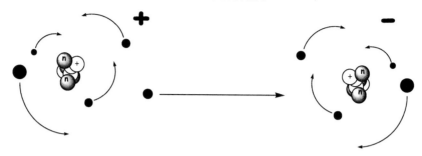

FIGURE 1.2. An electron is lost by the atom on the left (yielding a positive charge) and gained by the atom on the right (yielding a negative charge).

charge $(1-)$ and if an atom gains two electrons it develops a double negative charge $(2-)$. Charged atoms (and molecules) are called *ions*.

The processes of losing and gaining electrons are interrelated, as is also displayed in Figure 1.2. As one atom gains an electron, it is actually removing the electron from another atom which was willing to donate it. This activity is referred to as *oxidation* and *reduction*. Oxidation refers to the loss of an electron while reduction refers to the gain of an electron. Perhaps you were thinking that this may have something to do with antioxidant (antioxidation) nutrients, such as vitamins C and E and a whole host of others such as beta-carotene and lycopene. Well, were you? If you were, then you are accurate in your thought and have the mind of a scientist. We will get to free radicals and begin to talk about antioxidant protection later in this chapter. Also, you may have heard the term oxidation in reference to energy operations in our body (e.g., oxidation of fat). Again, you would be on the right track. But we are getting ahead of ourselves.

Many elements important to nutrition and the proper functioning of our body exist naturally in a charged state. These elements include sodium, chlorine, potassium, iodine, magnesium, and calcium. The charge associated with an atom will be displayed in superscript next to the element's symbol. As a rule, sodium (Na^+) and potassium (K^+) will give up one electron, while calcium (Ca^{2+}) and magnesium (Mg^{2+}) will give up two electrons. On the contrary, chlorine (Cl^-), flourine (F^-), and iodine (I^-) will take an electron from another atom. Actually, we tend to refer to chlorine, fluoride, and iodine as chloride, fluoride, and iodide with respect to this electrical state. Some of these charged atoms are commonly referred to as *electrolytes* because of their electrical state and properties, which will be discussed later on as well.

How do atoms combine with each other?

A couple millennia ago, the Greeks believed that water was one of the four elements of nature, along with fire, air, and earth, and that all things were made from combinations of these elements. Today, we of course know that there are a hundred or so basic elements. In fact, water is not a single element but a combination of atoms of two elements, hydrogen (H) and oxygen (O). When two or more atoms of the same or different elements combine together, *molecules* are formed. Therefore, water is a molecule. The chemical formula for a water molecule (H_2O) is probably the most widely quoted of all *chemical formulas*. A chemical formula is merely a molecule's element recipe. Thus, for each molecule of water, two hydrogen atoms (subscript 2 behind H) are bound to one oxygen atom (no subscript, so 1 is implied).

From our previous description of the size of atoms you can imagine then that an ordinary glass of water must contain millions of H_2O molecules. In fact, we can use water to tidy up our understanding of elements, atoms, and molecules. If we have an 8 ounce (oz) glass of pure water, we can say that the container is accommodating millions of molecules of water, and thus millions of atoms; however, only two elements are present, oxygen and hydrogen.

In general, atoms can link together or *bond* by two means. First, charged atoms can interact with oppositely charged atoms. Remember, as in so many aspects of life, opposites attract. Perhaps the best example of this kind of bonding is sodium chloride (NaCl) or common table salt. Here, the negatively charged chloride ions (Cl^-) are attracted and electrically stick to positively charged sodium ions (Na^+). You can also check your toothpaste for sodium fluoride (NaF) or toothpaste salt. By the way, the term *salt* is actually a general term that describes these types of electrical interactions.

$Na^+ \nearrow Cl^-$ $Na^+ \nearrow F^-$

sodium chloride (table salt)   **sodium fluoride (toothpaste salt)**

Another way that atoms can bond with each other is by sharing electrons. This is a fascinating event whereby atoms share electrons between them to form a stable union. In Figure 1.3 and throughout

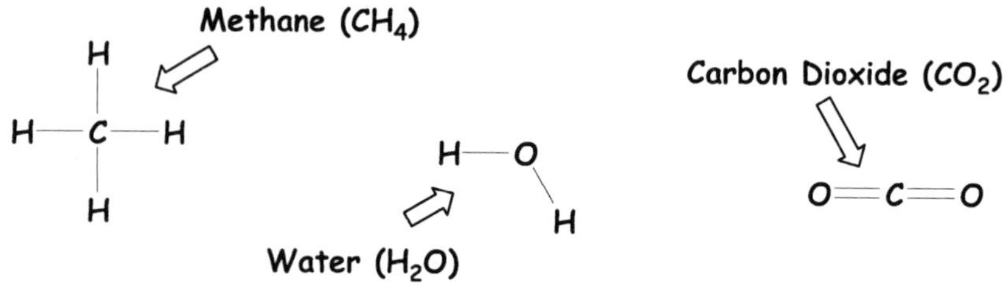

Methane (CH₄)

FIGURE 1.3. Methane and carbon dioxide are organic molecules while water is not.

this book you will see a straight line connecting atoms that are bonded in this manner. Probably the best examples of this type of bonding are the so-called *organic* molecules, which refers to those molecules that are based on carbon atoms. Organic also refers to that which is living. Therefore, the most important molecules of life must be carbon based. In fact, a large portion of this book discusses organic molecules, such as proteins, carbohydrates, fats, cholesterol, nucleic acids, and vitamins. These are all carbon-based substances.

What is the design of molecules?

One limitation of an ink-and-paper representation of molecules is that it often fails to truly capture the three-dimensional beauty of molecules. For example, DNA molecules exist in a spiral staircase design, while many protein molecules appear to be all bunched (or globbed) up. The three-dimensional design of a molecule helps determine what that molecule can do (its properties). Furthermore, we will see that many of the important molecules in our body are actually combinations of smaller molecules. For instance, proteins are made from amino acids, and fat molecules are made from fatty acids and glycerol.

How do molecules interact with one another?

Molecules in our body, or anywhere else in nature, can mingle among one another. If things are right, they can also interact. When molecules interact the process is called a *chemical reaction*. For instance, in the reaction below, A and B are substances that react *(reactants)*. As a result of this chemical reaction different substances are produced *(products),* namely, C and D. In a more realistic reaction, carbon dioxide (CO_2) reacts with water to form carbohydrate ($C_6H_{12}O_6$) and oxygen (O_2). This is photosynthesis, the process whereby plants make carbohydrates.

$$A + B \longrightarrow C + D$$
$$\text{or}$$
$$6\ CO_2 + 6\ H_2O \longrightarrow C_6H_{12}O_6 + 6\ O_2$$

The reaction arrow ($\longrightarrow$) separating the reactants and products merely shows which way the chemical reaction will proceed. A reaction may proceed in only one direction or it may be reversible, whereby the reaction will proceed in either direction. A reversible-reaction arrow looks like you might expect: $\longleftrightarrow$. If there is a number (coefficient) in front of reacting or produced substances this merely tells us how many molecules of a substance must react or be produced in order for the chemical reaction to make sense or be "balanced."

What are enzymes?

Life itself would be impossible without *enzymes*. Enzymes are proteins whose job is to regulate and accelerate most chemical reactions. You may remember from a high school or college chemistry lab that when you performed an experiment using two or more chemicals, another chemical was often added to help the reaction to take place or to speed it up. That chemical was an enzyme.

Enzymes are called *catalysts,* meaning they speed up the rate of a reaction between two or more chemicals. A given chemical reaction between two chemicals may take place without an enzyme, but the rate of the reaction may be incredibly slow. It might take hours, days, weeks, or even years to happen. This would be simply unacceptable, as the proper functioning of our body may require that same chemical reaction to take place numerous times in a fraction of a second. So enzymes speed up the rate at which chemical reactions occur. Another important feature of enzymes is that they are extremely specific. Most enzymes will work on only one reaction, just as a unique key will fit into a certain lock.

Is it possible for chemical reactions to be linked together?

In various situations in our body, many chemical reactions actually occur in series. One or more products of a chemical reaction become reactants in the next chemical reaction as part of a series. These reaction series are more commonly referred to as *pathways,* as depicted in Figure 1.4. We will discuss many pathways throughout our exploration.

ENERGY IS EVERYTHING

What is energy?

Energy may be best understood as a potential or presence that allows for some type of work to be performed. Some of energy's more recognizable forms are heat, light, mechanical, chemical, and electrical energy. Without energy we would not exist, and the universe if it existed would be a frigid, barren, motionless void.

According to the laws of thermodynamics, energy can be neither created nor destroyed. However, energy can be converted from one form to another. The total amount of energy in the universe remains constant while the quantity of the different forms can change relative to one another. For instance, you are probably reading this book by the light of a nearby lamp. Take a moment and turn off the lamp. Without touching the bulb, look at the thin filament inside. The filament transforms the electrical energy running from the wall socket and through the cord and eventually along the filament in the bulb into two other forms of energy—light and heat. As the filament illuminates, there is a reduction in electrical energy and an increase in

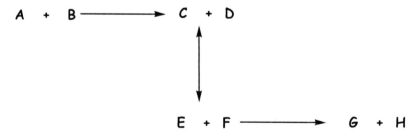

FIGURE 1.4. Here A and B are the initial reactants and G and H are the end products of the pathway.

light and heat energies. So energy is not lost but transformed to other forms.

A little bit closer to nutrition, food contains chemical energy in the form of carbohydrates, proteins, fats, and alcohol. Once inside our body the chemical energy of these substances can be transformed into mechanical energy to power muscular movement and other activities as well as heat to maintain our body temperature. Furthermore, we can store these energy molecules when we cannot immediately use them.

Is energy involved in chemical reactions?

In general, two types of chemical reactions take place—those that release energy *(energy releasing)* and those that require the input of energy *(energy requiring)*. When a chemical reaction takes place, the bonds between atoms are disrupted. This process releases energy as shown in Figure 1.5. Some of the released energy can be harnessed to create the new bonds found in the product(s).

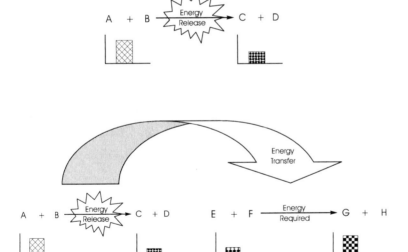

FIGURE 1.5. (Top) Energy is released from this chemical reaction. The bar graphs below the reactants and products present the energy in the bonds. There is less energy in the products thus energy was released in this reaction. (Bottom) Energy released by the first chemical reaction is utilized in the second chemical reaction.

If the energy associated with the bonds of the products is less than the energy associated with the initial energy in the reactants bonds, then the reaction can proceed without a need for outside energy input. In this situation, the fate of the leftover energy depends on whether the energy-releasing reaction was coupled with an energy-requiring reaction. In energy-requiring reactions, where the energy associated with the bonds of the products is greater than the energy associated with the reactants, the energy input is derived from a energy-releasing reaction coupled to it (see Figure 1.5).

Beyond those chemical reactions that either release or require appreciable amounts of energy there are many chemical reactions that take place without a release of or requirement for energy. Here the energy associated with the bonds of the reactants and products of chemical reactions is the same. These would be the reversible reactions we discussed earlier, where one enzyme catalyzes the reaction in both directions.

How does food energy become our body's energy?

On a daily basis we acquire energy from foods in the form of carbohydrates, protein, fat, and alcohol. However, we cannot directly use these molecules for energy. These substances must first engage in chemical reaction pathways that allow for us to capture their endowed energy in a form that we can use. Generally, when energy molecules are broken down some of their energy is captured in so-called "high-energy molecules." By far, the most important high-energy molecule is *adenosine triphosphate* or, more commonly, ATP. Figure 1.6 displays a simplified version of ATP. When energy is needed to power an event in our body an enzyme breaks the bonds between the phosphates releasing energy, which can be utilized to power that event. If ATP was "A" in Figure 1.5 (bottom) then its energy would be used in building new molecules in our body.

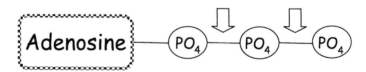

FIGURE 1.6. Adenosine triphosphate (ATP) is the principal "high-energy molecule" in our body. A lot of energy is harnessed in the bonds (arrows) between the phosphates (PO_4).

Interestingly, not all of the energy released in the breakdown of carbohydrates, protein, fat, and alcohol is incorporated in ATP. It has been estimated that we are able to capture only about 40 to 45 percent of the chemical energy available in those molecules in the form of ATP. The remaining 55 to 60 percent of the energy is converted to heat, which helps us maintain our body temperature (see Figure 1.7). The final product of the chemical reaction pathways involving carbohydrates, proteins, fat, and alcohol is primarily carbon dioxide (CO_2), which we then must exhale, and water (H_2O), which helps keep our body hydrated.

If we bear witness to the ATP molecule, we notice what looks like a *phosphate* tail (see Figure 1.6). Phosphate is made up of phosphorus (P) bonded to oxygen (O) and, as indicated in its name, ATP contains three phosphates. The energy liberated during the breakdown of energy nutrients is used to link phosphates together to make ATP. These phosphate links are thus little storehouses of energy. When energy is needed, special enzymes in our cells are able to break the links between adjacent phosphate groups. This releases the energy stored within that link, which can be harnessed to drive a nearby - *energy-requiring* reaction or process.

WATER SOLUBILITY DETERMINES HOW CHEMICALS ARE TREATED IN OUR BODY

Why do some things dissolve in water while others do not?

On the average, adults will maintain about 60 percent of their body weight as water. Since water is the predominant substance in the body, it is important to understand how other substances interact with

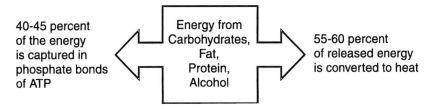

FIGURE 1.7. Only about 40 to 45 percent of the energy released from carbohydrates, protein, fat, and alcohol is captured in the phosphate bonds of ATP and other high-energy molecules; the remaining energy is converted to heat.

it. What we are really talking about is a substance's ability or inability to dissolve into water.

If a substance dissolves easily into water it is referred to as *water soluble*. Conversely, if a substance does not dissolve into water it is referred to as *water insoluble*. As a general rule, water-insoluble substances will dissolve in lipid substances, such as oil (fat). Therefore, we can call these substances either water insoluble, lipid soluble, or fat soluble. Examples of water insolubility are often obvious. We have all been frustrated by the inability of traditional salad dressings, such as vinegar and oil, to stay together and not separate into two layers. We have also witnessed oil tanker spills whereby the oil does not dissolve into the body of water but rather forms a layer on top of the water, posing a threat to the aquatic life. As many water-insoluble substances, such as the oil from the tanker or in the salad dressing, are less dense than water, they tend to float.

The key to understanding water solubility requires a closer look at the bonds between hydrogen and oxygen atoms in a water molecule. As Figure 1.8 demonstrates, two very small hydrogen atoms share electrons with one relatively large oxygen atom. Hydrogen atoms have but one proton in their nucleus, while oxygen atoms have eight protons. As a result, oxygen tends to pull the shared electrons closer

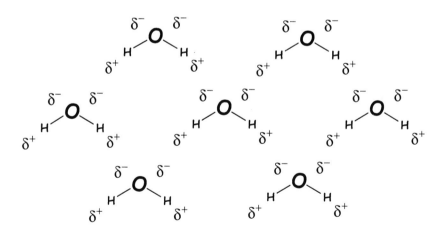

FIGURE 1.8. Water molecules are attracted to one another and other charged chemicals because of the partial positive charges on the H atoms and partial negative charges on the O atoms.

to it because it has a greater positive charge in its nucleus. This leaᵤ to a partial negative charge associated with oxygen atoms and a partial positive charge associated with hydrogen atoms. It is an electron tug-of-war, with hydrogen atoms having a weaker pulling force. It is important to see that the charges that develop are not full charges, as the electrons are technically still being shared. The charge is only a partial charge and will be designated with the Greek lowercase letter delta in superscript (δ^+ or δ^-).

Therefore, water is somewhat electrical in nature. Partially charged water molecule atoms can then interact with other water molecules due to opposite charge attraction. This is the glue that holds water together. This glue helps us understand the concept of surface tension, especially when the water level exceeds the capacity of a glass. The water molecules at the top of the glass are attracted to the other water molecules beneath them and they sort of hold on electrically, which keeps the too-full glass from overflowing, to a point.

Since atoms in a water molecule bear partial charges it only makes sense that they can interact with other substances that have a charge. This includes sodium (Na^+), potassium (K^+), and chloride (Cl^-). When these atoms (and other charged chemicals) are dissolved in water, the resulting fluid is able to carry an electric current. Scientists began to refer to them as *electrolytes* which means "electricity loving." Sodium and chloride are the electrolytes in sports drinks such as POWERade. These beverages are often called fluid and electrolyte replacements.

Lipids, such as fats and cholesterol, do not have a significant charge and as a result they are water insoluble. The partial charges of water atoms do not find lipid molecules electrically attractive. Therefore, the two substances do not mix. Or, from another perspective, the partial charges of water molecules are more attracted to water and other charged substances and basically ignore lipid substances.

Since lipid molecules fail to dissolve into water, they tend to clump together. As mentioned previously, because lipids are generally less dense than water, they tend to sit on top of water. This explains why some salad dressings separate with the oil on top. Also, it explains why oil spills lay on top of water and can be cleaned up by using a corralling device called a boom.

ACIDS AND BASES CONTRIBUTE
TO THE CHEMISTRY LAB OF OUR BODY

What are acids and bases?

The world is filled with *acids* and their counterparts, *bases*. These substances are in our foods and beverages, as well as throughout nature. An acid is any molecule that has the potential to release a hydrogen ion (H^+) when mixed into a water-based fluid. Therefore, when an acid is added to water, the free-hydrogen-ion content of the water will probably increase. Conversely, a base is any substance that when dissolved in water will bind free hydrogen ions also dissolved in the water-based fluid. A base will decrease the concentration of free hydrogen ions in that fluid. Therefore, acids and bases are opposites.

So we see that *acidity* simply refers to the amount of free hydrogen ions dissolved in water or a water-based fluid. Our body can be considered a container of water-based fluid, and, as will become more obvious soon enough, the concentration of hydrogen ions in our body fluid will greatly influence function and health.

How do we measure acidity or alkalinity?

Acidity, or alkalinity (basicity) for that matter, is measured on a basis of the hydrogen ion concentration on what is called the pH scale. The pH scale ranges from 0 to 14, with 0 being the most acidic and 14 being the most basic. Thus, a pH of 7 is said to be neutral because it splits the two extremes. The more acidic a fluid is the greater the hydrogen ion concentration and the lower the pH. The pH scale was conceived by Sören Sörensen who was a pretty good biochemist and an excellent brewer of beer! (So I am told.)

Back in the days before sophisticated pH meters, one could speculate as to whether a fluid was acidic or basic based on taste. Acidic substances tend to have a sour taste (lemon juice, orange juice), while more alkaline substances taste bitter.

So what is the big deal about pH? Our body has but a narrow pH range at which it can function appropriately. As noted on the scale in Figure 1.9, the pH of our circulating blood is about 7.4. This means that the pH of our body is slightly basic. If the pH falls below or above 7.4 these conditions are referred to as *acidosis* and *alkalosis,* respectively. Nearly all chemical reactions in our body are catalyzed by en-

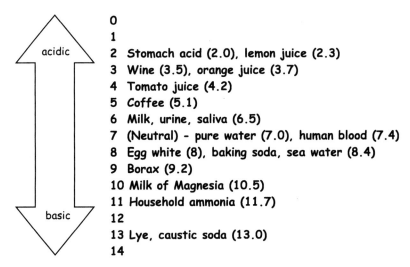

FIGURE 1.9. The pH of common substances, including human blood (7.4).

zymes, most of which function in our best interest at a pH around 7.4. Thus, when our pH falls or climbs, the efficiency of many enzymes is significantly affected. This can compromise normal function and possibly our vitality.

Inherent to our body are systems that help us maintain the pH of our body fluid (e.g., blood) around 7.4. These systems are called *buffering systems* and they act either to soak up excessive H^+ or to release H^+ when pH is subject to change. Thus pH can be maintained at the 7.4 ideal despite changing internal factors.

FREE RADICALS ARE BIOLOGICAL BULLIES; ANTIOXIDANTS ARE CELLULAR SUPERHEROES

What are free radicals and antioxidants?

Over the past decade or so, more and more attention has focused upon *free radicals* or *oxidants* and their counterparts, *antioxidants*. Once we understand free radicals, it is easy to appreciate the importance of nutrients associated with antioxidant activities such as vitamins C and E, β-carotene, lycopene, selenium, copper, iron, manganese, and zinc. A free radical is a substance that endeavors to interact with other molecules and either steal an electron from them or force an electron upon them. Most of the time it is the former. You will remember that earlier we called the process of losing an electron oxidation and the process of gaining an electron reduction. The major difference between proper oxidation and reduction and the damaging activity of free radicals is a matter of desire. You see, free radicals often interact with molecules that do not want to give up an electron. Therefore, free radicals are sort of biological bullies that will interact with other molecules without regard for the stability of these molecules. Typically free-radical substances include oxygen, such as the following:

- Superoxide (O_2^-)
- Hydrogen peroxide (H_2O_2)
- Hydroxyl radicals (OH^-)

One obvious feature of the free radicals just listed is that they closely resemble the oxygen (O_2) we breathe. So how abnormal could they be? The presence of free radicals in our body is not necessarily a disease and seems to be unavoidable. Free radicals are normally produced in the process of making ATP in cells and detoxifying some chemicals as well. In addition, certain immune processes purposely generate free-radical substances to attack foreign entities or debris in our body. However, free radicals can certainly lead to disease if their presence becomes too great and they are left to their own devices. This tends to happen when we allow free radicals access to our body via the foods we eat and the substances we breathe. Cigarette smoke is loaded with free-radical substances, probably greater than 100 different kinds.

Free radicals can cause damage within the human body by attacking extremely important molecules such as DNA, proteins, and special fatty acids. If these or other molecules are attacked by free radicals and have an electron removed from their structure (oxidation) it is like pulling a bottom card from a house of cards. The victimized molecule is rendered weak and unstable and subject to breakdown. An example of this oxidative damage can be demonstrated by leaving vegetable oil out in an open container exposed to sunlight. The presence of oxygen and energy from sunlight leads to the formation of oxygen-based free radicals, which attack the fat causing them to break down in smaller molecules. Some of these molecules can produce an offensive odor and taste. Throughout time we have accepted the presence of free radicals, and our body has evolved to meet the challenge. We are armed with a battery of antioxidants to keep the free radicals in check. The term *antioxidant* implies that these molecules will prevent free radicals from pulling electrons (oxidation) from other molecules. They may do so by donating their own electrons to a free radical. This pacifies a free radical and spares other molecules. Antioxidants are different from nonantioxidant molecules in that they remain relatively stable after giving up an electron. They are designed to handle this process.

Hey, you made it through Chapter 1. For many people these concepts may seem easy; however, for others, they may present more of a challenge. One thing is certain: if you have at least a general comprehension of these concepts, nutrition becomes a lot easier to understand. In Chapter 2 we discuss some of the finer aspects of the structure and function of our body.

Chapter 2

How Our Body Works

CELLS ARE LIFE

It is obvious that humans are not the only life-form or *organism* residing on this planet. In fact, we are only one of several million different species of organisms. Organisms include everything from mammals, birds, reptiles, and insects, to plants, bacteria, fungi, and yeast. But bear in mind that even though organisms such as a tomato plant and an octopus may seem completely different, they have numerous similarities which strongly suggest a common ancestry for all life-forms hanging out on Earth, which includes you and me.

Among the millions of species on this planet, the *cell* is the common denominator. Cells are the most basic living unit. In many species, such as bacteria and amoeba, the entire organism consists of a single isolated cell. But for plants and animals, including us, the organism exists as a compilation of many cells working together. In fact, every adult human is a compilation of some 60 to 100 trillion cells.

As a rule of nature life begets other life and thus all cells must come from existing cells. This is to say that in order to create a new cell, another cell has to divide into two cells. It also suggests that all life-forms on Earth may be derived from the same cell or type of cell. The process of cell division is tightly regulated and, as we will discuss in later chapters, when this regulation is lost and cells divide out of control, cancer can arise.

When you and I were conceived, an egg (ovum) from our mother was penetrated by our father's sperm. This resulted in the formation of the first cell of a new life. Therefore, everyone you know was only a single cell at first. That cell had to then develop and divide in two cells, which themselves divided to create four cells, and so on.

What are cells?

The term *cell* implies the concept of separation. Each cell has the ability to function on its own. In multicellular organisms such as humans, individual cells are also sensitive and responsive to what is going on in the organism as a whole. Therefore, these cells survive as independent living units and also cooperatively participate in the vitality of the organism to which they belong.

Human cells can differ in size and function. Some are bigger and some longer, some will make hormones while others will help our body move. In fact, there are roughly 200 different types of cells in our body. Although these cells may seem unrelated most of the general features will be the same from one cell to the next. Therefore, we can discuss cells by describing the features of a single cell. Unique characteristics of different kinds of different cell types (e.g., red blood cells [RBC] and muscle and fat cells) will be described as they become relevant later in this chapter and book.

A wall or, more scientifically, a plasma membrane encloses every cell in our body. As shown in Figure 2.1, the plasma membrane separates the inside of the cell from the outside of the cell. The watery environment inside the cell is called the *intracellular fluid*. Meanwhile, the watery medium outside of cells is called the *extracellular fluid*. Previously, it was noted that our body is about 60 percent water. Of this 60 percent, roughly two-thirds of the water is intracellular fluid while the remaining one-third is extracellular fluid, which would include the plasma of our blood.

What types of substances are found in the intracellular and extracellular fluids?

In our body fluids we would find small dissolved substances such as ions, amino acids, and the carbohydrate glucose, as well as larger proteins. The major ions (electrolytes) would include potassium (K^+), sodium (Na^+), chloride (Cl^-), calcium (Ca^{2+}), magnesium (Mg^{2+}), phosphate (PO_4^{3-}), and bicarbonate (HCO_3^-). As demonstrated in Figure 2.2, all of these and other substances will be found in both the intracellular and extracellular fluids. However, there are basic differences between the concentration of substances dissolved in

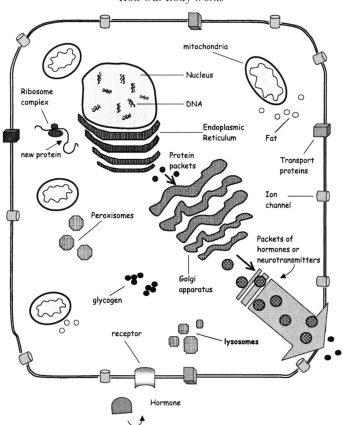

FIGURE 2.1. This is a model of a human cell. Cells contain DNA, the instructions for bonding proteins, and organelles that perform specific functions.

either fluid, and the plasma membrane is bestowed with the awesome responsibility of functioning as a barrier between the two mediums.

What would we expect to find inside of our cells?

Immersed in and bathed by the intracellular fluid are small compartments called *organelles*. The word organelle means "little organ." Two of the more recognizable organelles are the *nucleus* and *mitochondria*. Other organelles include *endoplasmic reticulum, Golgi apparatus, lysosomes*, and *peroxisomes* (see Figure 2.1). The various organelles are little operation centers within cells. Each type of

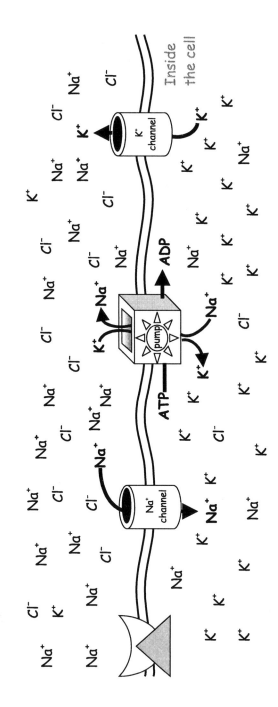

FIGURE 2.2. The concentration of sodium (Na+) and chloride (Cl−) is greater in the extracellular fluid while potassium (K+) is more concentrated in the intracellular fluid. These electrolytes move down their concentration gradients through channels and are pumped against their concentration gradient by energy (ATP)-requiring pumps.

24

organelle performs a different and specialized job (see Table 2.1). Each organelle has a membrane with many similarities to the plasma membrane. Therefore, as we discuss the nature of the plasma membrane below you can keep in mind that some of these features also pertain to organelle membranes as well.

Also within the intracellular fluid of certain cells we would expect to find some energy reserves in the form of *fat droplets* and *glycogen* (carbohydrate) (see Figure 2.1). The amount of glycogen and fat will vary depending on the type of cell. Another important component of cells is *ribosomes*. Ribosomes are the actual site where proteins are constructed.

Do individual cells and our body as a whole attempt to maintain an optimal working environment?

Just as you clean your apartment or house and determine what kind of stuff is found within your living area, so too will our cells clean and regulate the contents in their intracellular fluid. This allows each cell to maintain an optimal operating environment. Scientists often use the term *homeostasis* to describe the efforts associated with the maintenance of this optimal environment. Furthermore, just as it is the responsibility of each cell to maintain its own ideal internal environment, at the same time many of our organs work in concert to regulate the environment within our body as a whole (see Box 2.1). These or-

TABLE 2.1. Overview of Organelle Function

Organelle	Function and Specialized Features
Nucleus	Houses almost all of our DNA
Mitochondria	The site of most ATP manufacturing in cells; houses some DNA
Lysosomes	Involved in breaking down unnecessary or foreign substances; contains acidic environment and digestive enzymes
Endoplasmic reticulum	Involved in making proteins and lipid substances destined to be exported from a cell
Peroxisomes	Like lysosomes but with a different assortment of enzymes; site of detoxification
Golgi apparatus	The final packaging site for substances due to be exported from a cell

gans include the kidneys, lungs, skin, and liver. Many of our most basic functions, such as breathing, sweating, urinating, digesting, and the pumping of our heart, are actually functions dedicated to homeostasis. Therefore, homeostasis is the housekeeping efforts of all our cells working individually as well as together to provide an environment conducive to optimal function.

BOX 2.1. General Mechanisms of Homeostasis

- Regulation of the ion concentrations inside and outside of cells
- Blood pressure regulation
- Regulation of optimal levels of blood gases (O_2 and CO_2)
- Maintaining optimal body temperature
- Regulating blood glucose and calcium levels
- Maintaining an optimal pH level

What is the nature of the plasma membrane?

Each cell is enveloped by a very thin membrane measuring only about 10 nanometers (nm) thick. A nm is one-billionth of a meter—pretty thin indeed. The makeup of the plasma membrane is a very clever combination of mostly lipids and proteins with just a touch of carbohydrate. Interestingly, plasma membranes use the basic principle of water solubility to allow for its barrier properties. Actually, it is the lipid portion that provides this character. Molecules that are somewhat similar to triglycerides (fat) called *phospholipids* are arranged to provide a water-insoluble capsule surrounding cells. What that means is that water-soluble substances such as sodium, potassium, and chloride, carbohydrates, proteins, and amino acids are restricted from moving freely through the membrane. Some lipid substances and gases seem to freely move across the plasma membrane. The plasma membrane will also contain the lipid substance cholesterol. Cholesterol appears to increase the stability of the plasma membranes.

If we were to weigh all of the components of the plasma membrane we would find that it is about half protein. However, this is a bit misleading as the much smaller lipid molecules of the plasma membrane actually outnumber protein molecules by about fifty to one. Since the plasma membrane functions as a barrier between the outside and inside of the cell, there must be a means or doorways whereby many water-soluble substances can either enter or exit a cell. One of the roles of proteins in the plasma membrane is to function as doors, thereby allowing substances such as sodium, potassium, chloride, glucose, and amino acids to enter or exit a cell. This is shown in Figures 2.1 and 2.2.

Proteins are truly the more functional component part of the plasma membrane, as phospholipids and cholesterol provide more structural support. Let us go into a little more detail about just how some of the proteins function as doorways in our plasma membranes. Some of these proteins function as channels or pores that will allow the passage of only one specific substance across the membrane. This is like opening the stadium doors for fans before a concert. The concentration of fans outside the stadium is much higher than within and the natural flow is for the general movement of people into the stadium, an area of lower concentration.

Plasma membrane channels mostly allow the passage of ions such as sodium, potassium, chloride, and calcium down their concentration gradient. However, the movement will be in mass amounts resulting in a sudden and significant change in a cell's environment. As an example, *ion channels* are especially important in nerve and muscle cells, and drugs often prescribed for people with cardiovascular concerns are calcium-channel blockers, which will be discussed more in just a bit and also in Chapter 13.

We should stop for a moment and emphasize a very important concept. In nature, when provided the opportunity, things will tend to move from an area of higher concentration to an area of lower concentration. This type of movement is called *diffusion* and it can be applied to so many aspects of nature. The movement of substances across our plasma membranes is an excellent example of diffusion. Simply put, diffusion is when a substance moves from an area where it is found in higher concentration to an area of lower concentration. For example, muscle cells are told to contract by calcium. Thus when muscle cells want to relax (not contracted) they must pump out nearly all of the calcium. This sets up a huge diffusion gradient. In fact, the calcium concentration outside the muscle cell will be greater than ten times that inside during relaxation of that muscle cell. However, when that muscle cell is told to contract, calcium channels open, calcium diffuses, and that cell contracts. Calcium-channel blockers attempt to inhibit the opening of channels and the subsequent contraction of muscle cells in the walls of certain blood vessels. This is an attempt to relax the muscle and allow the vessels to dilate a bit. This then would lower the pressure associated with the blood (blood pressure).

Channels or pores are not the only types of proteins found in our plasma membranes. Other proteins can function as *carriers* that can physically relocate or "transport" substances across the membrane. Here again substances would be moving along their concentration gradient. These carrier proteins tend to transport larger substances than channels can, and the movement tends to occur only one or two substances at a time. Substances that utilize carrier proteins include carbohydrates and amino acids. Perhaps the most famous example of a carrier protein is the glucose transport protein (GluT) which is the primary concern in type 2 diabetes mellitus. We will spend much more time on glucose transporters later on.

Not all substances move across our plasma membrane down their concentration gradient. Like trout swimming upstream, substances moving across the plasma membrane in this manner go against the natural flow of nature. To perform this operation, certain membrane proteins can function as *pumps*. Quite simply, pumps will move substances across the membrane against their concentration gradient. Said another way, substances can be pumped across the membrane from the area with a lower concentration of that substance through the plasma membrane to the side with a higher concentration. As this goes against the natural flow of things, it will require energy to make it happen. (You can bet the trout are tired.) The energy is derived from splitting ATP. In fact, a very respectable portion of the energy that humans expend every day is attributed to pumping substances across cell membranes. We will go into much more detail about this later on in this chapter and other chapters.

Last, but certainly not least, not all proteins in the plasma membrane function in transport operations. Some proteins function as *receptors* for special communicating substances in our body such as *hormones* and *neurotransmitters*. Typically, receptors will interact with only one specific molecule and ignore all other substances. In a way, then, these proteins are involved in the transport processes. Here, however, the transported item is not a substance but information.

What is DNA?

DNA (deoxyribonucleic acid) is found in almost all the cells of our body. Within those cells DNA is for the most part housed in the nucleus, while a much smaller amount of DNA can be found in mitochondria. DNA contains the instructions (blueprints) for putting specific amino acids together to make proteins. You see, the human body contains thousands of different proteins, all of which our cells have to build using amino acids as the building blocks. Without the DNA's instructions, our cells would not know how to perform such a task.

DNA is long and strandlike and organized into large structures called *chromosomes*. Normally we have twenty-three pairs of chromosomes in our cells' nuclei. If we were to take a chromosome and find the end points of the DNA, we could theoretically straighten it out like thread from a spool. If we did so we would find thousands of small stretches called *genes* on the DNA. We have thousands of genes, which contain the actual instructions for building specific proteins.

To oversimplify one of the most amazing events in nature, when a cell wants to make a specific protein, it makes a copy of its DNA gene in the form of *RNA* (ribonucleic acid). You see, DNA and RNA are virtually the same thing. However, one of the most important differences is that the RNA can leave the nucleus and travel to the actual site of protein manufacturing in our cells, the ribosomes. Ribosomes are found in the endoplasmic reticulum of our cells or somewhat independently inside cells (see Figure 2.1). At this point both the blueprint instructions (RNA) and the amino acids are available. The ribosomes simply link or bond amino acids together in the correct sequence.

Where is ATP made in cells?

ATP is made in our cells by capturing some of the energy released from energy molecules when they are broken down in energy pathways. Most of the ATP made in our body is made in mitochondria (singular: mitochondrion). For this reason mitochondria are often referred to as the "powerhouses" of our cells. A relatively small portion of the ATP generated in our cells each day will be made in the intracellular fluid outside the mitochondria.

Each mitochondrion contains two membranes, an outer and an inner membrane. It is the inner membrane and the environment that it encloses that are principally involved in ATP formation. The inner membrane is folded to get more of the ATP-producing machinery into the mitochondria (see Figure 2.1). As you might expect, cells with higher energy demands will have more mitochondria. This is certainly true for heart and skeletal muscle cells and cells within our liver.

What does the term metabolism mean?

Each and every second of every day our cells are engaged in the operations that help keep them alive and well while at the same time also contributing to the proper functioning of our body as a whole. This requires each cell to perform an incredible number of chemical reactions every second. The term *metabolism* generally refers to the sum total of all chemical reactions in our body. More specifically, then, metabolism is the total of all reactions taking place in each cell added together.

In general, chemical reactions and/or pathways will release energy. Ultimately, this extra energy will be converted to heat. Since body temperature remains fairly constant, the heat produced in metabolism must be removed from our body. Therefore, our metabolism can be estimated by measuring how much heat is lost from our body.

The term metabolism is somewhat general. For instance, human metabolism refers to all the energy released from all the chemical reactions and associated processes in our body. However, if we wanted to describe just those chemical reactions within a specific tissue, such as muscle or bone, we would say "muscle metabolism" or "bone metabolism." We can be even more focused and use the term metabolism to describe only those reactions associated with a single nutrient or nutrient class. For example, if we were discussing the chemical reactions that involve only proteins or carbohydrates, we would be discussing protein or carbohydrate metabolism, respectively. Include a descriptor to focus the attention on a specific aspect of our general metabolism.

What does "tissue" mean, and do the tissues throughout our body work as a team?

Humans are truly a complex array of organs and other tissues designed to support the basic functions and vitality of our body. We are able to process inhaled air and ingested food and regulate body content. We selectively take what we need from the external environment and eliminate what we do not need. We think, move about, and reproduce. Many of these operations occur without us even being aware of them (see Box 2.1 and Table 2.2).

One other term we should be familiar with is *tissue*. Quite simply, tissue is comprised of similar or cooperating cells performing similar or cooperative tasks. These cells may be grouped together to form fascinating tissues such as bone, skin, muscle, nerves, and blood.

WE HANG OUR BODY ON THE BONY SKELETON

What is the skeleton?

The exquisite appearance of the human body is founded upon our skeleton. Our skeleton is a combination of 206 separate bones and supporting ligaments and cartilage. The bones of our skeleton are attached to muscles, which allow us to move about. Bones also provide protection. For instance, the skull and the vertebrae enclose the brain and spinal cord, respectively, thereby protecting the invaluable central nervous system (CNS). Twelve pairs of ribs extend from our vertebrae and protect the organs of our chest. Bone also serves as a storage site for several minerals, such as calcium and phosphorus, and is the site of formation for many of our blood cells.

By approximately six weeks of pregnancy the skeleton is rapidly developing and is visible in a sonogram. Bones continue to grow until early adulthood, complementing the growth of other body tissue. Up until this point, bones grow in both length and diameter. Around this time the longer bones of our body, such as the femur, humerus, tibia, and fibula, begin to lose the ability to grow lengthwise and our adult height is realized. Some of the bones of the lower jaw and nose continue to grow throughout our lives, although the rate of growth slows dramatically.

TABLE 2.2. Primary Functions of the Major Tissues and Organs in Our Body

Tissue/Organ	Function
Bone	Bone provides structure and the basis for the movement of limbs and our entire body. It also serves as a mineral storage. Bone is primarily composed of minerals and protein and smaller amounts of cells, nerves, and blood vessels.
Skeletal muscle	We have three kinds of muscle (skeletal, cardiac [heart], and smooth), which is largely water and protein and to a lesser degree carbohydrate and fat. Contraction of muscle results in movement of some type. Skeletal muscle is connected to bone and provides movement of our limbs and body.
Heart and blood	Our heart is mostly muscle (cardiac). Contraction of cardiac muscle establishes the blood pressure in our heart, which drives blood through our blood vessels. We have about 100,000 miles of blood vessels and our blood is, for the most part, a delivery medium.
Smooth muscle	Smooth muscle lines tubes in our body such as airways, blood vessels, digestive tract, reproductive tract, etc. Smooth muscle is responsible for regulating the flow of content (gases, fluids, semisolids) through those tubes.
Lungs	Serve as the site of oxygen and carbon dioxide exchange between our body and the air around us.
Liver	Perhaps the "hub" of nutrition, our liver is involved in maintaining blood glucose, regulating blood lipid levels, processing amino acids, making plasma proteins (e.g., clotting factors, transport proteins) and bile, and metabolizing and storing many vitamins, minerals, and other nutrients.
Kidneys	Regulate the composition of our body fluid. They do this by filtering and regulating the composition of our blood, which in turn regulates the composition of the fluid in between and inside of our cells.
Adrenal Glands	Our adrenals are steroid hormone-producing factories. They produce cortisol (stress hormone), aldosterone, a lot of DHEA, and lesser amounts of androstenedione, testosterone, and estrogens.
Thyroid gland	Produces the hormones thyroid hormone and calcitonin. Thyroid hormone is one of the most influential hormones in regulating our energy expenditure.
Brain and spinal cord	Our brain is an information-processing center and the spinal cord is the conduit for signals to leave (or be carried to) our brain to the rest of our body. Our brain initiates and regulates muscle activity, processes sensory information, and controls body temperature and appetite.
Skin	Site of heat removal and protective coating. Some vitamin D is produced in our skin.
Pancreas	Produces the hormones insulin and glucagon and digestive enzymes.
Pituitary gland	Produces many hormones, including thyroid stimulating hormone (TSH) and adrenocorticotropic hormone (ACTH).

As you may expect, the longest, heaviest, and strongest bone in our body is the femur or thigh bone. These bones extend nearly two feet in some of us, and provide much of the support we need against the force of gravity. Meanwhile, the three small bones in the inner ear are the smallest bones in our body. In addition, the tiny pisiform bone of the wrist is also very small, having the approximate size of a pea.

What is bone?

Our fascination with the fossil remains of dinosaurs and other ancient creatures may lead us to believe that bone is a hard, nonliving part of our body and part of the bodies of other animals, including those from long ago. Although bone is indeed solid and strong, allowing form, movement, and organ protection, it is living tissue and constantly changing.

Bone contains several different types of cells, which are supported by a thick fluid called the *matrix*. As simplified in Figure 2.3, within the matrix reside proteins, primarily collagen, and to a much lesser degree other related substances, such as some really unique carbohydrates. Also in the matrix are mineral deposits, largely a calcium- and phosphate-based crystal called *hydroxyapatite,* as well as calcium phosphate. Bone is roughly 60 to 70 percent mineral complexes and the remaining bone is largely protein (see also Figure 10.1), primarily collagen. Hydroxyapatite are like tiny, long, and flat sheets of

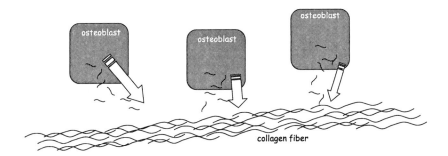

FIGURE 2.3. These bone cells (osteoblasts) are making collagen proteins that form into collagen superproteins, which are like rope, in the matrix of bone. Mineral complexes then adhere to the collagen. Collagen makes bone strong and minerals make it hard.

minerals that actually lie on top and along longer collagen fibers. These mineral deposits provide the hard and compression-resisting properties to bone. For the most part, it is also these mineral complexes along with some proteins that exist as fossils long after the death of an animal.

In addition to some cells, proteins, carbohydrates, and minerals, other tissue can be found in bone. For instance, small blood vessels run throughout bone and deliver substances to and away from bone. Some nerves can be found in bone as well.

Is bone constantly changing?

Bone is constantly being *turned over.* Specific cells within bone are constantly breaking down bone components such as proteins and mineral complexes. Meanwhile, other cells are constantly building bone. Although this may seem counterproductive its merit lies in the ability of bone to adapt or be remodeled according to the demands placed upon it. For example, one of the benefits of weightlifting is an increased stress placed on bone, which causes the bone to adapt by increasing its density. In this case, the efforts of cells that build bone will exceed the efforts of cells that will break down bone components. On the contrary, prolonged exposure to zero gravity (weightlessness) in outer space will decrease the stress placed upon bone resulting in a loss of bone density. In this situation, the efforts of cells that break down bone will exceed those efforts of cells that build bone components.

NERVOUS TISSUE IS ELECTRICAL AND EXCITABLE

What is nervous tissue?

Nervous tissue is comprised mostly of nerve cells or *neurons,* which serve as the basis for an extremely rapid communication system in our body and also as a thinking entity. The CNS includes the brain and spinal cord and represents the thinking and responsive portion of our nervous tissue. Links of neurons extend from the CNS to various organs and tissues in our body thus allowing the CNS to regulate their function. Also, links of neurons extend to our skeletal muscle thereby allowing the CNS to initiate and control our movement. Special neurons function as sensory receptors and are located in the skin and sensory organs (i.e., tongue, nose, ears, eyes) as well as deeper in tissue inside our body. These receptors keep the brain informed as to what is going on inside and outside our body. They register pain and sensation (sight, hearing, taste, smell, and touch) and relay that information to the brain where it is interpreted.

How do neurons work?

Neurons are often referred to as *excitable cells*. Excitable cells are able to respond to a stimulus by changing the electrical properties of their plasma membrane. Only muscle and nerve cells possess this ability and thus are deemed excitable.

The basis for excitability lies in the electrolytes (ions) that are dissolved into our extracellular and intracellular fluids. As mentioned before, the concentrations of the different electrolytes are not the same across the plasma membrane (see Figure 2.4). In general the concentrations of sodium (Na^+), chloride (Cl^-), and calcium (Ca^{2+}) are much greater in the extracellular fluid, while the concentration of potassium (K^+) is greater in the intracellular fluid. This means that these electrolytes have the potential to move across the plasma mem-

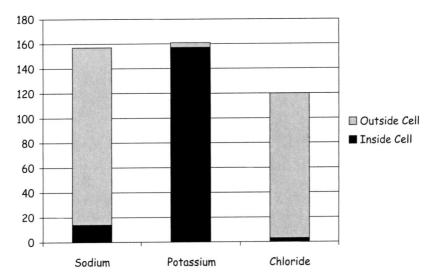

FIGURE 2.4. Difference in the concentration of sodium, potassium, and chloride across the plasma membrane of our cells. Cells must expend considerable energy (ATP) to maintain these differences through pumping operations.

brane, down their concentration gradient, when their respective ion channels open up.

When an excitable cell is stimulated, ion channels open in a specific and timely fashion. This allows electrolytes to move either into or out of the cell depending on the direction of their concentration gradient. The movement of the charged electrolytes changes the electrical nature of the plasma membrane at the site of the stimulus. Furthermore, when the cell is stimulated at one point on its plasma membrane, the excitability or impulse then moves along the plasma membrane like a ripple on a pond. Thus the excitability spreads and is often called a *nerve impulse* as shown in Figure 2.5.

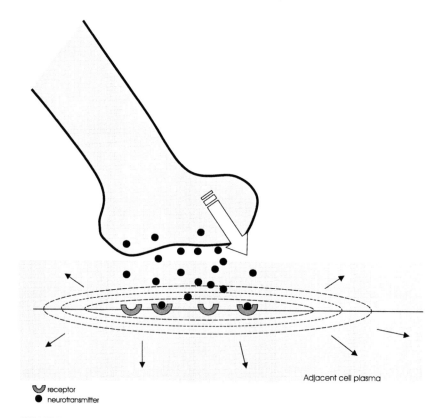

Adjacent cell plasma

⩗ receptor
● neurotransmitter

FIGURE 2.5. Neurotransmitters released at the end of the neuron will interact with receptors on the adjacent cell (muscle or nerve). This can result in excitability of that cell, which may stimulate muscle contraction or transmit a nervous impulse.

How do neurons become excited?

Neurons become excited in response to a stimulus. Sensory neurons are sensitive to specific stimuli in their surrounding environment. For example, sensory neurons found in human skin are sensitive to touch, pain, and change in temperature outside of the body. Meanwhile, sensory neurons located inside the body are sensitive to pain and changes in temperature inside the body. Sensory receptors in the ears, eyes, nose, and mouth register sound, light, smell, and taste, respectively. Once these neurons are excited by a stimulus, the excitability or impulse moves along that neuron toward the brain, where it is interpreted. Our brain initiates impulses as well. These impulses may travel throughout the brain for thinking and memory recall. Or these impulses may travel away from the brain toward destinations outside the CNS, such as skeletal muscle, the heart, and other organs.

How do neurons communicate?

Although some neurons are very long and may extend several feet or so, the trek of an impulse traveling either from a sensory neuron to the brain or from the brain to other parts of the body requires several neurons linked together. These neurons are lined up end to end, but they do not actually touch. An impulse reaching the end of one neuron is transferred to the next neuron by way of special communicating chemicals called *neurotransmitters*. (See Figure 2.5.)

Many different neurotransmitters are employed by nervous tissue, including serotonin, norepinephrine, dopamine, histamine, and acetylcholine. Many of these will be discussed in later chapters, as either they are derived from nutrients or nutrients play a very important role in putting them together. In fact, most neurotransmitters are made of amino acids. Furthermore, some neurotransmitters are very important in regulating how much and what types of foods we eat.

What is the brain?

The brain is an organ that is very densely packed with neurons. As an adult, the human brain weighs about three and a half pounds and is protected by the skull. The brain is designed to interpret sensory input and decipher other incoming information, to develop both short- and long-term memory, to originate and coordinate most muscular movement, and to regulate the function of many of our organs. So many neuron operations take place within the brain that the electrical activity can be measured by placing sensors on the skin of the head. The recorded output of this measurement is called an electroencephalogram (EEG). No other animal on this planet has such a developed brain relative to its body size. In fact, the human brain is so big that during pregnancy the size of the baby's head is a primary factor dictating the timing of birth. If babies were not born until the tenth or eleventh month of pregnancy, it would be extremely difficult for the head to fit through the mother's birth canal.

What is the spinal cord?

The spinal cord extends from the brain and serves mostly as a relay station connecting the brain to the rest of the body. For protection, the human spinal cord is encased by bony vertebrae. The region of the spinal cord closest to the brain connects the brain to regions of the body in that proximity. This would include the chest and arms. Moving further down the spinal cord and away from the brain, you begin to find the interconnections between the CNS and the lower portions of our body, such as our legs. However, as the nerve links extending from the lower extremities must move through the upper regions of the spinal cord in order to connect with the brain, damage to the upper region of the spinal cord will affect the lower as well as the upper areas of our body. Thus, if damage occurs lower in the spinal cord it may result in temporary or permanent paralysis of only the lower extremities. However, if the spinal cord is damaged higher up, it can result in paralysis of both lower and upper extremities.

When you would like to move a particular body part, the process (idea) originates in the brain in a region called the *motor cortex*. Motor means movement! Once initiated, the impulse is carried along a linkage of nerve cells to the skeletal muscle responsible for moving the limb or body part that you desire to respond. The whole process may only require a couple neurons connecting the brain to the muscle and occurs in a fraction of a second.

While the motor cortex of our brain is busy sending signals to our skeletal muscle, signaling it to move, another region of our brain is evaluating and refining the movement. This region is called the *cerebellum,* which is behind and lower than the more recognizable parts of the brain. It is also this region of the brain that is particularly sensitive to the effects of alcohol and explains why movement becomes less refined when we are intoxicated.

SKELETAL MUSCLE ALLOWS US TO MOVE

What is skeletal muscle?

Skeletal muscle is made up of very specialized cells that have the ability to shorten when they are stimulated. With the exception of reflex mechanisms, such as the knee tap by a physician, movement of our skeletal muscle is under the command of our brain, as mentioned earlier. Because muscle cells are very long they are often referred to as *muscle fibers* (see Figure 2.6). The fibers are bundled up like a box of dry spaghetti or straight wires in a cable. The muscle fiber bundles are themselves bundled up and are part of larger collection of similar bundles which make up a particular muscle. Skeletal muscle is so named because it is generally anchored at both ends to different

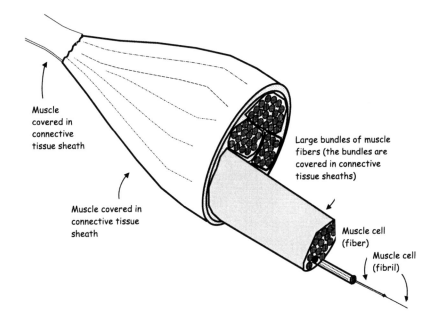

FIGURE 2.6. Cross section of a skeletal muscle. Muscle cells are bundled up in connective tissue sheaths, which in turn are gathered into larger bundles.

bones of our skeleton. When muscle contracts, it pulls on a specific bone, which moves the bone, thus moving a body part.

How does skeletal muscle work?

Like neurons, skeletal muscle fibers are also excitable. In fact, the excitability process of muscle cells is very similar to that of neurons, while the end result is different. Excitability in muscle fibers leads to the contraction of the muscle cell while neurons merely carry the electrical nerve impulse to another neuron or to skeletal muscle or other tissue and organs.

The inside of skeletal muscle fibers appears very different from other cells because of the contractile apparatus it contains. Each muscle fiber contains a tremendous amount of small fiberlike units called *myofibrils,* as shown in Figures 2.6 and 2.7. The prefix *myo* refers to muscle and *fibril* means little fiber. Each myofibril is a stalklike collection of proteins. The predominant proteins are *actin* and *myosin,* which are referred to as the thin and thick filaments, respectively. They are organized into a series of tiny contraction regions called a *sarcomere* (see Figure 2.7). Myofibrils are composed of thousands of sarcomeres situated side by side.

When skeletal muscle fibers become excited, calcium (Ca^{++}) channels open and calcium floods in and around the myofibrils and bathes the sarcomeres. Calcium then interacts with specific proteins associated with actin and induces sarcomere contraction. The contraction of one muscle fiber is really the net result of the shortening of all the tiny sarcomeres in each myofibril within that cell. Further, the contraction of the muscle itself is the net result of contraction and shortening of muscle fibers that make up that muscle.

Skeletal muscle cells have another unique characteristic. They contain an organelle called the *sarcoplasmic reticulum* which is actually a modified version of the endoplasmic reticulum found in other cells. This organelle stores large quantities of calcium. In fact, when a skeletal muscle cell is stimulated, most of the calcium that bathes the sarcomeres actually comes from the sarcoplasmic reticulum.

What powers muscle contraction?

In order for muscle fibers to contract, a lot of ATP must be used (see Figure 2.8). Some of the energy released from ATP is used to power the contraction. Interestingly, ATP is also necessary for a con-

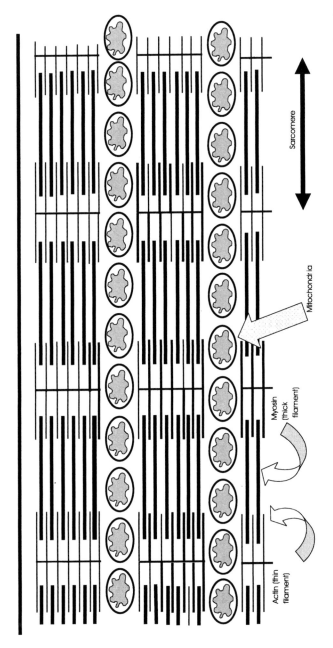

FIGURE 2.7. Inside a skeletal muscle cell are proteins involved in contraction. These are myosin (thick filaments) and actin (thin filaments). Mitochondria are the sites of aerobic ATP formation.

Sarcomere

Mitochondria

Myosin (thick filament)

Actin (thin filament)

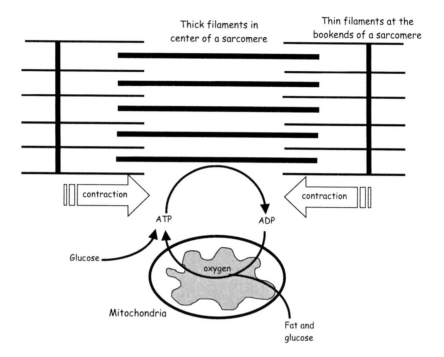

FIGURE 2.8. Muscle cell contraction is powered by ATP. The energy released by ATP allows myosin to pull actin filaments toward the center of the sarcomere. The net effect of all the sarcomere contraction results in the shortening of the whole muscle cell. Carbohydrate and fat are mostly used to regenerate the ATP as it is being used.

tracted muscle cell to "relax" as well. When the muscle is no longer being stimulated, ATP helps the thick and thin filaments to dissociate from each other so that each sarcomere can return to its prestimulated relaxed position. Also, ATP is necessary to pump calcium out of intracellular fluid of the muscle fiber. Calcium is either pumped out of the cell or more likely into sarcoplasmic reticulum organelles.

If ATP is deficient, muscle fibers become locked in a contracted state called *rigor. Rigor mortis* occurs when the human body dies as the integrity of muscle cell membranes decrease. This allows calcium to leak into the contracting regions of muscle fibers from the extracellular fluid and from within the sarcoplasmic reticulum. As a result, calcium bathes myofibrils and contraction is invoked. Usually there is enough ATP in these dying cells to power the contraction. The dying cell then remains locked in a contracted state.

THE HEART AND CIRCULATION
ARE A FANTASTIC DELIVERY SYSTEM

Some ancient philosophers believed that the heart was the foundation of our soul. Today we recognize the heart for its true function, that of a muscular pump. The adult heart is about the size of its carrier's fist and weighs about one-half pound (see Figure 2.9). It serves to pump blood through about 100,000 miles of blood vessels (see Table 2.3) to all regions of our body. Blood leaves the heart through arteries on route to tissue throughout the body. Arteries feed into smaller arterioles and subsequently tiny capillaries, which then thoroughly infiltrate tissue. Most blood vessel mileage is attributable to capillaries. These blood vessels are so numerous in tissue that nearly every cell in our body will have a capillary right next to it or very close. This is like having one river (artery) flowing into town that branches to the extent whereby every house has its own little stream (capillary).

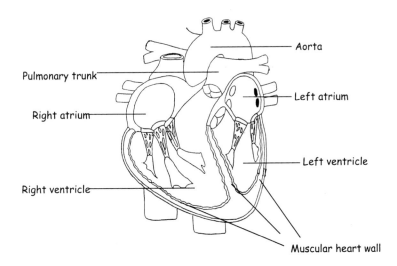

FIGURE 2.9. The anatomy of the heart. There are four chambers (right and left atria and ventricles).

TABLE 2.3. Select Hormones Related to Nutrition and Metabolism

Organ of Origin	Hormone	Principal Activity
Pituitary gland	Growth hormone (GH)	Increases growth of most tissue; increases protein synthesis and fat used for energy
	Prolactin	Increases milk production in female mammary glands
	Antidiuretic hormone (ADH)	Decreases water loss by our kidneys by increasing water reabsorption through our nephrons
Thyroid gland	Thyroid hormone (T_3/T_4)	Increases rate of metabolism in our cells; normal growth
	Calcitonin	Decreases blood calcium levels by increasing kidney loss and decreasing absorption in our gut
Parathyroid gland	Parathyroid hormone (PTH)	Increases blood calcium levels by decreasing urinary losses and increasing absorption in the gut
Adrenal gland	Aldosterone	Increases sodium reabsorption in kidneys (decreases urinary loss of sodium)
	Cortisol	Increases glucose production in the liver and release into blood; stimulates muscle protein breakdown; promotes inflammation; increases fat release from fat cells
	Epinephrine (adrenalin)	Increases heart rate and stroke volume; increases glucose production in liver and release into our blood, increases fat release from fat cells
Pancreas	Insulin	Increases glucose uptake into muscle and fat tissue; increases storage of glucose as glycogen; decreases fat release from fat cells and increases fat production; increases protein production
	Glucagon	Increases fat release from fat cells; increases glucose production in the liver and release into blood

As blood reaches the end of the capillaries and the tissue has been properly served, the blood will drain into larger venules. The venules will eventually drain into larger veins, which ultimately return blood to the heart. This is like the streams draining into larger creeks, which then drain back into the larger river.

Quite simply, our blood serves as a delivery system. It delivers O_2 nutrients and other substances to cells throughout our body. At the same time, blood also serves to remove the waste products of cell metabolism such as CO_2 and heat from our tissue. Capillaries are the actual sites of exchange of substances and heat between our cells and the blood.

Our heart consists of four chambers (two atria and two ventricles), left and right. The left half, consisting of the left atrium and ventricle, serves to receive oxygen-rich blood returning from the lungs and pump it to all the tissues throughout the body. The right half of the heart, consisting of the right atrium and ventricle, serves to receive oxygen-poor blood returning from tissue throughout our body and pumps it to the lungs. Therefore, our heart functions as a relay station for moving blood throughout our body in one large loop, hence the term circulation.

How does our heart work?

Our heart is composed mostly of muscle cells that are somewhat similar to skeletal muscle cells yet retain certain fundamental differences. Although most of the events involved in contraction of heart (cardiac) muscle are the same as skeletal muscle, the heart is not attached to bone. Furthermore, our heart does not require the brain to tell it when to contract (beat). However, the brain certainly can play both a direct and indirect role in regulating the beating of our heart. The stimulus that invokes excitability in the heart comes from a specialized pacemaker region within our heart, called the sinoatrial node (SA node). The human heart may beat in excess of 2 billion times throughout a person's life.

Unlike skeletal muscle, which pulls on bone when it contracts, the heart constricts in a wringing fashion when it contracts. As the heart contracts, the pressure of the blood inside the heart (ventricles) increases. As a result, blood is propelled out of the heart into the arteries. This increase in pressure provides the driving force that forces blood to surge through our blood vessels. The dynamics of blood flow will be discussed in more detail in the final chapter.

What is the composition of blood?

The blood is comprised of two main parts, the *hematocrit* and the *plasma,* which can be assessed clinically (see Figure 2.10). *Red blood*

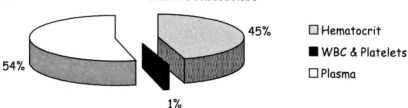

54%

45%

1%

☐ Hematocrit

■ WBC & Platelets

☐ Plasma

FIGURE 2.10. The components of our blood. The hematocrit is comprised of RBC. Roughly 90 percent of the plasma is water and the remaining 10 percent is largely proteins, electrolytes, and lipoproteins.

cells (RBCs) are the sole component of the hematocrit and function primarily as a shuttle transport for O_2. Hematocrit is the percentage of our blood that is RBC. A typical adult hematocrit may be 40 to 45 percent of total blood.

Plasma is about 55 percent of our blood. Of the plasma, about 92 percent is water while the remaining 8 percent includes over 100 different dissolved or suspended substances such as nutrients, gases, electrolytes, hormones, and proteins such as albumin and clotting factors. The remaining components of our blood are the *white blood cells* (WBCs) and *platelets,* which collectively make up about 1 percent of blood. WBCs are the principal components of the human immune system and provide a line of defense against bacteria, viruses, and other intruders. Some WBCs attack foreign invaders and useless materials while others manufacture antibodies and other immune factors. Last, but certainly not least, platelets participate in the clotting of blood.

What are red blood cells (RBCs)?

Red blood cells have the responsibility of transporting oxygen throughout the body. About 33 percent of the weight of an RBC is attributed to a specialized protein called *hemoglobin* and thus RBCs are often referred to as "bags of hemoglobin." Hemoglobin is a large and complex protein that contains four atoms of iron. Hemoglobin's job is to bind to oxygen so that it can be transported in the blood. There are about 42 to 52 million RBCs per mm^3 (or cc) of blood; and each RBC contains about 250 million hemoglobin molecules. Since each hemoglobin molecule can carry four O_2 molecules, the potential exists to transport one billion molecules of O_2 in each RBC.

There are two reasons for the need for such a large amount of hemoglobin in our blood. First, O_2 does not dissolve very well into our blood, which is water based. Second, the demand for O_2 is extremely high in our body. Therefore, hemoglobin increases tremendously the ability of the blood to carry O_2. Any situation that significantly decreases either the number of RBCs or the hemoglobin they carry can compromise O_2 delivery to our tissues and potentially compromise function and health.

How do we exchange O_2 and CO_2 with the atmosphere?

When the heart pumps, blood is propelled from the right ventricle into the *pulmonary arteries* for transport to the lungs. Upon reaching the lungs and the pulmonary capillaries, CO_2 exits the blood and enters into the airways of our lungs. It is then removed from our body when we exhale. At the same time, O_2 enters the blood from the airways of our lungs and binds with hemoglobin in RBCs. The oxygen-containing blood leaves the lungs and travels back to the heart. Thus every breath you take serves to exchange gases, bringing needed oxygen into your body while removing carbon dioxide.

How does the heart supply blood throughout our body?

As our heart contracts, blood is pumped from the left ventricle into the *aorta*. Blood moves from the aorta into the arteries, then arterioles, and finally tiny capillaries in our tissue. The blood leaving our left ventricle is rich with O_2 while the blood returning to our heart from tissue throughout our body has given up oxygen to working cells while acquiring CO_2. This blood is then pumped by the right ventricle to the lungs to reload the hemoglobin with O_2 and release CO_2.

What is cardiac output?

If we were to measure the amount of blood pumped out of our heart during one heartbeat, whether it be from the left or right ventricle, we would know our *stroke volume*. Then, if we multiply the stroke volume by our heart rate (heartbeats per minute) we would know the *cardiac output*.

Cardiac Output = Stroke Volume (mL) × Heart Rate (beats/min)

Cardiac output is the volume of blood pumped out of the heart, either to the lungs or toward body tissue, in one minute. It should not matter which of the two destinations we consider, as they occur simultaneously and will have a similar stroke volume of about 5 to 6 liters (or quarts) per minute.

During exercise both heart rate and stroke volume increase, which consequently increases cardiac output. For some of us, cardiac output may increase as much as five to six times during heavy exercise. This allows for more oxygen-rich blood to be delivered to working skeletal muscle.

Where does the cardiac output go?

If referring to the cardiac output of the right ventricle, there is only one place for it to go: the lungs. Said another way, 100 percent of the cardiac output from the right ventricle is destined for our lungs. However, the blood pumped out of the left ventricle has many destinations. Under resting and comfortable environmental conditions about 13 percent of the left ventricle's cardiac output goes to our brain, 4 percent goes to our heart, 20 to 25 percent goes to our kidneys, and 10 percent goes to our skin. The remaining cardiac output from the left ventricle (48 to 53 percent) will then go to the remaining tissue in our body, such as the digestive tract, liver, and pancreas.

During heavy exercise, a greater proportion of this cardiac output is routed to working skeletal muscle. This requires some redistribution or stealing of blood routed to other less active areas at that time, such as our digestive tract. Contrarily, during a big meal and for a few hours afterward, a greater proportion of this cardiac output is routed to the digestive tract, which steals a portion of the blood directed to areas having no immediate need, such as skeletal muscle.

What is blood pressure?

Whether blood is in the heart or in blood vessels, it has a certain pressure associated with it. In fact, blood moves through circulation from an area of greater blood pressure to an area of lower blood pressure. As mentioned earlier, when the heart contracts, the pressure of the blood in the ventricles increases. This establishes a blood pressure gradient that then drives the movement of blood through the blood vessels. This is somewhat like turning on a garden hose. When you turn on a garden hose, the water pressure is greatest close to the faucet (versus toward the open end of the hose). The result is that water moves from the area of greater water pressure toward the area of lesser water pressure and out the end of the hose.

We define *pressure* as a force exerted upon a surface and can measure it in mm Hg (mercury). If we apply this definition to our blood, we can say that blood pressure is the force exerted by blood upon the walls of a blood vessel. When blood pressure is measured at, for example, 120/80 or "120 over 80" this means that the pressure exerted by the blood is 120 mm Hg during heart contraction and 80 mm Hg when the heart is relaxing between beats. Often the term *systolic* is applied to the period when our heart contracts while *diastolic* refers to the period when our heart is relaxing. Blood pressure is typically measured in the large artery of the arm because of its accessibility.

OUR KIDNEYS ARE FILTERING SYSTEMS

What do our kidneys do?

Typically understated in function, our kidneys regulate the composition and volume of the blood. Our two kidneys, along with their corresponding ureters, the bladder, and the urethra, make up our urinary or renal system. Although our kidneys are less than 1 percent of our total body weight, they receive about 20 to 25 percent of our left ventricle's cardiac output. Together our kidneys will filter and process approximately forty-seven gallons of blood-derived fluid daily.

Each one of our two kidneys is home to about one million tiny blood processing units called *nephrons*. Each nephron will engage in two basic operations. First, they filter plasma into a series of tubes; second, they will process the filtered fluid. As you might expect, the filtered plasma-derived fluid not only contains water but also small substances dissolved within, such as electrolytes, amino acids, and glucose. Cells (e.g., RBCs, WBCs) and most proteins in our blood are too large and are not filtered out of the blood.

There are two possible fates for the components of the filtered fluid. They can either be absorbed back into our blood or they will not be reabsorbed and ultimately become a component of urine. Normally, the reabsorption of substances such as glucose and amino acids is extremely efficient. Contrarily, the reabsorption of water and electrolytes involves some regulation. For example, if the concentration of sodium is too high in the blood, then less sodium will be reabsorbed so that an optimal blood level is achieved. Conversely, if the level of sodium dissolved within the blood is low, then sodium reabsorption from the filtered fluid becomes very efficient and very little is lost in the urine. As you might expect, the processes engaged in reabsorbing glucose, amino acids, electrolytes, and other desired substances require a lot of ATP. Normal kidney operations make a significant contribution to our total daily energy use.

What is the composition of urine?

Of the forty-seven gallons of fluid filtered and processed by the nephrons daily, less than 1 percent actually becomes urine. Our urine is generally comprised of things our body has no need for, such as some by-products of cell metabolism, and also excessive quantities of things we normally need such as water and electrolytes. About 95 percent of urine is water, while the remaining 5 percent is substances dissolved within.

Do our kidneys do anything else?

Beyond regulating the composition of our blood, the kidneys engage in other operations involved in homeostasis. For instance, our kidneys are very sensitive to the amount of O_2 being transported in the blood. If they detect that the level of O_2 in our blood is too low, they will release a substance (hormone) into the blood that tells bones to make more RBCs. If there are more RBCs, then logically more O_2 can be transported in the blood. Furthermore, the kidneys are vital in the normal metabolism of vitamin D, which will be discussed later.

DIGESTION MAKES NUTRIENTS
AVAILABLE TO OUR BODY

What does "digestion" mean and what is it all about?

The term *digest* means to break down or disintegrate. Therefore, digestion serves to break down the food we eat into smaller substances that are suitable for absorption into our body. All of the activities of digestion take place in our digestive or gastrointestinal tract.

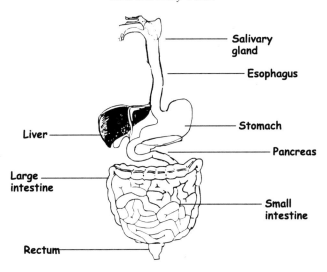

Salivary
gland

Esophagus

Stomach

Liver

Pancreas

Large
intestine

Small
intestine

Rectum

FIGURE 2.11. The digestive system includes the digestive tract and supporting organs, including our liver, pancreas, and gallbladder.

The digestive tract is a tube 22 to 28 feet long that actually passes through our body as shown in Figure 2.11. As food moves through the length of the digestive tract, it is really on the outside of the body. Only when a substance crosses the cell lining of the digestive tract and enters into our circulation is it actually inside our body, which is called *absorption.*

Digestion requires both physical and chemical operations. The teeth, along with the musculature of the mouth, stomach, and small intestine, work to physically grind, knead, and mix food with digestive juices. At the same time, the muscular lining of our digestive tract serves to propel the digestive mixture forward.

Chemical digestion involves the activities of *digestive enzymes* that will break down large complex food molecules into smaller substances appropriate for absorption. Proteins, carbohydrates, and lipids must be split into simpler molecules for absorption. Also, the vitamins and minerals found in foods must be liberated from other food molecules and complexes in order to be absorbed as well. *Bile* is also involved in chemical digestion; however, it functions not as an enzyme but more as a detergent. Bile is pivotal in the digestion and absorption of lipid substances.

What happens to food in the mouth?

Once food is in the mouth it is bathed in saliva. Saliva adds mois-ture to the food that is being chewed. This will improve the ease of swallowing. Each day we will produce about 1 to 1.5 quarts (liters) of saliva. Furthermore, saliva also contains both a carbohydrate and lipid digestive enzyme that begins the chemical digestive process. Once we swallow, food travels through the esophagus and gets de-posited in the stomach.

What is the stomach and what does it do?

The stomach, typically a bit less than a foot in length, functions as a food reservoir for swallowed food. The volume of our stomach de-pends on the quantity of food therein. An empty stomach may have a volume of only 1 to 3 ounces (~ 50 to 75 milliliters) whereas a full stomach can expand to volumes of 2 to 3 quarts (~ 2 to 3 liters).

The stomach is a very muscular organ. It churns food and mixes it with stomach juice. Stomach juice contains hydrochloric acid (HCl), which renders the stomach a very acidic environment (pH 1.5 to 2.5). A protein-digesting enzyme is also found in stomach juices. The pres-ence of this enzyme, along with the acidic environment, will begin pro-tein digestion. On the average, our stomach may produce about 2 to 3 quarts (~ 2 to 3 liters) of stomach juice daily. Beyond protein digestion, the acidic stomach juice also kills most bacteria in foods.

Our stomach is sealed at both ends by tight muscular enclosures called sphincter muscles. This prevents acidic juices from entering the esophagus at one end and also allows separation between the stomach and small intestine at the other end. If stomach juice is able to reflux into our esophagus it can produce a burning sensation com-monly referred to as *heartburn*. This is why chronic heartburn is rou-tinely treated with antacids, as they attempt to neutralize the acid in the stomach. Other drugs may be used that attempt to decrease acid production by the stomach.

What happens to food after it leaves the stomach?

The mixture of partially digested food drenched in acidic stomach juice is slowly sent into the small intestine. This portion of our diges-tive tract is the location of the majority of digestive enzyme activity and the absorption of nutrients. The wall of the small intestine presents a very sophisticated pattern of folds and projections. This design allows the small intestine to have an absorptive surface approximating the size of a tennis court. This allows for very efficient absorption.

When the food mixture is spurted into the small intestine, it hardly resembles what we ate. Yet most of the nutrients still need further digestion to reach their absorbable state. First, bicarbonate produced by the pancreas enters the small intestine and neutralizes the acidic food mixture draining from our stomach. Then digestive enzymes that are also produced by our pancreas and bile from the gallbladder and liver make their way to the small intestine as well. These factors, along with digestive enzymes produced by the cells that line the small intestine, will complete digestion.

What is bile?

Bile is made up of several substances, the most outstanding being *bile acids* (bile salts). During digestion, the small intestine is a watery place to be. Along with the water entering our digestive tract in foods and beverages, water is also the basis of digestive juices. Water-insoluble substances in our diet, such as fats, cholesterol, and fat-soluble vitamins, will clump together into droplets in the small intestine. This would decrease their digestibility and absorption. This is where bile comes in. Bile acts as an emulsifier or detergent interacting with lipid droplets so that many smaller lipid droplets result instead of fewer larger ones. The advantage to creating many smaller lipid droplets is that more contact occurs between lipids and lipid-digesting enzymes. If bile were absent, as in certain disorders, lipids would stay as larger droplets in the small intestine and for the most part remain undigested and unabsorbed and end up in the feces.

Bile is produced by the liver and oozes in the direction of the small intestine twenty-four hours a day, seven days a week. The liver is connected to the small intestine via a series of tubes or ducts. During periods of time in between meals, some of the bile drains into the gallbladder, where it is stored. Then during a meal the gallbladder squeezes the bile out and it heads to the small intestine. This allows for more bile to be present in the small intestine during digestion.

What is the colon?

By the time the digestive mixture reaches the large intestine or *colon* most of the nutrients have been absorbed. Although some water and electrolytes will be absorbed in the colon, its primary responsibility is to form the feces that will eventually leave the digestive tract. The colon is also home to a rich bacteria colony—as many as 400 different species of bacteria may be found. These bacteria provide some benefit to the body as they make some vitamins and fatty acids that can help nourish the body. Research is underway in an effort to better understand the relationship between the colon's bacteria and human health.

What is the composition of feces?

Human feces is a combination of water, bacteria, parts of cells that line the digestive tract, and undigested food components, such as fibers. The coloring of feces is attributable to several of the substances that are removed from the body in the feces. For instance, when the body breaks down hemoglobin, coloring pigments are produced. These substances become part of bile, which empties into the digestive tract. These add color to the feces.

HORMONES ARE MESSENGERS
TRAVELING IN OUR BLOOD

What are hormones?

There are two ways that one region of our body can communicate with another. The first is by way of nerve impulses and the second is by way of hormones. Hormones are produced by specific organs (glands) in the body including the pituitary gland, parathyroid gland, thyroid gland, hypothalamus, pancreas, stomach, small intestine, adrenal glands, placenta, and gonads (ovaries and testicles) (see Table 2.3). Hormones are released into our blood and circulate throughout our body. As they circulate they can interact with specific cells of a specific tissue and elicit a response within those cells.

Only cells that have a specific receptor for a hormone will respond to a circulating hormone. This is an extremely accurate operation. Some hormones may have receptors on cells of only one kind of tissue in our body, while other hormones may have receptors on cells of most tissues in our body. For example, the hormone prolactin stimulates milk production in female breasts. Therefore, the cells associated with the milk-producing mammary glands will have receptors for prolactin, while most other cells in our body will not have prolactin receptors. Growth hormone and insulin receptors, on the other hand, will be found on the cells of many kinds of tissues in our body.

Are there different classes of hormones?

Hormones may be grouped into one of two general categories: *amino acid-based hormones* and *steroid hormones*. The amino acid-based hormones include hormones that are proteins and those hormones that are derived from the amino acid tyrosine. Examples of protein hormones include insulin, growth hormone (GH), glucagon, and antidiuretic hormone (ADH). Examples of hormones made from the amino acid tyrosine are epinephrine (adrenalin) and thyroid hormone (T_3 and T_4). Steroid hormones are made from cholesterol and include testosterone, estrogens, cortisol, progesterone, and aldosterone.

Chapter 3

The Nature of Food

NUTRIENTS NOURISH OUR BODY

As a general rule, animals need to consume other forms of life or their products in order to survive. For us, this would include animals and their products (i.e., milk, eggs) and/or plants and their products (fruits, vegetables, cereal grains). Even eating some forms of microorganisms such as yeast can help us survive. In this day and age, as food manufacturers spend millions of dollars developing new forms of food, we still must adhere to this basic rule. It would be impossible to nourish our bodies with foods completely manufactured in a food science laboratory unless those foods contained the same substances that we have obtained throughout our existence by eating other life-forms on this planet.

We are able to obtain nourishing substances or nutrients by eating other life-forms or their products for a very simple reason: All life is believed to have a common ancestry or evolutionary background. Therefore we must expect many similarities in the chemicals that make up the various life-forms. We are able to eat other life-forms (and their products) to derive those chemicals that are important to both of us.

What are essential nutrients?

We exist at the upper end of the food chain, meaning that a large variety of life-forms are food to us, but we are not regular food for other life-forms. Plants, on the other hand, maintain a position at the other end of the food chain as they are food for many life-forms, including insects, fish, and mammals. Humans, for certain, are relatively needy from a nutritional perspective. We have an inescapable need or requirement for a whole bunch of substances that we cannot make. Thus, we must eat other life-forms that contain these substances. This brings forth one of the most important concepts of environmentalism. How much longer can the human population increase before we are globally unable to feed it? This problem is reflected in other top feeders such as sharks and other carnivores. Their total population can never exceed the availability of their food (e.g., herbivores), whose population also depends upon the availability of their food (e.g., plants).

Quite simply, a *nutrient* is a substance that in some way nourishes the body. It will either provide energy or promote the growth, development, and/or maintenance of the body. The list of nutrients is indeed long, probably a few hundred substances. However, not all of the nutrients are deemed essential. Essential nutrients are a subclass of nutrients and include only those nutrients that are absolutely vital and are not made in the body either at all or in sufficient quantities to meet human needs. We must have these essential nutrients in the foods we choose to eat; if we do not, signs of deficiency can develop over time.

We can reinforce our understanding of the difference between nutrients and essential nutrients with a couple of examples. Glycine is an amino acid, which is absolutely necessary to make proteins in our cells. However, we have the ability to make glycine and therefore, theoretically, it does not need to be part of our diet. Our body will gladly put the glycine we eat to work, so it is indeed a nutrient; it is just not an essential nutrient. Said another way, if glycine was lacking from our diet, it is unlikely that deficiency signs would develop because we can make plenty of it in our cells. Carnitine serves as another example as its presence is absolutely necessary for our cells to use fat effectively as an energy source. So carnitine in our diet is certainly nourishing; however, during normal conditions we can make plenty of carnitine in our body. Essential nutrients can be grouped together based on general similarities such as those that provide energy (carbohydrates, proteins, fats), vitamins, minerals, and water. This is presented in Table 3.1.

How much of the essential nutrients do we need?

If our diet fails to consistently provide adequate amounts of essential nutrients, over time signs of deficiency will result. To address this notion, a government committee of esteemed scientists developed the first set of Recommended Dietary Allowances (RDAs) in the early

TABLE 3.1. Essential Nutrients for Humans

Energy Nutrients	Vitamins	Minerals	Other
Protein, carbohydrates, and fat	Vitamins A, D, E, K, B_6, B_{12}, and C, thiamin folate, biotin, niacin, pantothenic acid	Calcium, zinc, copper, sodium, potassium, iron, phosphorus, magnesium, chromium, chloride, molybdenum, fluoride, selenium, manganese, iodide, chromium	Water

Note: Considerations of essentiality will be addressed later.

1940s. As you can see in Table 3.2, the RDAs are in essence a compilation of the nutrients known to be essential and diet recommendations for intake to allow for proper growth and general health of different populations of Americans are based upon age and gender, including pregnancy and lactation for females.

The RDA nutrients and their recommended intake quantities are periodically scrutinized and revised based on the most current research findings. An essential nutrient may be with an Adequate Intake (AI) quantity instead of RDA. Like RDAs, AI are also recommendations for a given nutrient, however there was not enough scientific information to designate a more confident RDA quantity. Currently there are RDAs and/or AI for vitamins A, D, E, K, C, B_6, and B_{12}, as well as thiamin, riboflavin, niacin, folate, biotin and pantothenic acid as calcium, phosphorus, magnesium, iron, zinc, iodine, selenium, copper, manganese, fluoride, chromium, and molybdenum. Last, sodium, potassium, and chloride have Estimated Minimum Requirements. These elements are found in most foods, either naturally or after processing, and are extremely well absorbed into the body after we eat them. Therefore, a deficiency in any of these essential nutrients is unlikely, providing there are no confounding factors.

How are the RDAs determined?

The RDAs are determined based upon in-depth research studies, including those performed to determine "balance." Balance studies are designed to determine how much of a specific nutrient humans need to eat in order to balance that which is normally lost daily from the

TABLE 3.2. Recommended Dietary Allowances (RDAs)

Median Heights and Weights

Age (years) or Condition		Weight		Height		Average Energy Allowance (kcal)	
		(kg)	(lb)	(cm)	(in)	(kg)	Per Day
Infants	0.0-0.5	6	13	60	24	108	650
	0.5-1.0	9	20	71	28	98	850
Children	1-3	13	29	90	35	102	1300
	4-6	20	44	112	44	90	1800
	7-10	28	62	132	52	70	2000
Males	11-14	45	99	157	62	55	2500
	15-18	66	145	176	69	45	3000
	19-24	72	160	177	70	40	2900
	25-50	79	174	176	70	37	2900
	51+	77	170	173	68	30	2300
Females	11-14	46	101	157	62	47	2200
	15-18	55	120	163	64	40	2200
	19-24	58	128	164	65	38	2200
	25-50	63	138	163	64	36	2200
	51+	65	143	160	63	30	1900
Pregnant	1st semester						plus 0
	2nd semester						plus 300
	3rd semester						plus 300
Lactating	1st 6 months						plus 500
	2nd 6 months						plus 500

Fat-Soluble Vitamins

	Age (years) or Condition	Vitamin A (RE)*	Vitamin D (μg/day)**	Vitamin E (mg or αTE)***	Vitamin K (μg)
Infants	0.0-0.5	400	5	4	2
	0.5-1.0	500	5	5	2.5
Children	1-3	300	5	6	30
	4-8	400	5	7	55
Males	9-13	600	5	11	60
	14-18	900	5	15	75
	19-30	900	5	15	120
	31-50	900	5	15	120
	50-70	900	10	15	120
	>70	900	15	15	120
Females	9-13	600	5	11	60
	14-18	700	5	15	75
	19-30	700	5	15	90
	31-50	700	5	15	90
	50-70	700	10	15	90
	>70	700	15	15	90
Pregnant	≤18	750	5	15	75
	19-30	770	5	15	90
	31-50	770	5	15	90
Lactating	≤18	1,200	5	19	75
	19-30	1,300	5	19	90
	31-50	1,300	5	19	90

Note: Some of the values listed as RDA are Adequate Intake (AI) Values set by the Nutrition and Food Board. AI are similar to RDA, but lack the same knowledge base.

*RE = 1 μg retinal, 12 μg β-carotene, 24 μg α-carotene, or β-cryptoxanthin

**1mg of vitamin D = 40 IU Vitamin D

***1mg∝TE= 1 mg ∝-tocopherol

TABLE 3.2 (continued)

Water-Soluble Vitamins

	Age (years) or Condition	Vitamin C (mg/day)	Thiamin (mg/day)	Riboflavin (mg/day)	Niacin (mg/day) NE*	Vitamin B6 (mg/day)	Folate (µg/day)	Vitamin B12 (µg/day)	Biotin (µg/day)	Pantothenic Acid (mg/day)	Choline (mg/day)
Infants	0.0-0.5	40	0.2	0.3	2	0.1	65	0.4	5	1.7	125
	0.5-1.0	50	0.3	0.4	4	0.3	80	0.5	6	1.8	150
Children	1-3	15	0.5	0.5	6	0.5	150	0.9	8	2	200
	4-8	25	0.6	0.6	8	0.6	200	1.2	12	3	250
Males	9-13	45	0.9	0.9	12	1.0	300	1.8	20	4	375
	14-18	75	1.2	1.3	16	1.3	400	2.4	25	5	550
	19-30	90	1.2	1.3	16	1.3	400	2.4	30	5	550
	31-50	90	1.2	1.3	16	1.3	400	2.4	30	5	550
	50-70	90	1.2	1.3	16	1.7	400	2.4	30	5	550
	>70	90	1.2	1.3	16	1.7	400	2.4	30	5	550
Females	9-13	45	0.9	0.9	12	1.0	300	1.8	20	4	375
	14-18	65	1.0	1.0	14	1.2	400	2.4	25	5	400
	19-30	75	1.1	1.1	14	1.3	400	2.4	30	5	425
	31-50	75	1.1	1.1	14	1.3	400	2.4	30	5	425
	50-70	75	1.1	1.1	14	1.5	400	2.4	30	5	425
	>70	75	1.1	1.1	14	1.5	400	2.4	30	5	425
Pregnant	≤18	80	1.4	1.4	18	1.9	600	2.6	30	6	450
	19-30	85	1.4	1.4	18	1.9	600	2.6	30	6	450
	31-50	85	1.4	1.4	18	1.9	600	2.6	30	6	450
Lactating	≤18	115	1.4	1.6	17	2	500	2.8	35	7	550
	19-30	120	1.4	1.6	17	2	500	2.8	35	7	550
	31-50	120	1.4	1.6	17	2	500	2.8	35	7	550

Note: Some of the values listed as RDA are Adequate Intake (AI) Values set by the Nutrition and Food Board. AI are similar to RDA, but lack the same knowledge base.
*1 NE = 1 mg niacin = 60 mg of tryptophan

Minerals

	Age (years) or Condition	Calcium (mg/day)	Phosphorus (mg/day)	Magnesium (mg/day)	Iron (mg/day)	Zinc (mg/day)	Selenium (µg/day)	Copper (µg/day)
Infants	0-0.5	210	100	30	0.27	2	15	200
	0.5-1.0	270	275	75	11	3	20	220
Children	1-3	500	460	80	7	3	20	340
	4-8	800	500	130	10	5	30	440
Males	9-13	1300	1250	240	8	8	40	700
	14-18	1300	1250	410	11	11	55	890
	19-30	1000	700	400	8	11	55	900
	31-50	1000	700	420	8	11	55	900
	50-70	1200	700	420	8	11	55	900
	>70	1200	700	420	8	11	55	900
Females	9-13	1300	1250	240	8	8	40	700
	14-18	1300	1250	360	15	9	55	890
	19-30	1000	700	310	18	8	55	900
	31-50	1000	700	320	18	8	55	900
	50-70	1200	700	320	8	8	55	900
	>70	1200	700	320	8	8	55	900
Pregnant	≤18	1300	1250	400	27	12	60	1000
	19-30	1000	700	350	27	11	60	1000
	31-50	1000	700	360	27	11	60	1000
Lactating	≤18	1300	1250	360	10	13	70	1300
	19-30	1000	700	310	9	12	70	1300
	31-50	1000	700	320	9	12	70	1300

Note: Some of the values listed as RDA are Adequate Intake (AI) Values set by the Nutrition and Food Board. AI are similar to RDA, but lack the same knowledge base.

TABLE 3.2 (continued)

Minerals (continued)

	Age (years) or Condition	Iodine (µg/day)	Chromium (µg/day)	Fluoride (mg/day)	Manganese (mg/day)	Molybdenum (µg/day)
Infants	0-0.5	110	0.2	0.01	0.003	2
	0.5-1.0	130	5.5	0.5	0.6	3
Children	1-3	90	11	0.7	1.2	17
	4-8	90	15	1	1.5	22
Males	9-13	120	25	2	1.9	34
	14-18	150	35	3	2.2	43
	19-30	150	35	4	2.3	45
	31-50	150	35	4	2.3	45
	50-70	150	30	4	2.3	45
	> 70	150	30	4	2.3	45
Females	9-13	120	21	2	1.6	34
	14-18	150	24	3	1.6	43
	19-30	150	25	3	1.8	45
	31-50	150	25	3	1.8	45
	50-70	150	20	3	1.8	45
	>70	150	20	3	1.8	45
Pregnant	≤18	220	29	3	2	50
	19-30	220	30	3	2	50
	31-50	220	30	3	2	50
Lactating	≤18	290	44	3	2.6	50
	19-30	290	45	3	2.6	50
	31-50	290	45	3	2.6	50

Note: Some of the values listed as RDA are Adequate Intake (AI) Values set by the Nutrition and Food Board. AI are similar to RDA, but lack the same knowledge base.

body and the amount needed to maintain respectable levels of that nutrient in body tissue. When these studies were performed, scientists observed that there was quite a bit of variability among the balances of different individuals. A hypothetical representation of a particular nutrient's balance is depicted in Figure 3.1. In this figure we see that the RDA for this nutrient is set to include about 99 percent of the people sampled. Therefore, generally speaking, the RDAs will provide more of the nutrient than needed for balance for most individuals. From this we can certainly understand that the RDAs are not really personal recommendations but are more appropriate for making recommendations for populations. For example, the RDA for vitamin C for adult women is 60 mg, which would allow for adequate replacement of vitamin C losses for about 98 percent of adult women.

It should be noted that the recommendation for energy was not set to include 98 percent of the population, but only 50 percent (see Figure 3.1). If the recommendation was set to include 98 percent of the population this might lead to weight gain for most people using the recommendation for energy as a guideline. The most practical way to determine your energy needs is to experiment at home. Determine any fluctuations in body weight over time while altering your food energy intake. Ultimately, you find the energy intake that produces neither weight loss nor gain.

Beyond balance studies, other research studies involving the relationship between the essential nutrients and the body are reviewed to help determine the RDA. For example, the RDA for many nutrients during the years of rapid growth and during pregnancy must take into account not only balance but also the provision of additional amounts of a nutrient to allow for these periods of rapid growth. RDA determinations do not take into consideration disease, medications, or exercise training.

Alcohol is another energy-providing substance and may be classified as a nutrient because it provides energy. However, it is not an essential nutrient because it is not necessary for growth, development, and the maintenance of health. In fact, many nutritionists will not even recognize alcohol as a nutrient because of the health risks associated with overconsumption.

Are the RDAs used for food labeling?

To protect the public against misleading statements on food labels, U.S. Congress has made it mandatory by law that food manufacturers

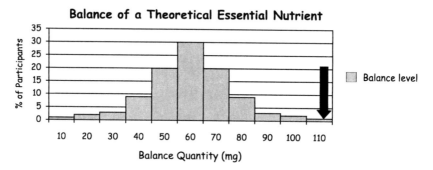

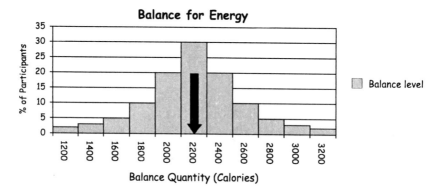

FIGURE 3.1. Based upon balance studies the RDA (arrows) for an essential nutrient would include roughly 98 percent of the general population (top). Here, the RDA for the theoretical nutrient would be about 110 mg. Meanwhile, the recommendation for energy (bottom) is set at an average energy needed for balance so that it does not generally promote excessive energy consumption.

follow specific guidelines on their food labels. Food labels contain the *Nutrition Facts,* which in most cases provide at least the following information:

- A listing of ingredients in descending order by weight
- Serving size
- Servings per container
- Amount of the following per serving: total calories, total protein, calories contributed by fat, total fat, saturated fat, cholesterol, total carbohydrate, sugar, dietary fiber, vitamin A, vitamin C, calcium, iron, sodium

As many individuals try to plan their nutrient intake, the nutrition facts also include the *daily value* (DV). The DV uses reference nutrition standards to indicate how a single serving of a food item relates to the standards. The DV is based upon current nutritional recommendation standards, which are based on the guidelines that follow.

- A maximum of 30 percent total Cal from fat, or < 65 g total
- A maximum of 10 percent total Cal from saturated fat, or < 20 g
- A minimum of 60 percent total Cal from carbohydrate
- 10 percent of total Cal from protein
- 10 g of fiber per 1,000 Cal
- A maximum of 300 mg of cholesterol
- A maximum of 2,400 mg of sodium

Also, the DV for other nutrients, such as vitamins A and C, thiamin, riboflavin, niacin, calcium, and iron, are founded upon RDA-based standards. However, these standards are not as specific for gender and age as the RDAs and therefore one quantity will apply to all people. The DV is expressed as a percentage and is based on a 2,000 and/or a 2,500 Cal intake, which approximates most American's recommended energy intake. Therefore a food providing 250 Cal per serving will be listed as either 13 percent or 10 percent DV for a 2,000 and 2,500 Cal diet intake, respectively. Beyond the nutrition facts, food manufacturers must also follow federal guidelines for other statements they choose to make on a food label. Some of the statements are listed on Table 3.3.

What is in my food besides food?

Many if not most manufactured foods contain food additives used to improve taste, texture, appearance, shelf life, safety, or nutritional value of the product. Some of the general food additive categories include: antioxidants, antimicrobials, coloring agents, emulsifiers, flavoring agents, sweeteners, pH controllers, leavening agents, texturizers, stabilizers, enzymes, and conditioners. All food additives were tested for safety and received approval by the Food and Drug Administration (FDA). This process can take years.

TABLE 3.3. Guidelines for Food Label Claims

Claim	Requirement
Fat free	Must contain less than 0.5 g per serving
Saturated fat free	Must contain less than 0.5 g per serving
Cholesterol free	Must contain less than 2 mg per serving
Sugar free	Must contain less than 0.5 g per serving
Sodium free	Must contain less than 5 mg per serving
Calorie free	Must contain less than 5 Cal per serving
Low fat	Must contain no more than 3 g of fat per serving
Low sodium	Must contain less than 40 mg per serving
Low calories	Must contain less than 40 Cal per serving
Low cholesterol	Must contain less than 20 mg per serving
High or good source	One serving must contain at least 20 percent or more of the recommendation for that nutrient
Reduced, less, or fewer	Must contain at least 25 percent less of a nutrient, per serving, as compared to the same nutrient in a reference food
More or added	Must contain at least 10 percent more of the DV for a nutrient as compared to a reference food
Light or lite	The food must contain at least 50 percent less fat than a similar, unmodified food which in its unmodified form contains more than 50 percent of its Cal from fat
Lean (meat, fish, poultry)	Must contain less than 10 g of fat, 4 g of saturated fat, and 95 mg of cholesterol per 100 g of the food
Extra lean	Must contain less than 5 g of fat, 2 g of saturated fat, and 95 mg of cholesterol per 100 g of the food
Fresh	Food must be unprocessed, in raw state, and never frozen

NUTRITION SUPPLEMENTS ARE
A MULTIBILLION-DOLLAR INDUSTRY

What are nutritional supplements?

Nutritional supplements are substances that are either common or uncommon to natural foods, but in some way they should contain one or more ingredients that would exist in a potentially edible food. These substances are either extracted from a natural food or they are made in a laboratory. Nutritional supplements probably began as an honest attempt to fill nutritional voids in the human diet. For example, a supplement may help an individual who does not eat dairy foods meet their calcium needs. However, from honest intentions the supplement business has evolved into a multibillion-dollar industry. Nutrition supplements are sold in supermarkets, drugstores, and stores typically found in shopping malls. These stores sell everything from recognized nutrients such as protein and amino acid preparations, essential fatty acids and fish oil supplements, and vitamins and minerals, to more obscure substances such as bee pollen, ginseng, choline, para-amino-benzoic acid (PABA), ginkgo biloba, conjugated linoleic acid (CLA), and carnitine. Well over 100 unique substances are marketed as nutrition supplements. Nutrition supplements are not as stringently regulated by the U.S. federal government as are intact foods or drugs. Therefore, the boundaries and guidelines for nutrition supplements are not as well defined as those for foods or drugs. As we move through the ensuing chapters we will mention different supplements as they apply to different topics of normal and applied nutrition topics.

Who needs a nutritional supplement?

Many nutritionists contend that if a person's diet is well balanced, containing multiple servings of fruits, vegetables, and dairy products, and includes adequate protein, essential fatty acids, and fiber, that individual is probably at least meeting the recommendations established for essential nutrients. Therefore, he or she would not be in need of a nutrition supplement. Also, if that individual's average daily intake for one or more essential nutrients was below recommendations, a nutritionist might try to encourage the inclusion of certain foods containing the desired nutrient rather than recommending a nutritional supplement. In many cases the simple addition or substitution of one or more food items in a diet can make the difference. However, unrelenting food preferences, food intolerance and allergies, or limited availability of certain foods can certainly necessitate the consideration of a nutrition supplement.

While vitamins and mineral preparations were the biggest selling nutrition supplements for many decades, today more and more of the market belongs to those supplements geared toward performance or physical appearance. Among the best sellers today are supplements purported to increase energy expenditure, increase muscle mass, and decrease body fat. Among these are supplements containing ephedrine, caffeine, creatine, and androstenedione. Therefore, personal quests for enhanced muscular size and potential enhancement of athletic performance may lead someone to purchase one or more nutrition supplements.

What should you know before you buy a supplement?

Before purchasing a nutritional supplement the consumer should have an understanding of the proven properties of the substance. The testimonial of friends and articles written in a popular magazine should not always be trusted for accuracy. Freelance writers who may not have an educational background in the health sciences but can write a very believable article often author these pieces. Your most accurate source of nutritional information is people educated in nutrition/medical-related fields, preferably with a higher educational degree (PhD, MD, DO) and who study the most current nutrition research. Make sure the author of a given book or article, or an individual presenting a seminar, is well educated in that field. Ask for credentials from reputable universities and colleges that actually have campuses.

If you are thinking about purchasing a supplement to enhance a particular aspect of your life, such as athletic performance or disease prevention/treatment, make sure the substance has been tested under circumstances similar to those to which you want to apply the supplement. For example, just because a certain vitamin is essential for normal energy metabolism does not mean that a supplemental dose of that vitamin will enhance your energy level during exercise. In another example, the nutrition supplement conjugated linoleic acid has been shown to decrease fat levels and the potential for cancer. However, nearly all the studies to date involved rodents and other animals or extracted cells. Therefore, the true effect on humans is not known because it has not been thoroughly tested in people. Furthermore, the original research should have been published in an established scientific publication, such as the *Journal of the American Medical Association, Journal of Physiology, New England Journal of Medicine, Journal of Nutrition, Medicine and Science in Sports and Exercise,* and the *American Journal of Clinical Nutrition.* These journals are peer reviewed, meaning that before a research article is published it is thoroughly evaluated by scientists who are experts in that field. Ask for this kind of information when you visit your local supplement supplier. Do not rely exclusively on the manufacturer's insert or brochure. Remember: they are trying to sell the product.

Often we read articles in certain "health" magazines that convince us of the benefits of a certain substance only to find an advertisement and ordering information for that supplement five pages later. It makes you wonder if it was really a credible article or just clever advertising designed to appear as a credible article. This is especially true when the same company that published the magazine sells the supplement. This happens a lot, especially in the bodybuilding arena. Be wary of magazine articles that seem trustworthy but have the word "ADVERTISEMENT" written at the top of the page in tiny print. Remember it is easier to believe something to be true, such as the need for a particular supplement, when there is a positive claim involved or a claim that is in line with what you are seeking. Also keep in mind that many of these substances have not undergone thorough scientific experimentation to test the purported properties and many may even have detrimental effects. Again, this goes back to the idea that nutrition supplements are not as stringently regulated as drugs.

Does "natural" always mean healthy?

Just as many drugs prescribed today are derived from chemicals naturally found in certain plants and animals, so too will some nutritional supplements come with druglike properties. Plants and animals make chemicals to support their own existence and some of these chemicals can indeed be toxic to other life-forms when ingested in significant quantities. So before you drink a tea made from a jungle tree bark, taste the jam made from exotic wild berries, or mix a powder made from the glands of an extraordinary fish into a glass of drinking water, make sure you know it is safe. For instance, fish oil supplements can decrease the ability of your blood to clot, which is potentially beneficial for people at risk of a heart attack. In this sense it is a "blood thinner." Should fish oil and related supplements be considered drugs? This is where the gray area exists for nutrition supplements and drugs. When do you stop calling a nutrition supplement a supplement and start calling it a drug? Another example is ephedrine (ma huang) from the ephedra plant. Ephedrine is a chemical that can mimic some of the actions of epinephrine (adrenalin). It can enhance the energy expenditure of some people by having a stimulatory effect on parts of the body, such as the heart. Several deaths have been attributed to ephedrine toxicity. At what point do we begin to recognize this chemical as a drug? It is likely that, by the time that you read this book, ephredrine will be restricted from supplement marketing. So we will see what happens.

Because a substance is *natural* does not always mean it is healthy. Remember the root of the word *natural* is nature. Humans are but a very small component of nature. Ultimately, the earth is not here for us, as we are perhaps temporary inhabitants. Therefore, many aspects of nature will not be compatible with our health or existence. This is especially true for chemicals produced by plants. As mentioned above, plants cannot run or hide from predators. Therefore, in order to survive, plants make a host of substances with which to defend themselves. Some of these substances are poisonous to insects, while others can impair the normal functions of the animals that eat them. In fact, the main insecticide in Round-Up is naturally produced by some plants. These concepts also apply to humans. While some of these substances in smaller amounts may have health-promoting properties, too much can be dangerous. We need to be very careful.

What are nutraceuticals and functional foods?

The latter portion of the twentieth century was a time of great strides in modifying the way many nutritionists and health care practitioners viewed nutrition. For decades we made nutritional recommendations based upon what needed to be avoided or limited in our diet choices. The nutritional "bad guys" were fat, which evolved to saturated fat-rich foods, cholesterol, sodium, and arguably sugar. Today it is quite clear that the other side of the nutrition coin, or "what we should eat," is probably as significant as "what we should not eat." *Nutraceuticals* are substances found in natural foods that seem to have the potential to prevent disease or be used in the treatment of various disorders. Meanwhile, *functional foods* are the foods in which one or more nutraceuticals can be found. Nutraceutical substances include some of the more recognized nutrients such as vitamins C and E and the mineral calcium, but also include such substances as genestein, β-carotene, capsaicin, allium compounds, lycopene, and so on (see Tables 3.4 through 3.6).

As you may have already surmised it is possible for a nutraceutical to be an essential nutrient. However, keep in mind that the nutra-

TABLE 3.4. Examples of Nutraceutical Substances Grouped by Natural Food Source

Plants		Animal	Microbial
β-glucan,	Allicin	Conjugated Linoleic Acid (CLA)	*Saccharomyces*
Ascorbic acid	*d*-limonene	Eicosapentaenoic acid (EPA)	*Boulardii*
γ-tocotrienol	Genestein	Docosahexenoic acid (DHA)	(yeast)
Quercetin	Lycopene	Spingolipids	*Bifidobacterium bifidum*
Luteolin	Hemicellulose	Choline	*Bifidobacterium longum*
Cellulose	Lignin	Lecithin	*Bifidobacterium infantis*
Lutein	Capsaicin	Calcium	*Lactobacillus acidophilus*
Gallic acid	Geraniol	Ubiquinone (coenzyme Q_{10})	(LC1)
Perillyl alcohol	β-ionone	Selenium	*Lactobacillus acidophilus*
Indole-3-	α-tocopherol	Zinc	(NCFB 1748)
Carbonol	β-carotene		*Streptococcus salvarius*
Pectin	Nordihydro-		(subs. *Thermophilus*)
Daidzein	capsaicin		
Glutathione	Selenium		
Potassium	Zeaxanthin		

Source: Wildman, R.E.C., *The Handbook of Nutraceuticals and Functional Foods* (CRC Press, 2001, p. 15).
Note: The substances listed in this table include those that are either accepted or purported nutraceutical substances.

ceutical properties of certain essential nutrients may not be why they are essential in the first place. For instance, vitamin C is essential for making important molecules in our body such as collagen, yet its nutraceutical roles may be more related to its antioxidant activities. We will spend more time discussing nutraceutical compounds in the later chapters. We are going to be hearing more and more about nutraceuticals for years to come.

Table 3.5. Examples of Foods with Higher Contents of Specific Nutraceutical Substances

Nutraceutical Substance/Family	Foods of Remarkably High Content
Allyl sulfur compounds	Onions, garlic
Isoflavones	Soybeans and other legumes, apios
Quercetin	Onion, red grapes, citrus fruits, broccoli, Italian yellow squash
Capsaicinoids	Pepper fruit
EPA and DHA	Fish oils
Lycopene	Tomatoes and tomato products
Isothiocyanates	Cruciferous vegetables
β-glucan	Oat bran
CLA	Beef and dairy
Resveratrol	Grapes (skin), red wine
β-carotene	Citrus fruits, carrots, squash, pumpkin
Carnosol	Rosemary
Catechins	Teas, berries
Adenosine	Garlic, onion
Indoles	Cabbage, broccoli, cauliflower, kale, Brussel sprouts
Curcumin	Tumeric
Ellagic acid	Grapes, strawberries, raspberries, walnuts
Anthocyanates	Red wine
3-n-butyl phthalide	Celery
Cellulose	Most plants (component of cell walls)

Source: Wildman, R.E.C., *The Handbook of Nutraceuticals and Functional Foods* (CRC Press, 2001, p. 16).
Note: The substances listed on this table include those that are either accepted or purported nutraceutical substances.

TABLE 3.6. Examples of Nutraceuticals Grouped by Mechanisms of Action

Anticancer	Positive Influence on Blood Lipids	Antioxidation	Anti-inflamm atory	Osteogenetic or Bone Protective
Capsaicin	β-glucan	CLA	Linolenic acid	CLA
Genestein	γ-tocotrienol	Ascorbic acid	EPA	Soy protein
Daidzein	δ-tocotrienol	β-carotene	DHA	Genestein
α-tocotrienol	MUFA	Polyphenolics	Capsaicin	Daidzein
γ-tocotrienol	Quercetin	Tocopherols	Quercetin	Calcium
CLA	ω-3 PUFAs	Tocotrienols	Curcumin	
Lactobacillus acidophilus	Resveratrol	Indole-3-carbonol		
Sphingolipids	Tannins	α-tocopherol		
Limonene	β-sitosterol	Ellagic acid		
Diallyl sulfide	Saponins	Lycopene		
Ajoene		Lutein		
α-tocopherol		Glutathione		
Enterolactone		Hydroxytyrosol		
Glycyrrhizin		Luteolin		
Equol		Oleuropein		
Curcumin		Catechins		
Ellagic acid		Gingerol		
Lutein		Chlorogenic acid		
Carnosol		Tannins		
Lactobacillus bulgaricus				

Source: Wildman, R.E.C., *The Handbook of Nutraceuticals and Functional Foods* (CRC Press, 2001, p. 17).
Note: The substances listed in this table include those that are either accepted or purported nutraceutical substances.

Chapter 4

Carbohydrates Are
Our Most Basic Fuel Source

CARBOHYDRATES POWER OUR BODY

The term carbohydrate was coined long ago as scientists observed a consistent pattern in the chemical formula of most carbohydrates. Not only were they composed of only carbon, hydrogen, and oxygen but also the ratio of carbon to the chemical formula of water is typically one to one ($C:H_2O$). Carbohydrate means "carbon with water." For example, carbohydrates glucose and galactose have the following chemical formula:

$$C_6H_{12}O_6 \text{ or } (CH_2O)_6$$

Where do carbohydrates come from?

To create energy-providing carbohydrates from the non-energy-providing molecules H_2O and CO_2 is a talent bestowed only to plants and a handful of bacteria. In a process called *photosynthesis,* plants couple H_2O and CO_2 by harnessing solar energy. Along with carbohydrates, O_2 is also a product of this reaction:

$$6\,CO_2 + 6\,H_2O \longrightarrow C_6H_{12}O_6 + 6\,O_2$$

Humans are unable to perform photosynthesis and thus we eat plants and plant products such as fruits, vegetables, and bread products to obtain a rich supply of carbohydrates. Beyond plants and their products, milk and dairy are also good sources of carbohydrates. In fact, milk is the only good animal source of carbohydrate. It should be mentioned that although humans cannot perform photosynthesis, we do possess the ability to make some carbohydrate in our body.

However, in order to do so, we must use molecules that already possess energy, as we will discuss soon enough.

Are there different types and classes of carbohydrates?

As you might guess, numerous different kinds of carbohydrates are found in nature; our discussion will be limited to those carbohydrates found in greater amounts in our diet and those important to our body. The simplest carbohydrates are the monosaccharides, which include glucose, fructose, and galactose. Other examples of monosaccharides include xylose, mannose, and ribose, but these may not be as familiar to you. There are over 100 different monosaccharides found in nature.

Glucose and fructose can be found in foods both independently or as part of larger carbohydrates. Fructose is what makes honey and many fruits sweet and is used commercially as a sweetener (i.e., high fructose corn syrup). On the other hand, while some galactose is found in certain foods, it is mostly found as part of larger carbohydrates.

Monosaccharides are as small as carbohydrates get. Said another way, monosaccharides cannot be split into smaller carbohydrates. All other carbohydrates are made up of monosaccharides linked together. For instance, disaccharides are composed of two monosaccharides linked together. The three disaccharides found in our diet, including their monosaccharide building blocks, are listed in Table 4.1.

Looking at Table 4.1 we see that glucose is one-half of the disaccharides lactose and sucrose and both halves of maltose. Maltose, or malt sugar, may be part of our diet in seeds or alcoholic beverages. Sucrose is derived from the sugarcane plant, which helps us understand why we call it "sugar." Lactose is the primary carbohydrate found in milk and dairy products. Nutrition scientists often refer to monosaccharides and disaccharides as "simple sugars" because of their relatively small carbohydrate size and their sweet taste.

Monosaccharides not only serve as building blocks for disaccharides but also for some larger forms of carbohydrates as well. The

TABLE 4.1. Disaccharide Building Blocks

Disaccharide	Monosaccharide Involved
Lactose	Glucose + galactose
Sucrose	Glucose + fructose
Maltose	Glucose + glucose

most recognizable larger carbohydrate is starch. Starch is found in varying degrees in plants and their products. It consists of large straight and branching chains of the monosaccharide glucose (see Figure 4.1). Plants make starch to store their energy in much the same way we store fat. Plant fibers, on the other hand, are also composed of straight and branching chains of monosaccharides, but their building-block monosaccharides are not limited only to glucose. Fibers are discussed later in this chapter.

In the human diet, we can also find a small amount of carbohydrates, called oligosaccharides, constructed from just a few monosaccharides (three to ten) linked together. Since these are found in relatively small amounts, they are not as essential to discuss. However, a few of these carbohydrates (e.g., raffinose and stachyose) will require mention, not necessarily for their nutritional value but for their effects within the digestive tract.

What do carbohydrates do in our body?

Carbohydrates play quite a few roles in the human body, but perhaps none as important as being an energy source for all cells. All cells in the body will use glucose to some degree. Meanwhile, cells of the CNS as well as RBCs and certain other types of cells in our body will exclusively use glucose under normal situations. Carbohydrates also provide limited yet readily available energy store called *glycogen*. Carbohydrates are also a modest yet vital component of cell membranes. Certain carbohydrates are also key portions of indis-

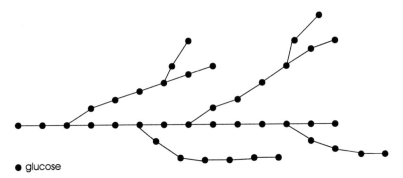

● glucose

FIGURE 4.1. Schematic of the highly branching links of glucose that make up starch (plants) and glycogen in animals. Glycogen is more highly branched than starch.

pensable molecules. For example, molecules such as DNA and RNA contain the carbohydrate ribose. Ribose is a monosaccharide that can be made in our cells from glucose. Also, very complex carbohydrates called glycosaminoglycans (GAGs) are very important in connective tissue, such as in our joints. The GAGs include chondroitin sulfate and hyaluronic acid, which are becoming popular nutrition supplements for joint inflammatory disorders.

CARBOHYDRATES ARE ABSORBED AS MONOSACCHARIDES

How much carbohydrate do we eat?

Carbohydrate consumption varies among populations on this planet. In America about half of the energy we eat comes by way of carbohydrates. About half of this carbohydrate is in the form of starch and the other half in the form of simple sugars. Sucrose makes up about half of the simple sugars we eat. In other areas of the world such as Africa and Asia sucrose consumption makes a lesser contribution while whole grains (e.g., wheat and rice), fruits, and vegetables make a greater contribution.

Sucrose consumption in the United States has risen steadily over the past century. The average consumption of sucrose, either by adding it as table sugar at home or by eating manufactured foods and beverages with sucrose as an ingredient was about 45 lb per person in the early 1990s. While sucrose consumption continues to rise, carbohydrate intake (as percentage of total Cal) has decreased over the past several decades. This decrease is largely due to the coinciding rise in fat consumption over the past century.

The carbohydrate content of certain types of food is listed in Table 4.2. Looking at this table we see that "sweets" such as candies and cakes are among those with the highest content of carbohydrate. Furthermore, nearly all of the carbohydrate in these foods comes by way of sucrose, which is added as a recipe ingredient. Fruits may be somewhat deceiving, according to Table 4.2, as their carbohydrate content is listed as roughly 5 to 20 percent. However, keep in mind that their water content makes up most of the remaining weight. Therefore carbohydrate is the major "dry" material in fruits. Cereal grains and products such as rice, oats, pastas, and breads also have a relatively

TABLE 4.2. Carbohydrate Content of Select Foods

Food	Carbohydrate (% of weight)
Sugar	100
Ice cream, cake, pie	40-50
Fruits and vegetables	5-20
Nuts	< 10
Peanut butter	< 10
Milk	5
Cheese	1
Shellfish and other fish	< 1
Meat, poultry, and eggs	< 1
Butter	0
Oils	0

high carbohydrate content. Conversely, animal foods such as meats, fish, and poultry (and eggs) are virtually void of carbohydrate. Animal flesh (skeletal muscle) does contain carbohydrate (glycogen) which is lost during the processing of the meat. Milk and some dairy products (yogurt, ice cream) are the only significant animal-derived carbohydrate providers.

Later in this book we will look more closely at some of the most popular diets today. These include those marketed by Dr. Atkins and Sugar Busters! On these diets, the followers eat very low amounts of carbohydrate. Therefore foods such as desserts, pastas, rice, breads, fruits, etc., are excluded or used very sparingly. Meanwhile, carbohydrate-void foods, such as meats, fish, oils, butter, etc., are consumed without concern. In addition many low-carbohydrate manufactured foods such as pasta, sodas, and breads are marketed for followers of these diets. The production of these foods requires some fancy food science, as explained later.

What are the recommendations for carbohydrate consumption?

Carbohydrate does not have an established RDA. However as part of the latest recommendations the National Research Council stated that more than half of our energy intake should come by way of carbohydrates. In support, most nutritionists do agree that the more carbohydrate the better, providing upward of 50 to 65 percent of the energy we eat. It is also recommended that most carbohydrates should come by way of fruits, vegetables, whole grain products, and lower-fat milks and dairy products. These carbohydrate sources will not only make a lower-fat contribution to our caloric intake, but also provide vitamins, minerals, fibers, and other nutraceutical compounds. However, as of late, popular diets have professed the benefits of a lower carbohydrate intake. We will spend time discussing the pros and cons of these types of diets later on.

In light of the human body's ability to make some glucose from certain substances, the question has been raised as to whether we need to eat carbohydrates at all. It does seem that at least 50 to 100 g of carbohydrate per day is necessary to prevent ketosis. Ketosis is a metabolic situation that occurs when fat becomes the primary energy source for longer periods of time. Ketosis is discussed in Chapter 5.

How are dietary carbohydrates digested?

Normally, just about all nonfiber dietary carbohydrate will be absorbed across the wall of our small intestine. As monosaccharides are the absorbed form of carbohydrate, disaccharides and starch must be broken down into monosaccharides. Carbohydrate digestion begins in the mouth as chewing breaks up food and mixes it with saliva. Saliva contains *salivary amylase,* which is an enzyme that begins to break down starch. The activity of salivary amylase is short lived due to the rather brief period of time that food stays in the mouth. As the swallowed food/saliva mixture reaches the stomach the acidic juice reduces the activity of salivary amylase, which halts carbohydrate digestion.

Chemical digestion of carbohydrates picks up again in the small intestine as the pancreas delivers *pancreatic amylase* along with a battery of other digestive enzymes. Pancreatic amylase resumes the assault upon starch molecules, breaking them into smaller links of glucose. The cells that line the small intestine will have the final say in carbohydrate digestion. They will produce enzymes that handle the smaller carbohydrates, such as disaccharides and the branch points of starch. The enzymes that split sucrose, maltose, and lactose into monosaccharides are called sucrase, maltase, and lactase, respectively.

Once monosaccharides are liberated they can move into the cells lining the wall of the small intestine. They can then move out the back end of these cells and then into tiny blood vessels (capillaries) in the wall of the small intestine. These capillaries drain into a larger blood vessel that leaves the intestines and travels to the liver (see Figure 4.2). It should be mentioned that the absorption of glucose and galactose requires energy (ATP) but fructose does not.

What is lactose intolerance?

By early childhood most of the world population, especially people of African, Asian, and Greek descent, lose the ability to produce sufficient amounts of the digestive enzyme lactase. This results in poor lactose digestion. The undigested lactose is not absorbed and continues to move through the small intestine. As lactose continues through the digestive tract it falls victim to bacteria in the colon. Bacteria easily break down lactose for energy and produce gases and other substances in the process. The gases that are produced can lead to bloating, cramping, and flatulence. Also, as lactose moves through

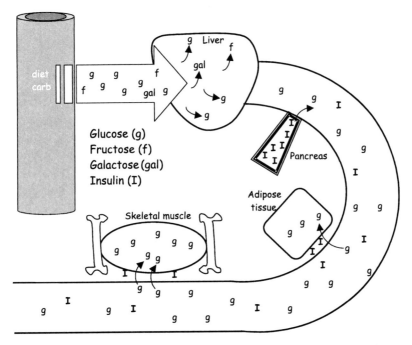

FIGURE 4.2. When blood glucose levels become elevated the pancreas releases insulin which promotes the uptake of glucose in muscle and fat cells.

the digestive tract it will hold onto water, which can soften feces and possibly produce diarrhea. These discomforts are collectively referred to as *lactose intolerance*.

It is interesting to ponder whether it is natural for humans to become lactose intolerant. Humans may be the only mammal that continues to consume milk after being weaned from their mothers' milk. We consider milk essential in our quest to meet our calcium needs and also we use milk as an ingredient in many recipes. Since lactose intolerance affects the greater majority of the population to some degree, and considering other mammals, it is easy to argue that perhaps it is more natural for us to lose the ability to produce adequate lactase. To deal with lactose intolerance many people add a product called Lactaid (lactase enzyme) to their milk to predigest the lactose. Lactaid milk is also available. This appears to be an effective method of adapting to lactose intolerance.

Why do beans produce gas in our digestive tract?

Legumes are plants that have a single row of seeds in their pods. What we commonly call legumes, such as peas, green beans, lima beans, pinto beans, black-eyed peas, garbanzo beans, lentils, and soybeans, are often the seeds of legume plants. Stachyose, raffinose, and other similar carbohydrates can be found in most legumes and these shorter links of monosaccharides are generally resistant to our carbohydrate digestive enzymes. These carbohydrates tend to contain three to five monosaccharides and their design tends to be a disaccharide linked to one or two monosaccharides. These interesting carbohydrate arrangements are not readily digested by the digestive enzymes. So, similar to lactose in lactose intolerant people, these carbohydrates will stay intact in our small intestine and carry into our colon. In the colon, bacteria break down these carbohydrates producing gases which lead to bloating, cramping, and flatulence. A product available in stores called Beano is an enzyme preparation that will digest these carbohydrates when it is ingested just prior to the legume-containing meal.

How are sweeteners related to carbohydrates?

All of the sugars mentioned, either as monosaccharides or disaccharides, elicit a sweet taste and are thus referred to as natural sweeteners (see Table 4.3). Therefore, simple sugars can be added to foods

TABLE 4.3. Sweetness of Sugars and Alternatives

Type of Sweetener	Sweetness (Relative to Sucrose)	Typical Sources
Simple Sugars		
Lactose	0.2	Dairy
Maltose	0.4	Germinating (sprouted) seeds
Glucose	0.7	Corn syrup
Sucrose	1.0	Table sugar
Fructose	1.7	Fruit, honey, sweetener (HFCS in soft drinks)
Sugar Alcohols		
Sorbitol	0.6	Diet candies, sugarless gums
Mannitol	0.7	Diet candies, sugarless gum
Xylitol	0.9	Sugarless gum, diet candies
Artificial Sweeteners		
Aspartame (NutraSweet)	200	Diet soft drinks, powdered sweeteners
Acesulfame-K 200	200	Sugarless gum, diet drink mixes
Saccharin	500	Diet soft drinks, powdered sweeteners
Sucralose	600	Diet soft drinks, sugarless gum, cold desserts

to enhance their sweetness. However, since these sweet molecules also come with an energy value, food manufacturers and people often try to substitute natural sweeteners with an alternative sweetener that does not carry the same energy content. Also, simple sugars in food can adhere to our teeth and promote the formation of dental caries. Many candies and gums are manufactured with alternative sweeteners to reduce their potential to promote tooth decay.

Saccharin has long been a controversial sweetener, as the FDA proposed a ban in 1977. This movement was due in large part to reports of experimental animals consuming saccharin and their increased cancer risk. However, the methods used in these studies raised some concerns regarding the applicability to people. Laboratory animals were fed very large doses of saccharin over an extended period of time. The saccharin in their diet would be the equivalent of humans drinking improbably high quantities of saccharin-sweetened diet sodas every day for months. In any regard, the cancer-promoting potential of saccharin is still questionable in levels that would be typically consumed by people and therefore products containing saccharin may carry a warning on their labels. Saccharin is 500 times as sweet as sucrose.

Aspartame, also known as NutraSweet, is a dipeptide that thinks it is a disaccharide. A dipeptide is two amino acids linked together. Typically, amino acids alone or together are not known for their sweetening abilities. However, when these two amino acids (phenylalanine and aspartic acid) are linked together along with methanol the result is a very potent sweetener. Since aspartame consists of amino acids, the building blocks of proteins, it has an energy value. However, because aspartame is about 200 times sweeter than sucrose, a little bit goes a very long way as a sweetener. Thus its energy value is nominal and certainly not a concern for those who count their calories.

You will find NutraSweet in food substances that are served chilled, not heated. Examples include diet drinks, gelatins, and diet gums. Aspartame is subject to breakdown when heated and therefore it is not ideal for use in baked sweets. Recently some concern has been expressed regarding consumption of NutraSweet and the development of neurological abnormalities such as headaches, dizziness, nausea, and other side effects. Many individuals have filed complaints with the FDA about NutraSweet. Some scientists think that these people may be more sensitive to one of the components of NutraSweet (or its metabolites) when it is broken down in the body. Furthermore, Acesulfame or Sunette is one of the latest sweeteners approved by the FDA and has an intensity of sweetness similar to NutraSweet. Acesulfame is used as a sweetener in many countries other than the United States and it appears to be stable in cooking processes, contrary to NutraSweet. Meanwhile, Sucralose is the new kid on the block, receiving FDA approval in 1998. Only these four sweeteners are approved at this time; however, other FDA approvals are pending.

Does a diet higher in sucrose cause acne, hyperactivity, or diabetes?

Over the years, many theories have evolved about the relationship between higher consumptions of sucrose and various diseases and conditions. First, dietary sugar does not appear to promote the development of diabetes mellitus, at least not directly. Diabetes mellitus can be largely categorized into two groups: those individuals that have a reduction in ability to make insulin (type 1) and those individuals that appear to make insulin, but whose muscle and fat cells appear to be less sensitive to its presence (type 2). In most cases of type 2 diabetes mellitus, one of the most significant underlying factors is an excessive body weight in the form of fat. If a person eats excessive amounts of sugary foods, which by simple excess of energy intake will lead to fat accumulation, obesity, and subsequent diabetes, then perhaps an argument can be made. However, sugar would then be an indirect factor, not a direct factor.

For many years researchers tried to link hyperactivity in children to a high-sugar diet. Much of the work completed in this area failed to show that a relationship exists. Hyperactivity or attention deficit hyperactivity disorder (ADHD) is currently believed to stem from a deficit in an individual's inhibitory processes in the brain. As many as two million children were diagnosed with ADHD in 1994, although some researchers believe that a significant percentage of those individuals did not actually have ADHD. Current treatment involves psychological treatment and/or taking an amphetamine-like substance called Ritalin (methylphenidate).

High-sugar foods do not seem to contribute to acne development either; acne appears to be more related to hormones circulating in the blood. In many situations, acne results from a clogging of pores that connect oil-releasing glands to the surface of our skin. When pores become clogged, they may eventually become infected, inflamed, and rise up. Many dermatologists recommend keeping the face clean without overwashing. Overwashing can irritate and dry the skin. Dry, tight skin from excessive washing may narrow or close pore openings, doing more harm than good.

It appears that perhaps the only direct cause-and-effect relationship between dietary sugar and disease is tooth decay. The mouth is exposed to the outside environment and is the entry point for food. Thus, the mouth becomes a natural home for bacteria. When sugary foods adhere to the teeth, bacteria can break down the sugar and produce acids that erode the outer layer of teeth, creating cavities. Brushing the teeth physically removes the sugar and much of the bacteria adhered to them. Also, some toothpastes contain baking soda, which, as a base, may help neutralize the acid produced by bacteria.

THE LEVEL OF CIRCULATING BLOOD GLUCOSE
IS TIGHTLY REGULATED

Once monosaccharides are absorbed, where do they go?

As mentioned, monosaccharides (glucose, fructose, and galactose) are absorbed into the body by crossing the wall of the small intestine and entering circulation via a special blood vessel called the *portal vein*. The portal vein connects the digestive tract to the liver. Thus, the liver gets the first shot at the absorbed monosaccharides. The liver is able to pull nearly all of the galactose and fructose from our blood as well as a respectable portion of the glucose (see Figure 4.2). However, much of the glucose continues past our liver and enters the general circulation where other tissue in our body will have a shot at it. This increases the concentration of glucose in the blood from a normal level (70 to 110 mg) to 150 to 160 mg of glucose per 100 mL of blood or higher.

Do all carbohydrate-containing foods cause a similar rise in blood glucose?

As glucose is half of the disaccharides and the only monosaccharide in starch, we can certainly expect the concentration of blood glucose to rise after eating a carbohydrate-containing meal. But by how much, and will different foods having the same amount of carbohydrate result in the same increase in blood glucose? Would factors such as rate of digestion and absorption need to be considered as well? This kind of information surely would be of interest to some people, such as those with diabetes mellitus as well as endurance athletes (as discussed in Chapter 11).

For the longest time, scientists assumed that because starch was more structurally complex than simpler sugars, starchy foods would be digested more slowly and therefore absorbed more slowly and evenly after a meal. If the glucose was absorbed more slowly and evenly, this would result in a lower rise in blood glucose levels (glycemic effect). Oppositely, foods containing simpler sugars (e.g., soda, candy) would be digested and absorbed more rapidly, leading to a greater rise in blood glucose. Surprisingly though, in the 1970s, scientists found that the glycemic effect of pure glucose and starches similar to those found in bread, rice, and potatoes were not substantially different in their glycemic effects.

In the glycemic index experiments just mentioned involving glucose and starch, the scientists compared extracted starch to glucose. But what about intact food? Surely other components of an intact food would influence the glycemic effect of a given food. This led to the development of the *glycemic index* (GI). The GI for a food is its glycemic effect relative to a standard carbohydrate source (white bread) (see Box 4.1). Those foods with a glycemic effect similar to white bread include syrups, candy, colas, sport drinks, and potatoes.

How does our body respond to the rise in blood glucose?

The concentration of glucose in the blood is very tightly regulated. When the blood concentration of glucose climbs above the normal level, the pancreas releases the hormone insulin (see Figures 4.2 and 4.3 and Box 4.2). Insulin will bind to receptors on muscle cells and fat cells, which results in glucose movement into these cells. Because skeletal muscle and fat cells together make up greater than half of our total body mass, the net effect is a fairly rapid return to a more normal blood glucose concentration. Insulin increases the movement of glucose in these cells by increasing the number of glucose transport pro-

---

BOX 4.1. Foods Grouped by Relative Glycemic Index*

Higher Glycemic Index (> 85)	Glucose, sucrose, maple syrup, corn syrup, honey, bagel, candy, corn flakes, carrots, crackers, molasses, potatoes, raisins, sport drinks with simple carbohydrates (Gatorade, POWERade), sport drinks with carbohydrate polymers (GatorLode)
Medium Glycemic Index (60-85)	All-bran cereal, banana, grapes, oatmeal, orange juice, pasta, rice, whole-grain rye bread, yams, corn, baked beans, potato chips
Lower Glycemic Index (< 60)	Fructose, apple, applesauce, Cheerios, kidney beans, navy beans, chickpeas, lentils, dates, figs, peaches, plums, ice cream, milk, yogurt, tomato soup

Source: Adapted from Williams, M. H., *Nutrition for Health Fitness and Sport,* Fifth Edition (WCB McGraw-Hill, 1999, p. 102).
*GIs listed are relative to glucose.

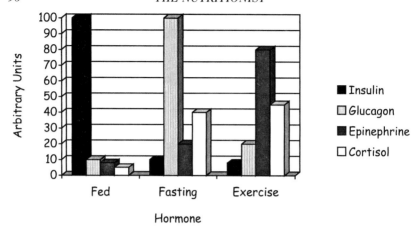

FIGURE 4.3. Relative levels of the major metabolic hormones during and right after a meal (fed), greater than 8-12 h after a meal (fasting), and during sustained moderate to higher intensity exercise. (Glucagon levels may increase during exercise if blood glucose levels decline.)

BOX 4.2. Actions of Insulin, Glucagon, Cortisol, and Epinephrine in Carbohydrate Metabolism

Insulin	• Increases the uptake of glucose by our muscle and fat cells
	• Increases the synthesis of glycogen in our muscle and liver
	• Increases fatty acid synthesis from excessive diet carbohydrate
	• Decreases fat breakdown and mobilization from our fat tissue
Glucagon	• Increases glycogen breakdown in our liver
	• Increases liver glycogen-derived glucose release into our blood
	• Increases glucose manufacturing in our liver
	• Increases fat breakdown and mobilization from our fat tissue
Epinephrine (Adrenalin)	• Increases glycogen breakdown in our liver and skeletal muscle
	• Increases liver glycogen-derived glucose release into our blood
	• Increases fat breakdown and mobilization from our fat tissue
Cortisol (Stress Hormone)	• Increases muscle protein breakdown to amino acids which can circulate to the liver and be used for glucose production
	• Increases liver glycogen-derived glucose release into our blood
	• Increases fat breakdown and mobilization from our fat tissue

teins on their plasma membranes. It is also this system that fails most people with type 2 diabetes mellitus.

All cells in our body will continuously pull a little bit of glucose from our blood throughout the day to help meet their constant need for energy. However, after a meal, the liver, muscle, and fat cells will take much more glucose out of the blood than they immediately need. This allows blood glucose levels to return to a normal, fasting concentration.

What will the liver, muscle, and fat cells do with the extra glucose they removed from the blood?

Not only will insulin promote the uptake of glucose in our muscle and fat tissues, it will also dictate how these tissues and our liver deal with the extra glucose. Insulin promotes the metabolic processes in these cells that allow them to immediately use glucose for energy as well as store the extra energy in glucose.

Even though carbohydrates contribute approximately one-half of the energy in our diet, our body composition is not reflective: a little less than 1 percent of our total body weight is attributable to carbohydrate. This means that carbohydrate is stored with limitations, most of which is in our liver and skeletal muscle as glycogen. Glycogen is composed of large branching links of glucose and is very similar to plant starch. Other tissues, such as fat cells and the heart, also contain a little glycogen; however, their contribution to our total body glycogen stores is very small. Our liver can manage about 6 to 8 percent of its weight as glycogen for about 100 g total. Only about 1 percent of the weight of skeletal muscle cells is attributable to glycogen. However, since the total amount of skeletal muscle in our body far exceeds our liver, it will contribute much more to our total glycogen stores. Skeletal muscle may contain about 350 to 400 g, which is about four-fifths of our total glycogen stores. As you may expect, people with more muscle resulting from exercise training will have more body glycogen due to increased muscle mass but also increased glycogen content in the muscle.

Since the potential to store glucose as glycogen is somewhat limited, we require another means of storing the energy present in extra glucose. Therefore, during the same time that our liver and skeletal muscle is busy making glycogen, our liver and fat tissue will also work to convert some of the extra glucose to fat. The fat that is made in our fat cells is stored within those cells. Meanwhile, the fat that is made in the liver is transported in the blood to fat cells and to a lesser degree other tissue such as muscle, breast tissue, etc. Interestingly, scientists have determined that our ability to convert excessive carbohydrate to fat might not be as efficient as we once thought. In fact, the conversion of excessive carbohydrate to fat may actually be a minimal operation in most adults. It now seems that consuming a high carbohydrate diet may increase our body fat content not necessarily by increasing the production of fat from carbohydrate, but more likely by decreasing our use of fat as a daily energy source as we are forced to use more carbohydrate.

Can eating a high carbohydrate diet make us fatter?

This is a point we need to be clear on. Eating too much energy makes us fat. The major focus here is the energy imbalance, not the carbohydrate content of the diet. Although it is true that eating a high carbohydrate diet in conjunction with eating excessive energy will certainly support weight (fat) gain, so too will excessive fat and/or protein.

One of the reasons that carbohydrates have been bashed as of late is because of the effects of insulin upon stored fat. Insulin hinders the release of fat from adipose tissue. Therefore many dieters believe that carbohydrates, or more specifically insulin, are working against them. However, this function of insulin is very important in the normal scheme of things. It keeps the fat tissue from breaking down and releasing fat during and for a couple hours after a meal. At this time absorbed food energy nutrients are circulating in our blood so there would be no need to break down our fat stores. Insulin will also promote the formation of fat from excess diet energy. So, the combination of decreased fat breakdown and increased fat production may lead people to believe that insulin makes them fat!

Before we dismiss this concept, that insulin is working against people in their quest to lose body fat, we should recognize that some people have elevated insulin and glucose levels during fasting. More times than not this occurs in people who have a higher level of body fat and low levels of activity. Thus eating a higher carbohydrate diet may indeed work against them to some degree. Eating a lower carbohydrate diet may allow for more fat to be used for energy, particularly during the first week or so of mild energy restriction. We discuss this more in Chapter 8.

What is diabetes mellitus?

For many people, the fine regulation of the level of blood glucose becomes impaired. This results in chronic high blood glucose concentrations medically known as *hyperglycemia*. The impairment may be due to a decreased ability of the pancreas to produce insulin. This is type 1 diabetes mellitus. The lack of insulin allows glucose levels to remain elevated even in a fasting state. Furthermore, after a meal blood glucose levels can climb exceptionally high (see Figure 4.4). In the past, type 1 diabetes mellitus has also been called insulin-dependent diabetes mellitus because medical treatment involves insulin therapy via injection. Recently, automated pumps for insulin delivery have become popular, and insulin nasal sprays may become common therapy in the future. Type 1 diabetes mellitus has also been referred to as juvenile (or child-onset) diabetes because diagnosis is much more common in children. However, type 1 diabetes mellitus is the most correct terminology.

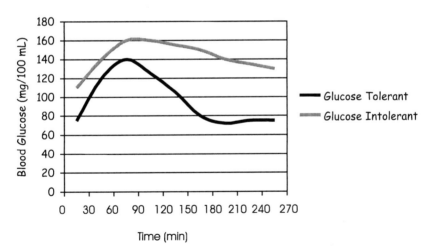

FIGURE 4.4. Glucose levels during an oral glucose tolerance test (OGTT). Two fasting people were provided with 75 g of glucose and their blood glucose was measured every thirty minutes for four hours. Note that even after four hours the glucose-intolerant person's blood glucose was still elevated.

For most other people diagnosed with diabetes mellitus, blood glucose regulation is impaired despite their ability to produce insulin. In fact, many of these individuals may actually produce more insulin than what seems normal. This type of diabetes mellitus is most appropriately referred to as type 2 diabetes mellitus. However, type 2 diabetes mellitus has also been known by other names. In the past it has also been referred to as non-insulin-dependent diabetes mellitus, as medical treatment did not absolutely require insulin injections. However, because insulin injections may be prescribed from time to time this terminology can be confusing. Also, this type of diabetes has been referred to as adult-onset diabetes mellitus. Again, this can be confusing as more and more cases of type 2 diabetes mellitus are being diagnosed in children.

It seems that in type 2 diabetes mellitus, muscle and fat cells become less sensitive to insulin. What has become very clear to researchers, physicians, and nutritionists is that there is a strong relationship between obesity and this form of diabetes mellitus. In fact, nearly 90 percent of all individuals diagnosed with type 2 diabetes mellitus are also recognized as obese. In support of this relationship, most obese type 2 diabetics regain the ability to regulate their blood glucose as they reduce their body fat level. Although the relationship seems clear enough, the mechanism has been somewhat elusive to scientists. However, today, some evidence suggests that swollen fat cells themselves may release (and/or not release) chemicals that contribute to decreased sensitivity to insulin.

What happens to carbohydrate storage in between meals?

The complete digestion and absorption of a meal can take several hours, depending upon its size and composition. Therefore, carbohydrate or more specifically glucose from that meal may be available for several hours as well. However, once this ends, a new blood glucose scenario begins to take shape. Cells throughout the body will continue to help themselves to glucose in the blood to help meet their energy needs. The net effect is that our blood glucose concentration will begin to decrease. When the concentration of glucose in the blood begins to decline, the pancreas responds again. However, this time it responds by releasing the hormone glucagon into our blood (see Figure 4.3). Glucagon works in a manner that is generally opposite to insulin. It will labor to increase blood glucose concentration, thereby returning it toward normal levels. To accomplish this, glucagon promotes the breakdown of liver glycogen to glucose. This glucose is then released from the liver into circulation. Glucagon will also promote another activity in our liver that will generate glucose. The process is called gluconeogenesis, which literally means to create new glucose if you read its root words right to left. In this process, certain amino acids, lactate (lactic acid), and glycerol from our circulation will be taken up by our liver and used to make glucose. Like the glucose generated from glycogen breakdown, this glucose can also be released into our blood to maintain blood glucose levels.

During a fasting period, a little epinephrine (adrenalin) and cortisol is also released into circulation from our adrenal glands (see Figure 4.3 and Box 4.2). Among epinephrine's many roles will be its influence upon the liver and skeletal muscle. It will support the effects of glucagon in the liver that were just mentioned. In skeletal muscle, the slightly elevated epinephrine will lightly promote the breakdown of glycogen to glucose. Contrary to the glucose produced from the breakdown of liver glycogen, this glucose is not released into the blood. Rather, this glucose becomes a supportive energy source for those muscle cells while fat is the major energy source. However, when this glucose is used for energy in those cells, a little bit of lactate may be produced. This lactate can enter circulation, reach the liver, and be converted to glucose. This glucose can then be released into the blood. Therefore, our skeletal muscle can modestly contribute to maintaining our blood glucose concentration during fasting.

Cortisol also supports the breakdown of glycogen and the conversion of amino acids, lactate, and glycerol to glucose in our liver. Because cortisol also promotes the breakdown of our body protein, especially skeletal muscle protein, it ensures a supply of amino acids for conversion to glucose in our liver (see Figure 4.5). Cortisol is often regarded as the "stress hormone" and, as will be discussed later, fasting, especially prolonged fasting, is a form of stress.

What happens to carbohydrate stores during exercise?

The hormone picture that develops during exercise is similar to the one discussed regarding a fasting period; however, there are relative differences. Epinephrine is released from our adrenal glands as a direct effect of exercise. Quite simply, the greater the exercise intensity,

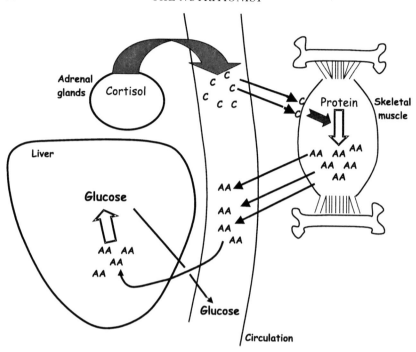

FIGURE 4.5. During fasting and endurance exercise (at least moderate intensity) cortisol causes the breakdown of muscle protein and some amino acids can be used to make glucose in the liver.

the greater the epinephrine release. Epinephrine stimulates the breakdown of muscle cell glycogen (see Box 4.2 and Figure 4.3). This makes glucose available for the muscle cells hard at work. Epinephrine also promotes the breakdown of glycogen to glucose in the liver. Some of this glucose will then circulate to working muscle to provide support. Cortisol may also be released in response to moderate to intense exercise, particularly as the exercise becomes prolonged (i.e., endurance cycling and running). Cortisol will also support the breakdown of glycogen as well as gluconeogenesis in our liver.

Meanwhile, glucagon will be released from the pancreas if blood glucose levels decrease during exercise. This is probably not a factor during most types of exercise. However, in the later stages of endurance exercise blood glucose levels may decline some, as working muscle relies more heavily on this energy source.

FIBER IS AN IMPORTANT NUTRACEUTICAL FAMILY

What is fiber?

A simple definition of fiber is: a carbohydrate or related substance in the human diet that is generally resistant to human digestive activities. Fiber comes from plant sources and is mostly in the form of cellulose, hemicellulose, pectin substances, gums, mucilages, and lignin. Since plants lack the bony skeletal design that provides much of an animal's shape and form, fibers provide much of the structural support to plant cell walls and the plant in general. Plants also use certain fiber as the foundation for their scar tissue. It is important to remember that while humans and other mammals prefer to produce proteins (i.e., collagen) as the structural basis of their bodies, plants will make and use carbohydrates. The fiber content of some foods is presented in Table 4.4.

About how much fiber do we eat and what are the recommendations?

It is estimated the average American woman and man eats about 12 grams and 18 grams of dietary fiber daily, respectively. Meanwhile the World Health Organization (WHO) recommends 25 to 40 grams of dietary fiber daily. It is likely that we evolved on a high-fiber diet due to the unavailability of processing techniques. Some have estimated that our fiber consumption may have been as high as 50 grams daily when fiber-rich foods were more bountiful in our diet. Some populations in Africa have been noted to retain high-fiber intakes.

TABLE 4.4. Fiber Content of Various Foods

Food	Fiber (% weight)
Almonds, wheat germ	3
Lima beans, whole wheat flour, oat flakes, pears, pecans, popcorn, walnuts	2
Apples, string beans, broccoli, carrots, strawberries	1
White flour	< 1

What is the fate of fiber in our digestive tract?

Contrary to starch, fiber is not broken down well by our digestive enzymes. This is partly explained by the manner in which the monosaccharides are linked together. Whereas salivary and pancreatic amylase are very efficient in breaking the links between monosaccharides in starch, these enzymes are generally ineffective at breaking the links between monosaccharides in fiber. Plants build these bonds in a special way.

As plant fibers are generally resistant to human digestive processes, they will stay intact throughout the small intestine. Then when these fibers reach the colon they will add bulk to the feces and also make them more moist, which allows for easier transit of the feces through the remaining colon. Meanwhile, bacteria will find certain fibers irresistible and they will digest a significant portion of the carbohydrates traveling through the colon. Bacteria are able to break the links between the monosaccharides of plant fibers, making them an available energy source. Bacteria will generate substances such as CO_2, methane gas (CH_4), and hydrogen gas (H_2) as products of their metabolism. These gases often lead to uncomfortable bloating and flatulence associated with higher fiber intakes. Also, other molecules, such as short-chain fatty acids, are produced by bacteria, which can be absorbed into the body. These fatty acids yield a small amount of energy and perhaps medical benefits.

What are the medical benefits of a high-fiber diet?

The more insoluble fibers, consisting of mostly cellulose and hemicellulose, appear to have a beneficial effect upon feces formation and evacuation. Bran is an excellent source of these insoluble fibers. This explains the popularity of bran breakfast cereals, muffins, and other products among individuals experiencing constipation and diverticulosis.

Diverticulosis is a situation in which there is an out-pouching of the inner wall of the colon. This disorder is believed to be the result of increased pressure within the colon. In turn, this increased pressure is most likely the result of the highly refined diet that people choose to eat in the United States. A refined diet results in less fiber or "roughage" and thus less digestive leftovers or "residue" making its way into the colon. Less content in the colon results in a smaller diameter and greater pressure exerted upon its walls from within. It is a matter of physics, as there is an inverse relationship between the radius (r) of a collapsible tube and pressure (P) as follows:

$$P = 1/r^4$$

So you see, if the radius of the colon increases due to increased content then the internal pressure decreases, and vice versa. Researchers have clearly shown that those populations in the world that eat more fiber have a lower incidence of diverticulosis. Diverticulosis can lead to a medical concern called *diverticulitis.* Here the out-pouchings become impacted with bacteria and debris, leading to irritation, inflammation, pain, and sometimes bleeding.

Soluble fibers include pectins, gums, mucilages, and some hemi-celluloses and are purported to reduce blood cholesterol and be beneficial to diabetics. Soluble fibers may bind to cholesterol in the digestive tract rendering them unavailable for absorption. Also there is evidence to suggest that the short-chain fatty acids produced in the colon by bacterial breakdown of soluble dietary fibers may reduce cholesterol formation in the liver. These two factors may lead to reductions in the level of cholesterol in blood; this will be explored more thoroughly in the final chapter.

Soluble fibers may also slow the movement of food from the stomach to the small intestine. This may slow the entry of diet-derived glucose into the bloodstream, thereby lessening the after-meal rise in blood glucose for people diagnosed with diabetes mellitus. Recently, however, the American Diabetes Association has stated that this effect may not be as significant as was once thought.

Are there any disadvantages to eating a high-fiber diet?

Some scientists have speculated that there may be some considerations when consuming a high-fiber diet. First, as mentioned previously, bacteria produce by-products of their metabolism, including gases, which may lead to bloating and cramping. Also, because fiber can attract water, it is possible that a high-fiber diet may result in the removal of more water from the body than desirable. Therefore, a higher fiber diet should be complimented with a higher water intake. In addition, research has shown that certain types of fiber and associated molecules, such as oxalates and phytate, can interact with nutrients in the digestive tract and hinder their absorption. These nutrients include iron, copper, zinc, magnesium, and calcium. Many nutritionists recommend that individuals taking a vitamin/mineral supplement should do so with the meal containing the least amount of fiber-rich foods.

Chapter 5

Fats and Cholesterol
Are Not All Bad

THE BASICS OF FATS AND CHOLESTEROL

Over the past couple of decades fat and cholesterol have taken a beating in the press, being labeled as the nutritional bad boys. We are told to avoid them as much as possible. Yet one cannot help but wonder whether fats and cholesterol have been simply misunderstood. Without question, certain types of fats in excess can have a negative impact upon certain risk factors for heart disease; however, other types of fat are not really a problem, while others still contain fatty acids essential to our health. Interestingly, with the rebirth of the low carbohydrate diet, fat has become a sought-out component of some people's diets in a quest for weight loss. Furthermore, the storage of excessive energy in the body as fat versus carbohydrate or protein certainly holds tremendous merit, which is often overlooked.

Along with fat bashing, strong anticholesterol campaigns have been launched. However, keep in mind that cholesterol is used in our cells to make many really important chemicals such as hormones, bile acids, and vitamin D. Therefore, it is important to understand fats and cholesterol completely before we label them as "bad."

What are lipids?

Fats and cholesterol belong to a special group of molecules called *lipids*. The members of this club have something pretty significant in common: they are relatively insoluble in water. This might not seem like a big deal, but keep in mind that most of our planet's surface is water and, more important to our topic, most of our body is water as well. Because of their inability to dissolve into water, the human body must make special efforts to accommodate lipids both during digestion and also inside of the body. During digestion, an emulsifying substance called *bile* is called to action to facilitate lipid digestion and absorption. As for fat and cholesterol inside of the body, they require special transport shuttles to circulate. Fat also has its own cell type specifically designed for storage. These cells are called *adipocytes,* or more commonly "fat cells," and large collections of adipocytes are called *adipose tissue.* Adipose tissue is found under the skin (subcutaneous fat) and in deeper deposits such as in the abdomen, around vital organs, and throughout skeletal muscle.

What is the difference between fat, oils, and triglycerides?

Fats and oils are terms commonly used to refer to food sources of *triglycerides.* Often fat and oil are considered to be different based on appearance: fat is solid at room temperature and oil is liquid. However, they are really two of the same thing, generally speaking. They are both collections of triglycerides. In accordance and to make this book easier to read, we will use "fat" to include all sources of triglycerides.

A triglyceride molecule is a combination of three *fatty acids* linked to a *glycerol* molecule backbone (see Figure 5.1). Although a triglyceride molecule will always have this general design, there can be great variability in the type and combinations of fatty acids that link to glycerol. Only one glycerol molecule exists, but like monosaccharides there are numerous different types of fatty acids in nature. Also,

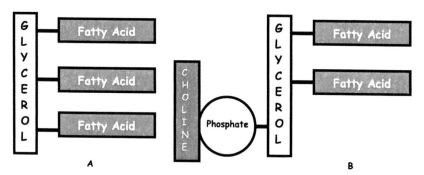

FIGURE 5.1. (A) Triglyceride (fat) and a phospholipid molecule is a glycerol backbone with three fatty acids attached. Thus, a monoglyceride and a diglyceride would contain only one and two fatty acids, respectively. (B) Phospholipids are diglycerides with phosphate and something else attached in place of the third fatty acid. This one is lecithin (phosphotidylcholine).

if a triglyceride involves three fatty acids then monoglycerides and diglycerides will have one and two fatty acids attached to glycerol, respectively. Technically, they can be considered fat as well.

What is cholesterol and can we make it in our body?

Perhaps no other substance in foods or in our body receives more bad press than cholesterol (see Figure 5.2). However, it is important to realize that cholesterol is absolutely vital to our existence. Cholesterol can be made in many cells, and under normal situations we seem to make all that we need. In fact, we will make about 1 g of cholesterol each day. The liver is by far the most productive organ when it comes to making cholesterol. Cholesterol is a necessary component of cell membranes and many vital substances in the body are made from cholesterol. These substances include bile components, vitamin D, testosterone, estrogens, aldosterone, progesterone, and cortisol.

What foods provide us with triglycerides and cholesterol?

As displayed in Table 5.1, fats and oils and thus triglycerides are present in both animals and plants. Oil is a natural component of many plant tissues and their seeds. Oils can be extracted from seeds or plant tissue through a process called *pressing,* which literally squeezes out the oil. Other methods of extraction are also utilized by food manufacturers. Common oils include sunflower, safflower, corn, olive, coconut, canola, and palm oil. Contrarily, butter is made from the fat in milk, while lard is hog fat, and tallow is the fat of cattle or sheep. Other animal flesh will contain fat, including poultry and their eggs.

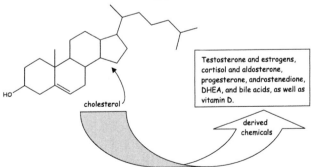

FIGURE 5.2. The cholesterol molecule and its derivatives (steroid hormones and other cholesterol-derived molecules).

TABLE 5.1. Approximate Fat and Cholesterol Contents of Various Foods (by Weight)

Foods	Fat (%)*	Cholesterol (%)
Animal Foods		
Beef	32	< 1
Bologna	29	1
Butter	82	2
Chicken, white meat	4	< 1
Cheese, cheddar	32	1
Cheese, cottage (4%)	4	1
Codfish	< 1	Trace
Egg, whole	12	4
Egg, white	< 1	Trace
Halibut	3	Trace
Hamburger	13	< 1
Lamb chops	36	1
Mackerel	6	Trace
Margarine	82	–
Milk (whole)	3	< 1
Milk (skim)	Trace	Trace
Pork chops	21	1
Pork sausage	46	1
Salmon	4	Trace
Plants Foods		
Avocados	13	–
Bread (white)	4	< 1
Cereals and grains	1-2	–
Crackers	1	–
Fruits	< 1	–
Leafy vegetables	< 1	–
Legumes	< 1	–
Margarine	82	–
Root vegetables	< 1	–

*Percentage of a food's mass that is attributable to fat. To determine grams of fat in a food simply multiply the percentage by the weight (grams) of the food.

Cholesterol is not a necessary substance for plants, therefore they do not need to make it. Contrarily, mammals will make cholesterol to help meet their body needs. As a result, cholesterol intake in the diet is attributed only to consumption of animal foods or foods that have animal products in their recipe.

How are triglycerides and cholesterol digested?

Digestion is a watery affair and has been loosely compared to white-water rafting. In addition to the water-based fluids we drink, liters of water-based fluid enter the digestive tract daily. Dissolved in those fluids that our body provides are digestive enzymes. This means that our digestive enzymes are water soluble, while their task is to interact with and break down water-insoluble lipids for absorption. This presents an interesting yet readily solved problem.

When lipids are present in the small intestine the natural course would be for these substances to clump together. This is analogous to oil clumping together in the kitchen sink when we do dishes or the separation of oil from the watery portion of traditional salad dressings. If lipids remain clumped together in the small intestine, surely the efficient digestion of these substances would be hindered. To solve this potential problem, bile is delivered to the small intestine and serves as an emulsifier or detergent during lipid digestion. Here, components of bile coat smaller droplets of lipid, rendering them water soluble, as depicted in Figure 5.3. Bile activity keeps larger lipid droplets from reforming. So instead of having a few very large droplets of lipids we have many tiny droplets instead. When lipids are

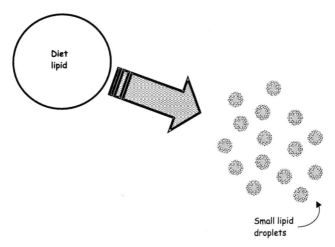

FIGURE 5.3. Small lipid droplets are created due to the mixing actions of the stomach and small intestine. Bile components coat the little lipid droplets making them water soluble and rendering fats, cholesterol, and other lipids easier to digest and absorb.

present as tiny droplets, digestive enzymes have no problem attacking them and efficiently doing their job.

Although a triglyceride-digesting enzyme called *lingual lipase* is present in saliva, the job of digesting triglycerides is mostly handled by another lipase enzyme delivered by the pancreas. Pancreatic lipase detaches two fatty acids from glycerol, which results in a monoglyceride and two fatty acids (see Figure 5.4). In turn, the remaining fatty acid may be detached by yet another enzyme from some of the monoglycerides. This would then produce glycerol and a fatty acid. Thus, the products of triglyceride digestion are fatty acids, monoglycerides, and glycerol, which are now small enough to move into the cells lining the small intestine. Meanwhile, some of the cholesterol in our diet is actually linked to other molecules, with the most prevalent attachments being fatty acids. These are often referred to as *cholesterol esters*. Other digestive enzymes *(cholesterol esterase)* will liberate cholesterol so that it can be absorbed.

The efficiency of the digestion and absorption of the lipids we eat is > 90 percent. However, in the absence of bile, much of the dietary lipid would escape digestion and absorption. Bile is made in the liver

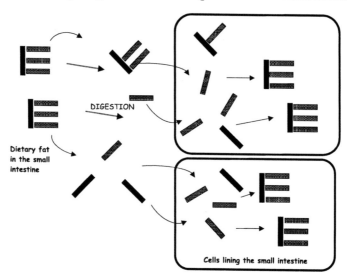

FIGURE 5.4. Triglycerides are digested to fatty acids, monoglycerides, and some glycerol, all of which move into the cells lining the small intestine. Triglycerides are put back together inside these cells and put into chylomicrons to enter circulation (lymphatic).

and stored in the gallbladder during nondigestive times. Disorders involving the liver or gallbladder can lead to reduced bile production and/or delivery to the small intestine. Recently, certain drugs and dietary supplements have been marketed to reduce the absorption of fat from the diet. For instance, the supplement chitin is a special complex carbohydrate produced by insects. Chitin is marketed as a fat binder, thereby reducing fat absorption and allowing for weight loss to occur. It will be interesting to see if this is well tolerated by humans and whether chitin will also reduce the absorption of essential fatty acids, fat-soluble vitamins, and other health-beneficial fat-soluble substances.

When fat-containing food particles arrive in the small intestine, bile is squeezed out of the gallbladder and travels to the small intestine through a duct. Some people may have had their gallbladder removed for medical reasons. Since bile is made in the liver and the gallbladder merely functions as a temporary storage depot for that bile, this is not a serious concern. In most cases, the liver sends adequate amounts of bile directly to the small intestine during digestion, which compensates for the missing gallbladder. However, if fat is not well digested and absorbed, a lower-fat diet may be necessary. The presence of increased amounts of fat in feces can be used to gauge the efficiency of fat digestion and absorption. Feces will become more pale and greasy in appearance when proper absorption does not occur. In addition, bacterial metabolism of some of the fat may result in some discomforting symptoms as well.

How are triglycerides and cholesterol absorbed?

Absorbing lipids into the body requires special consideration. Since the blood is mostly water, how can these water-insoluble substances be introduced into this watery medium? Cells lining the wall of the small intestine reassemble triglycerides and package them up along with cholesterol into protein-containing shells called chylomicrons. Chylomicrons are ejected from those cells and enter the blood by first circulating through the lymphatic vessels. Chylomicrons are very large and therefore unable to squeeze through the holes in the walls of the capillaries, so they must then drain into lymph vessels in the wall of the small intestine instead. However, within minutes, chylomicrons will circulate to a duct in the chest that gives them access to the blood (see Figure 5.5). Each chylomicron

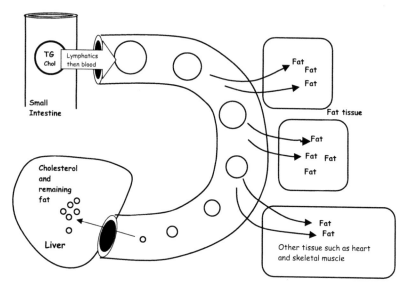

FIGURE 5.5. Chylomicrons are made in the cells that line the wall of the small intestine. They carry a lot of fat and a lesser amount of cholesterol from the diet. They enter lymphatic circulation and then the blood. They deposit nearly all of their fat before being removed by the liver.

will then circulate for about a half hour, delivering its lipid bounty to tissue throughout the body, as will soon be discussed.

What are fat substitutes?

Fat tends to impart a smooth texture and tastier quality to many foods. For example, most of ice cream's taste and mouth-feel are the result of its rich fat content. However, along with the positive attributes associated with fat in foods, there are some potential negative attributes as well. Fat enhances the energy content of a food. Furthermore, a diet rich in fatty foods contradicts nutritional recommendations. Therefore, food manufacturers have long searched for fat substitutes that would provide the desirable mouth-feel and taste of fat but not the energy content or fat itself.

Earlier substitutes were fairly successful but unable to completely capture the true characteristics of fat. These include plant gums, cellulose, Paselli SA2, N-Oil, Sta-Slim 143, and Maltrin. Researchers have developed several newer fat substitutes, some of which are used in food production today, while others are still awaiting FDA approval. Olestra and Simplesse are two substitutes that offer much promise. Olestra consists of several fatty acids attached to a molecule of sucrose; it was approved for use in savory snack foods, such as chips in 1996. The fatty acids provide many of the desirable qualities of fat to be experienced by the mouth. However, since olestra is not digested and absorbed, it comes without an appreciable energy expense. Some scientists have raised concerns associated with the large-scale use of olestra in foods. One concern is that olestra might bind to vitamin E and other fat-soluble vitamins in the digestive tract and decrease their absorption. To accommodate this concern, these substances are added to olestra-containing products. Also, some nutritionists have expressed concern that olestra can cause digestive discomforts, such as cramping or diarrhea. Although excessive intakes of olestra may have this effect, lower and more typical consumption of olestra-containing products probably does not cause any more digestive problems than regular snacks.

Simplesse is the product of milk and egg proteins, mixed and heat-treated until fine mistlike protein globules are formed. These protein globules seem to taste and provide a mouth-feel similar to fat. On the contrary, however, this substitute yields much less energy than fat. Simplesse's application is limited to cool or cold items, such as cheese, cold desserts, mayonnaise, yogurt, and salad dressings. Heat will break down the fine protein globules, therefore Simplesse is inappropriate for baked or fried items.

FATTY ACIDS CAN VARY IN LENGTH, DEGREE, AND TYPE OF SATURATION

Can fatty acids vary in length?

For the most part, the length of fatty acids can vary by as much as twenty carbon atoms or so. If a fatty acid has four carbon atoms or less, it is referred to as a short-chain fatty acid. Furthermore, if a fatty acid chain has six to twelve or greater than twelve carbon atoms, it would be referred to as a medium-chain fatty acid or a long-chain fatty acid, respectively. Most fatty acids in nature have an even number of carbons, yet some fatty acids have an odd chain length.

What are saturated and unsaturated fatty acids?

If a fatty acid is linked to glycerol, the second carbon closest to the link is referred to as the "alpha carbon" (see Figure 5.6). Meanwhile, the carbon furthest from the linkage with glycerol is called the "omega (ω) carbon." This is because the first letter of the Greek alphabet is alpha and the last letter is omega. No matter how many carbons are in your fatty acid chain, these carbon atoms will always be addressed in this manner. Looking at a fatty acid not linked to glycerol, the alpha carbon would be the first carbon atom adjacent to the carbon bonded to two atoms of oxygen.

Fatty acids can differ in their degree of saturation. Saturation refers to whether all of the carbon atoms between the alpha and omega carbon atoms are bonded to two atoms of hydrogen. If this is the case, then the carbons are saturated with hydrogen and that particular fatty acid would be called a saturated fatty acid (SFA) (see Figure 5.6). However, if at one or more points adjacent carbon atoms are bonded to only a single hydrogen atom each, the fatty acid would then be unsaturated (see Figure 5.6). By nature, when two adjacent carbon atoms in a fatty acid are linked to only one hydrogen atom each, the carbon atoms must bond to each other twice. Chemists call this a *double bond*. If a fatty acid has only one point of unsaturation or one double bond, it is referred to as a *monounsaturated* fatty acid (MUFA); if there is more than one double bond, then it is a *polyunsaturated* fatty acid (PUFA).

What are **trans** *fatty acids and what is the big deal?*

Taking a closer look at double bonds, we see that there can be some variation here as well. If the hydrogen atoms attached to the carbon atoms of a double bond are positioned on the same side of the double bond, it is a *cis* arrangement (see Figure 5.7). If the hydrogen atoms bonded to the carbon atoms are on opposite sides of the double bond, it is referred to as a *trans fatty acid. Cis* fatty acids are the more prevalent form in which fatty acid double bonds occur in the body and in our natural food sources.

Interest has been growing regarding the presence of *trans* fatty acids in our diet and their potential impact upon health. Although *cis* versus *trans* may seem like a very minor point in regard to fatty acid design, these contrasting forms can impart different properties to a fatty acid.

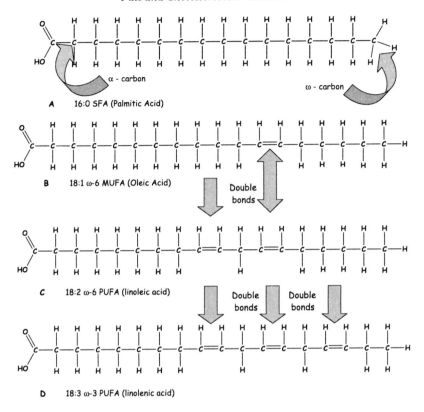

FIGURE 5.6. A saturated fatty acid (A) showing the alpha (α) and omega (ω) carbons. The monounsaturated (B) and polyunsaturated fatty acids' (C and D) unsaturated points are indicated.

Cis double bonds cause a kinking or bending of the fatty acid, while *trans* double bonds do not. This makes unsaturated fatty acids with *trans* double bonds similar to saturated fatty acids in that they do not bend or kink.

It is certainly possible for a PUFA to contain both *cis* and *trans* double bonds. As you might expect, the *cis* double bond will kink the fatty acid chain while the *trans* double bond will not. Furthermore, as it is possible for a PUFA to contain both *cis* and *trans* double bonds, it is also possible for a PUFA to contain all *trans* double bonds. Again, in this situation, despite multiple double bonds, the fatty acid would not kink. This makes it physically similar to a SFA of the same length.

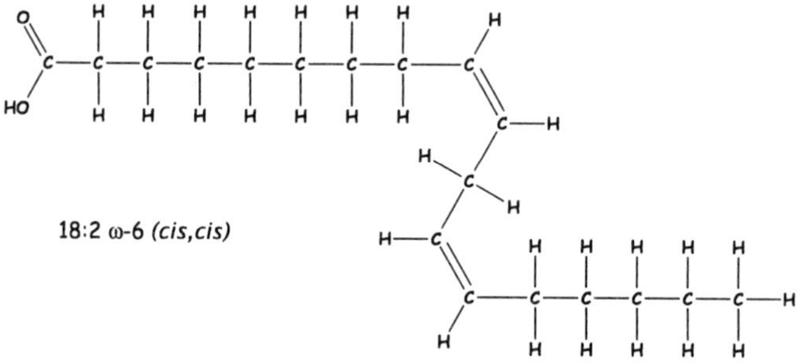

FIGURE 5.7. The top fatty acid is the same as drawn in Figure 5.6 C and it demonstrates its true three-dimensional design. The bottom fatty acid is the same as the top fatty acid, except that the double bonds are *trans* instead of *cis*. The *trans* double bonds fail to effectively kink the fatty acid chain.

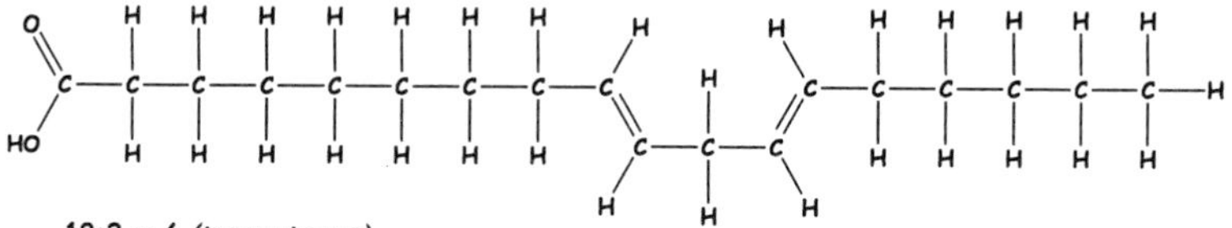

What foods contain trans fatty acids?

Trans fatty acids can be found in most fat sources although their prevalence is very low. Bovine food sources are probably the greatest contributors of *trans* fatty acids to the human diet. For instance, beef, butter, and milk triglycerides may contain 2 to 8 percent of their fatty acids as *trans* fatty acids. Interestingly, cows and cattle are not responsible for this *trans* fatty acid content. It is actually the bacteria in their unique stomachs that produce the *trans* fatty acid. These fatty acids are then absorbed by the cow (cattle) and make their way into the tissues and milk of these animals.

In addition, *trans* fatty acids can be created during the processing of oils (i.e., margarine and other hydrogenated oils) which will be described soon. Typically, about half are of the *trans* fatty acids in the human diet are derived from animal sources while the remaining half is derived from processed oils either consumed plain or used in recipes.

The potential impact of *trans* fatty acids on human health is not entirely clear. Some research evidence suggests that a diet rich in these fatty acids may raise blood cholesterol levels in a manner similar to saturated fatty acids. We will spend more time on why this may influence blood cholesterol levels in Chapter 13.

Since fatty acids can vary in both length and saturation, how can we identify specific ones?

As fatty acids can vary in length and saturation, scientists needed to devise a system that allowed them to discuss and write about them in an abbreviated, specific manner. In fact, they devised a couple of systems, but I will describe only the system that is most commonly used in the general population. To specify a particular fatty acid, first count the number of carbon atoms to determine its length. Then count the number of double bonds, if any. For instance, if a fatty acid is eighteen carbons long with one double bond it is simply referred to as 18:1. Likewise, if a fatty acid is sixteen carbon atoms long with no double bonds, we would refer to it as 16:0. State the length first, then colon (:), then the number of double bonds.

Although this system seems simple enough, describing an unsaturated fatty acid requires one to two more steps. First, we must indicate the position of the double bond(s). We can do this by counting from the omega end the number of carbons to the first carbon of the first double bond. For instance, if the first double bond starts at the third carbon atom in, it is an omega-3 (ω-3) fatty acid (see Figure 5.6). Likewise, if the first double bond appears at the sixth or the ninth carbon atom in, those fatty acids would be ω-6 and ω-9 fatty acids, respectively. For the most part, when addressing polyunsaturated fatty acids indicate only the position of the first double bond because subsequent double bonds seem to occur in series after one saturated carbon atom (see Figure 5.6). For example, an 18:3 ω-3 fatty acid will have three double bonds positioned at the third, sixth, and ninth carbon atoms in from the omega end. (Table 5.2 lists common fatty acids and their abbreviations.)

Can different kinds of fatty acids be part of the same triglyceride molecule?

There are probably no definite rules as to the selection of fatty acids that make up a triglyceride molecule. One triglyceride molecule may be composed of one saturated, one monounsaturated, and one

TABLE 5.2. Common Fatty Acids

Fatty Acid	Abbreviation
Acetic acid	2:0
Butyric acid	4:0
Caproic acid	6:0
Caprylic acid	8:0
Capric acid	10:0
Lauric acid	12:0
Myristic acid	14:0
Palmitic acid	16:0
Palmitoleic acid	16:1 ω-9
Stearic acid	18:0
Oleic acid	18:1 ω-9
Linoleic acid	18:2 ω-6
Linolenic acid	18:3 ω-3
Arachidic acid	20:0
Arachidonic acid	20:4 ω-6
Eicosapentaenoic acid (EPA)	20:5 ω-3
Docosahexaenoic acid (DHA)	22:6 ω-3

Note: These are some of the most common fatty acids found in foods and in the body.

polyunsaturated fatty acid, all of the same, or varying lengths. However, the types of fatty acids found within triglyceride molecules will be strongly influenced by the nature of the plant or the animal from which you obtained the triglyceride source. For instance, the triglycerides in olive oil largely contain the MUFA oleic acid (18:1 ω-9) (about 82 percent), while about two-thirds of the fatty acids in butter are SFA of a varied assortment in length.

The presence of certain types of fatty acids in either a plant or an animal largely depends upon the nature of the plant or animal and the purpose of the fat for that life-form. For instance, fish that live in deeper water will tend to be better sources of ω-3 PUFA because these fatty acids are found in the cell membranes of these fish and play a protective role against the increased pressure and decreased temperature experienced at greater depths. Also, fish manipulate the level of fat and the types of fatty acids to help regulate their buoyancy. For plants, they often house fat in their seeds (offspring) to serve as an energy source during development.

What do we mean by saturated and unsaturated fats?

Regardless of the origin of a triglyceride source (plant or animal), the triglycerides will contain a mixture of fatty acids. When we say that a fat source is *saturated,* we are indicating that the majority of the fatty acids within the source are saturated. For instance, we often refer to butter and beef fat as saturated fats. This is because the majority of their fatty acids are saturated. Table 5.3 lists the approximate percentages of fatty acids for each food source.

Why are oils liquid at room temperature while fats are solid?

In general, if the majority of fatty acids in a triglyceride source are saturated, then it most likely will be solid at room temperature. Contrarily, if a triglyceride source contains a greater percentage of unsaturated fatty acids, especially PUFA, then this source will most likely be liquid at room temperature. Despite their names, palm oil and palm kernel oil are more solid are room temperature.

TABLE 5.3. Approximate Fatty Acid Composition of Common Triglyceride Sources

Type of Fat	SFA (%)	MUFA (%)	PUFA (%)
Butter fat	66	30	4
Beef fat	52	44	4
Lard	41	47	12
Coconut oil	87	6	2
Palm kernel oil	81	11	2
Palm oil	49	37	9
Vegetable shortening	28	44	28
Peanut oil	18	49	33
Margarine	17	49	34
Soybean oil	15	24	61
Olive oil	14	77	9
Corn oil	13	25	62
Sunflower oil	11	20	69
Safflower oil	10	13	77
Canola oil	6	62	32

What is margarine?

As researchers identified the relationship between a diet high in saturated fat and cholesterol and the risk of heart disease a few decades ago, food manufacturers began to offer solidified oils to replace butter. Plant oils tend to have less saturated fatty acids and will not contain cholesterol. More specifically, plant oils have much lower amounts of three types of saturated fatty acids (16:0, 14:0, and 12:0), which are the SFAs that seem to raise blood cholesterol levels.

Margarine was produced by food manufacturers to replace butter at the table and in recipes. Margarine is made by adding hydrogen to unsaturated fatty acids in plant oils. This makes them a little more saturated and transforms them from a liquid to solid state. Scientists called this process *hydrogenation,* which certainly seems like a logical name. During hydrogenation some of the PUFAs are converted to MUFAs and some of the MUFAs are converted to SFAs (see Table 5.4). This converts the liquid oil to semisolid or to solid fat. The degree of the transformation depends upon how much hydrogenation is allowed to take place. Margarines that come in stick form are typically more hydrogenated than softer tub margarine. Hydrogenation occurs when the oils are heated up in a container and hydrogen gas is applied. The most popular plant oil used for hydrogenation is soybean oil.

As mentioned above, some of the *trans* fatty acids in our diet come by way of hydrogenated oils. When energy (heat) is applied to plant oils during hydrogenation, a small number of the *cis* double bonds can be converted to *trans* double bonds. A similar situation occurs if oils are used over long periods for cooking, such as in restaurants. Cookies, crackers, and other snack foods that utilize hydrogenated vegetable oil may contain up to 9-10 percent of their fatty acids as *trans* fatty acids.

TABLE 5.4. Hypothetical Margarine Made by Hydrogenating Corn Oil

Fat Source	SFA (%)	MUFA (%)	PUFA (%)
Corn oil	13	25	62
Margarine (from corn oil)	17	49	34

Note: During hydrogenation some of the PUFAs become MUFAs and some of the MUFAs become SFAs.

FAT IS OUR MOST SIGNIFICANT
MEANS OF STORING ENERGY

What does fat do in our body?

Fat (triglyceride) is an energy source for many of our cells (in particular muscle and liver) and is our primary means of storing the excessive energy from the foods we eat. Although some fat can be found in several cell types in our body (e.g., skeletal and cardiac muscle cells), by and large most of the fat stored in our body is housed in fat cells. Collections of fat cells (adipocytes) are commonly referred to as fat tissue or adipose tissue. Because a larger percentage of the fatty acids stored in adipose tissue is saturated, the fat tissue is more solid than liquid. This can result in the dimpling appearance in the layer of fat found beneath our skin (subcutaneous fat).

Storing excess energy as fat rather than as protein or carbohydrate has great advantages. First, we are able to store more than twice the amount of energy in 1 g of fat as we can in 1 g of carbohydrate or protein. Second, stored fat, by virtue of its water insolubility, will have less water associated with it than would stored carbohydrate and protein. The net effect of storing excess diet energy as fat versus carbohydrate or protein is that our body weight and volume is minimized. The teleological advantage is that it allows the human body to be lighter, smaller, and contain less vital water. This in turn allows human beings to more easily hunt and gather, migrate, defend themselves, and seek out partners with whom to mate.

Are we born with all of the fat cells we will ever have?

It would appear that we are not born with a full complement of fat cells as some scientists once thought. The number of fat cells in the body seems to increase at various stages throughout growth, but by the time adulthood is reached the total number of these cells seems to be somewhat fixed. This means that if our body fat mass does not change, we probably would not produce new fat cells as adults. However, there is a body of research evidence that leads scientists to think that even during adulthood we can increase our fat cell numbers by chronic overconsumption of energy. In adipose tissue there is a small number of so-called preadipocytes or fat stem cells. When these cells are signaled, they will produce new fat cells. As you may have guessed, the signals are chemicals, many of which are released by existing fat cells when they become swollen with an increased bounty of stored fat.

For a long time fat tissue and their cells were viewed as somewhat inert containers of energy storage. However, today we know that fat tissue functions as a gland with the capability to release a variety of factors relative to its size and endowed energy. As mentioned previously, some of these factors may promote the formation of more fat cells. Perhaps some of the most interesting released factors are those that circulate to the brain and provide insight to our energy storage status. One of the most important factors seems to be the hormone *leptin*. Fat cells release more and more leptin into our circulation when fat cells accumulate more fat. Leptin then signals the brain to reduce appetite.

Beyond energy storage, does fat have other functions in our body?

Fat tissue provides some protection to various tissues in the body. For instance, fat tissue around our internal organs provides some cushioning. This helps protect the organs against external trauma. Furthermore, the subcutaneous layer of fat storage also provides some cushioning, which protects muscle. Subcutaneous fat is not well vasculated, meaning that there is not a tremendous number of blood vessels in that tissue. Meanwhile, skeletal muscle is heavily endowed with blood vessels which provide O_2 and energy nutrients during activity and exercise. In the absence of subcutaneous fat it would be easier to rupture smaller blood vessels in skeletal muscle, which then would be evident in bruises. As an example, prior to competition, bodybuilders will be very cautious not to bang into things or play contact sports (e.g., touch football, roller hockey). As they attempt to "lean out" for the competition, they reduce their subcutaneous fat to nadir levels, which would allow them to bruise more easily. This then would impact their aesthetic presentation during the bodybuilding competition.

Subcutaneous fat not only helps protect skeletal muscle from trauma but it also helps conserve our body heat. This is because fat tissue is a relatively good insulating tissue. Maintaining our body temperature right around 98.6°F (37°C) allows cell operations to function optimally. Too little subcutaneous body fat may allow for greater heat losses daily and may partly explain why a leaner person may have a higher energy expenditure than another person having the same body weight but who is less lean.

While most of the fat tissue in an adult's body is somewhat pale (white adipose tissue), infants tend to have a fair amount of *brown adipose tissue* (BAT). This type of fat tissue is a little different from white adipose tissue as it contains a lot more blood vessels. This is one reason why it appears darker in color. BAT is especially important for infants to help them maintain their body temperature. When infants are born, they are fairly lean and it is easy for heat to leave their bodies. BAT has the ability to increase some of its metabolic events, which results in the generation of extra heat. BAT is able to uncouple the process of ATP formation via the breakdown of energy nutrients. Although this may seem somewhat "futile" when it comes to making ATP, it does allow for the generation of heat which will help maintain the body temperature of the baby. For adults, this may seem like a great way of burning unwanted fat, but scientists have revealed that as babies become children and then teens, the amount of BAT is reduced and becomes almost nonexistent by adulthood.

Does fat have a structural function in our body?

Our cell membranes contain molecules, called *phospholipids,* that seem to have structural similarities to triglycerides (see Figure 5.1). Like triglycerides, phospholipids contain a glycerol backbone to which fatty acids are attached. However, phospholipids contain only two fatty acids, not three as in triglycerides. The third fatty acid is replaced by phosphate combined with another molecule, such as choline or inostiol. When choline is found in the phospholipid, the molecule is called phosphotidylcholine, which is commonly referred to as lecithin.

The true purpose of phospholipids is to provide the basis for the water-insoluble properties of our cell membranes. In turn, then, the barrier-like properties of membranes allow each cell to regulate somewhat the movement of water-soluble substances into and out of cells and their internal organelles. In addition, phospholipids in the plasma membrane of cells may contain special fatty acids which can be detached and modified when the need arises. Modified versions of these special fatty acids can be released from a cell and have an effect on neighboring cells. These special fatty-acid-derived substances are an extraordinary class of molecules called the *eicosanoids,* which will be discussed in more detail soon (see Figure 5.8).

How much fat do we need in our diet?

At this time there is no established RDA for fat intake. However, scientists agree that there is indeed an absolute requirement for fat in our diet, however small it may be. Many nutritionists feel that a diet containing as little as 5 percent of its energy as fat, derived from a variety of food sources, may be more than adequate. These food sources would include not only plants but also fish and other marine life.

The need for dietary fat is not necessarily for energy purposes. Fat is really needed in our diet as a means of providing two essential fatty acids, *linoleic acid* (an ω-6 PUFA) and *linolenic acid* (an ω-3 PUFA). Good sources of linoleic acid are corn oil, soybean oil, cottonseed oil, sunflower oil, and safflower oil. Good plant sources of linolenic acid are soybean, canola, linseed, and rapeseed oils as well as some leafy vegetables. Marine mammals (e.g., whale, seal, walrus) and the oil derived from cold-water fish (cod-liver, herring, menhaden, and salmon oils) provide *eicosapentaenoic acid* (EPA) and *docosahexaenoic acid* (DHA). EPA and DHA are fatty acids that are made from linolenic acid in marine animals. A lot of interest in the ω-3 PUFA was created when researchers reported that there is a lower incidence of heart disease in Greenland. Diet patterns showed high fatty-fish consumption in these people, which leads to greater ω-3 PUFA intake and a reduced incidence of heart disease.

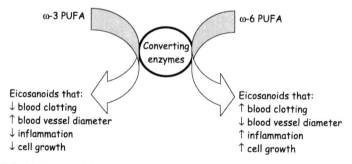

FIGURE 5.8. Essential fatty acids are used to make eicosanoid molecules. Those eicosanoids that are made from ω-6 PUFA are associated with events related to heart disease, cancer, and arthritis, while those derived from ω-3 PUFA are associated with reducing the risk and incidence of heart disease, cancer, and arthritis.

Is all of the fat stored in our fat cells derived from fat in our diet?

When we eat a meal containing fat, it is absorbed and circulates within chylomicrons. As it circulates, fat is slowly transferred from chylomicrons to fat cells primarily, and skeletal muscle cells, the heart, and other organs and tissue (e.g., breast tissue) secondarily (see Figure 5.5). In order to transfer diet-derived fat into our tissue, an enzyme must be present in that particular tissue. The enzyme is called *lipoprotein lipase* (LPL) and just like lingual lipase and pancreatic lipase, LPL also removes fatty acids from triglycerides. The fatty acids liberated by LPL move out of the chylomicrons and enter the nearby cells. Scientists have studied LPL for years and it now seems that differing levels of LPL activity in different locations of adipose tissue may partly explain why people seem to accumulate more fat stores in some regions of their bodies and not as much in other areas.

As mentioned previously, fat cells will store loads of fat, and insulin promotes this activity. On the contrary, skeletal muscle cells and the heart have a limited ability to store fat. However, the amount of fat that skeletal muscle can store may actually be increased some due to aerobic training (i.e., running, biking). The importance of this fat is performance related. During exercise, when circulating epinephrine levels climb, this fat is readily available for working muscle cells. In addition, aerobic exercise training also promotes adaptations in muscle cells, making them better fat burners during and in between exercise bouts. More on the relationship between exercise and fat burning and storage will be discussed in later chapters.

While diet-derived fat is being deposited in tissue throughout the body, liver and fat cells can take excessive glucose and amino acids and convert them to fat. As you may have guessed, insulin promotes this activity as well. The fat made in fat cells is stored within those cells, while the fat made in the liver is packaged up and relocated mostly to fat cells for storage.

How and when do we remove fat from our fat cells?

The fat stored in fat cells is available to us when we exercise and/or when food energy is not being absorbed (fasting). Just as insulin promoted the storage of fat when energy was coming into our body, the process of mobilizing fat from fat cells is promoted by the hormones released into our blood when we are fasting and/or exercising (see Figure 5.9). The hormones glucagon, epinephrine, and cortisol all promote the release of fat from fat stores.

In order for fat to be released from fat cells, fat is first broken down to fatty acids and glycerol, which then enter our blood and circulate. However, because of their general water insolubility, the fatty acids will hitch a ride aboard a protein in the blood called *albumin*. On the contrary, glycerol is fairly water soluble and can dissolve into blood.

The circulating fatty acids are removed by cells, especially skeletal muscle and our heart, liver, and other organs. The fatty acids are then used by those tissues for energy. However, keep in mind that cells of the CNS and RBCs cannot use fatty acids for energy and will continue to use glucose. During exercise, fatty acids become a major fuel source for working muscles. Glycerol, on the other hand, can be removed from the blood by the liver and used to make glucose. This process will certainly be important in order to maintain a desirable blood glucose level during prolonged exercise and fasting.

Fat Cells (Adipose Tissue)

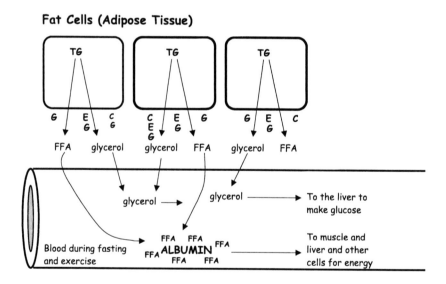

FIGURE 5.9. Circulating glucagon (G), epinephrine (E), and cortisol (C) tell our fat cells to break down their triglyceride (TG) to free fatty acids (FFA) and glycerol.

FAT AND CHOLESTEROL NEED SPECIAL HELP
TO GET AROUND IN OUR BODY

How are lipids shuttled around in our blood?

Not only will our liver make a fair amount of cholesterol on a daily basis, but it will also receive cholesterol from diet-derived chylomicrons. Like fat, most cholesterol is housed in the liver for only a short period of time as it is destined for other tissues throughout the body. Once cholesterol reaches other tissues, it can be used to make some of the substances listed previously or to become part of cell membranes. Some of the cholesterol in our liver is also used to make bile salts, a key component of bile.

So far it has been mentioned that dietary lipids require a special transportation vehicle, and now it has been noted that the liver will also package up fats and cholesterol and send them out into the blood. In both situations the lipids are shuttled around in the blood as part of *lipoproteins*. Generally speaking, lipoproteins are a protein-containing shell encasing the lipid substances in need of transportation (see Figure 5.10).

Lipoproteins can be divided into four general classes based upon their densities. Because they differ in this regard, we can quantify the different lipoprotein classes (see Figure 5.10). In order of increasing density our lipoproteins are chylomicrons, *very low density lipoproteins* (VLDL), *low density lipoproteins* (LDL), and *high density lipoproteins* (HDL). Looking at the composition of these lipoproteins in Figure 5.10, we see that the greater the lipid to protein ratio, the lower the density. This makes perfect sense because lipids are less dense than proteins.

The proteins that help make up the lipoprotein shell are called *apoproteins* (apolipoproteins). Not only do they make the lipoprotein more soluble in water, but they will also function in helping the lipoprotein be recognized by specific tissues throughout our body. This means that the apoproteins interact with specific receptors for the different lipoproteins on certain tissue. This allows a lipoprotein either to unload some of their lipid cargo or to be removed from the blood and broken down. For instance, the receptor for LDL is located in the liver tissue and also in other tissue throughout the body. When a specific apoprotein on LDL docks on the LDL receptor, this allows LDL to be removed from the blood.

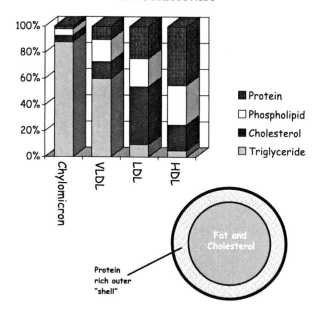

FIGURE 5.10. Lipoproteins are lipids encased in a water-soluble protein shell (bottom). Our blood contains several types of lipoproteins, which can be separated based upon their density (lipid to protein ratio). Chylomicrons are the biggest and have the highest ratio, opposite to HDL.

What is the general activity of the lipoproteins?

The activity of lipoproteins is fairly complex and extremely fascinating (see Table 5.5). Chylomicrons are made by the cells lining our small intestine and transport diet-derived lipids throughout the body. Chylomicron composition reflects our dietary lipid intake; therefore, they contain mostly fat. As chylomicrons travel throughout our circulation they unload most of their fat in fat cells and other cells such as muscle cells, as described previously. Once most of the fat has been removed, the remaining small chylomicron, often called a chylomicron remnant, is recognized and removed from the blood by the liver where it is broken down. Any cholesterol and leftover fat becomes the property of the liver.

As mentioned earlier, not only will the liver receive cholesterol and some fat from chylomicrons, but it is also a primary cholesterol- and triglyceride-producing organ in the body. Fat and cholesterol in excess of the liver's needs are packaged up into VLDL and released

TABLE 5.5. The Most Abundant Lipoproteins

Lipoprotein Class	Site of Production	General Activity	Fate
Chylomicrons	Small intestine	Transport dietary fat and cholesterol from digestive tract. Much of the fat is deposited in fat and muscle tissue.	Chylomicron remnants containing cholesterol and remaining fat are removed from the blood by the liver.
Very low density lipoproteins (VLDL)	Liver	Delivery of fat and cholesterol from the liver to tissue throughout the body.	As they circulate they deposit fat in fat tissue and other tissue and become LDL.
Low density lipoproteins (LDL)	Derived from VLDL in circulation	Deposit cholesterol in tissue throughout the body.	Eventually removed from the blood by the liver and to a lesser degree other tissue.
High density lipoproteins (HDL)	Produced by the liver and small intestine	Circulate and pick up cholesterol from tissue throughout the body.	Eventually removed from circulation primarily by the liver.

into our circulation. As VLDL circulate throughout our body, they unload a lot of their fat, mostly in fat cells. As a result their lipid to protein ratio decreases, which renders them more dense, and they classify as LDL (see Figure 5.11). Therefore, LDL are derived from circulating VLDL.

LDL has two fates. One fate is to continue to circulate throughout the body and deposit cholesterol in various tissue. The second fate is to be recognized by tissue, removed from the blood, and broken down. Many tissues throughout our body can do this, but the liver handles more than half of the task. The longer LDL circulate, the more opportunity there is for cholesterol to be deposited throughout our body.

The last type of lipoprotein is HDL. In regard to heart disease, if LDL wears the villain's black hat then HDL wears the hero's white hat. HDL is made in our liver and to a lesser extent in our intestines. It is HDL's job to circulate and pick up excess cholesterol from tissues throughout our body and return it to the liver. The whole process is very interesting because in order for circulating HDL to return the

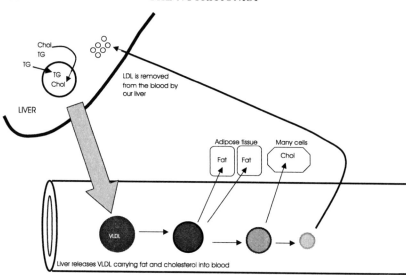

FIGURE 5.11. VLDL releases its fat to tissue (mostly adipose tissue) yielding LDL, which continues to circulate and deliver cholesterol to tissue. LDL is then removed from blood mostly by the liver.

cholesterol to our liver, some of the cholesterol is first passed to circulating LDL. The LDL is then subject to removal from our circulation and broken down. HDL will also deliver cholesterol to the liver as well.

What information can we derive from a blood cholesterol test?

It is important to remember that when health professionals refer to our *blood cholesterol* levels, they are describing the total cholesterol content of our blood. This is the sum of the cholesterol in all of the lipoproteins circulating in our blood at the time it was drawn. Typically, our blood is drawn after an overnight fast so there should not be chylomicrons in the blood. Chylomicrons will circulate only for a couple hours after a meal. The fractions of total cholesterol are the amount of cholesterol found in each type or class of lipoproteins. Thus LDL-cholesterol is the cholesterol only found in LDL. And likewise HDL-cholesterol is the cholesterol found only in HDL. With regard to atherosclerotic heart disease, the blood cholesterol-related

TABLE 5.6. Lipid Profile Example

Blood Lipid or Ratio	Measurement (mg/100 mL)	Normal Range (mg/100 mL)
Triglyceride (TG)	137	0-210
Cholesterol (total)	163	50-200
HDL-cholesterol	42	30-90
VLDL-cholesterol	27	5-40
LDL-cholesterol	94	50-140
Cholesterol:HDL-chol	3.9 (ratio)	3.7-6.7
LDL-chol:HDL-chol	2.2 (ratio)	

risk factors include having a total cholesterol level greater than 200 mg per 100 mL of blood, a higher LDL-cholesterol, a low HDL-cholesterol level, and an LDL to HDL ratio greater than 4:1 (see Table 5.6 for a sample lipid profile).

Chapter 6

Proteins Are Our Structural and Functional Basis

PROTEINS ARE COMBINATIONS OF AMINO ACIDS

The name protein is derived from the Greek term *proteos,* which means "primary" or "to take place first." Protein was first identified in a laboratory about a century ago at which time scientists described it as a nitrogen-containing part of food that is essential to human life. We now know that all proteins are collections of amino acids. Said another way, amino acids are the "building blocks" of proteins. Although the final functional form of some proteins may contain minerals or other nonprotein components, the basis for these proteins is still amino acids.

What are amino acids?

There are probably hundreds of different amino acids found in nature, but only twenty are incorporated into the proteins found in living things (see Table 6.1). This means that these twenty amino acids are the basis of protein found in birds, lizards, plants, bacteria, fungi, yeast, and so on. This is a very profound and also convenient situation. First, it allows us to further appreciate that, despite the obvious structural and functional differences between the different life-forms on this planet, there is common ground and more than likely common ancestry. Second, it somewhat simplifies human nutrition as we are able to obtain all of the amino acids we need to make our body proteins by eating the proteins of other life-forms.

All amino acids have the same basic design, as shown in Figure 6.1. There is both a nitrogen-containing amino portion and carboxylic acid portion attached to a centralized carbon atom. The presence of both an amino and an acid portion on each molecule led to the

TABLE 6.1. The Twenty Amino Acids Used to Make Proteins

Essential Amino Acids	Nonessential Amino Acids
Tryptophan	Alanine
Valine	Proline
Threonine	Tyrosine
Isoleucine	Cysteine
Leucine	Serine
Lysine	Glutamine
Phenylalanine	Glutamic acid
Methionine	Glycine
Arginine*	Asparagine
Histidine*	Aspartic acid

*Essential during growth

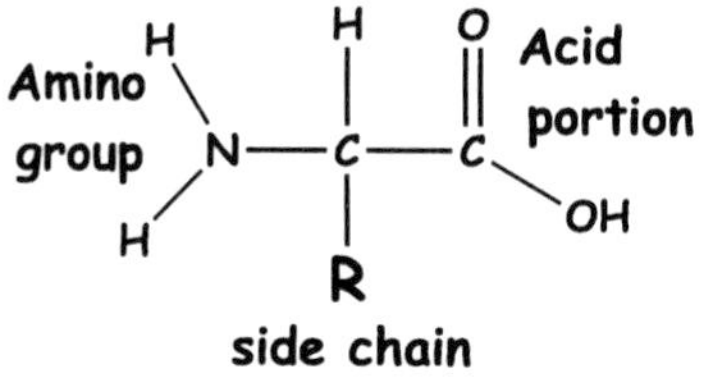

FIGURE 6.1. Basic components of amino acids. An amino acid contains a central carbon atom (C) with the following attachments: (1) amino group, (2) carboxyl (carboxylic acid) group, (3) hydrogen (H), and (4) "R" group or side chain.

name *amino acid* for this family of molecules. There is also a hydrogen atom attached to the central carbon, as well as a mysterious "R" group. The R group denotes the portion of an amino acid that will be different from one amino acid to the next. The R portion of an amino acid may be as simple as a hydrogen atom, as in glycine, or much more complex to include carbon chains and rings, acid or base groups, and even sulfur (S). The structure of the twenty amino acids used to make protein is shown in Figure 6.2.

How big are proteins and what do they look like?

Some proteins contain just a few amino acids linked together, while others contain hundreds of amino acids. Scientists often refer to the links of amino acids in the following manner:

- Peptides are two to ten amino acids including dipeptides, tri-peptides, etc.
- Polypeptides are 11 to 100 amino acids.
- Proteins are > 100 amino acids.

Other scientists will describe protein size based upon the weight of the protein molecule (molecular weight) and sometimes use the term Daltons as a unit of weight.

Some smaller proteins will exist as a somewhat straight chain of amino acids; however, most proteins will exist in a complex three-dimensional design (see Figure 6.3). Links of amino acids will contort themselves based upon the sequencing of the amino acids. Some amino acids are attracted to other amino acids in the chain while others are repulsed. This is due to either opposing or similar charges that are part of the side chains of amino acids. Also, as the amino acid chain bends, twists, and warps about three dimensionally, certain amino acids will form bonds to other amino acids. This helps stabilize the three-dimensional design and it will be the final structure that determines the functional properties of a protein. It is interesting that many proteins are actually all globbed up, somewhat like crumpled paper or loosely packed yarn. In fact, the names of some proteins, such as hemoglobin and immunoglobin, probably reflect their globbed (globular) nature. On the contrary, many proteins have more of a filament design, meaning that they are much longer than they are wide. Many of these proteins are like stretched out coils. This is the case with collagen. In fact, numerous collagen proteins will associate side by side to form a ropelike fibrous superprotein. Further still, it is possible for a protein to demonstrate both globular and filament attributes as is the case with muscle proteins actin and myosin.

What role do proteins play in the human body?

Protein and individual amino acids function in our body in a number of ways. Proteins can function as

- enzymes (regulate chemical reactions),
- structural proteins (yield form to cells and tissue),
- contractile proteins (provide basis for muscle contraction),
- antibodies (help protect us from foreign entities),
- transport proteins (help transport substances in our blood),
- protein hormones (i.e., insulin, glucagon, and growth hormone),
- clotting factors (allow our blood to clot to stop a hemorrhage), and
- receptors on cells.

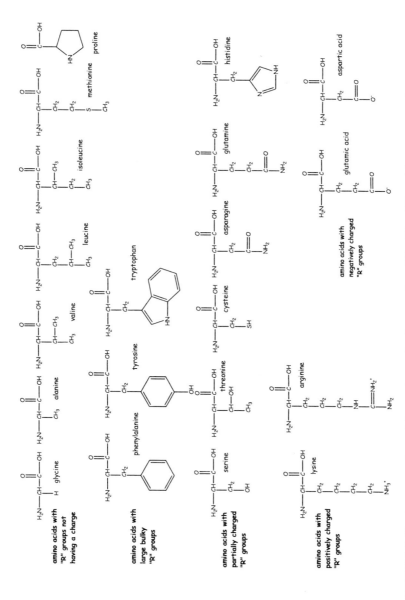

FIGURE 6.2. The twenty amino acids used to make the proteins of life. The "R" or side groups can be neutral or big and bulky or charged. The sequence of amino acids in a protein will then determine the final shape.

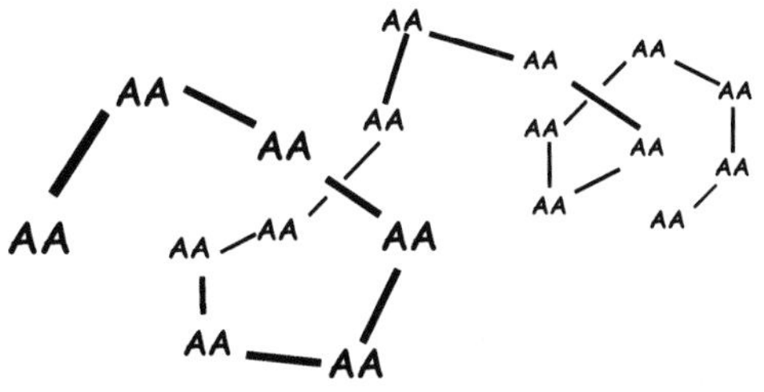

FIGURE 6.3. The specific sequence of amino acids will determine the final three-dimensional structure of the protein.

Individual amino acids can be used to make certain hormones and neurotransmitters such as epinephrine, serotonin, norepinephrine, and thyroid hormone (see Table 6.2). In fact, most neurotransmitters are derived from amino acids. Amino acids are also used to make other important substances such as choline, carnitine, nucleic acids, and the vitamin niacin. Last, amino acids can be used by some tissue as an energy source or can be converted to glucose or fat depending upon our current nutritional state (i.e., fasting, fed, exercise).

PROTEIN IS FOUND IN ALL NATURAL FOODS AND ENTERS OUR BODY AS AMINO ACIDS

What foods contain protein?

Because protein is vital to life, all organisms will contain protein. However, the protein content of organisms will vary. In general, foods of animal origin will have a greater protein content than plants and plant-derived foods, as demonstrated in Table 6.3. Among the foods that have the highest protein content (percent of energy) are water-packed tuna and egg whites. This is why these foods are popular with bodybuilders and others alike. Another popular protein source is milk. The principal proteins in milk are caseins and whey. Meanwhile, the predominant protein in egg whites is albumin (e.g., ovalbumin and conalbumin). Cereal grains produce a vast array of proteins (including albumins); however, the most interesting proteins may be gliadin and glutenin. When these proteins are mixed with water, such as when we make dough, gluten is formed. Gluten provides the structural basis for the network that traps gases produced by yeast

TABLE 6.2. Select Substances Made from Amino Acids

Amino Acid	Substances
Tryptophan	Serotonin
Lysine and methionine	Carnitine
Methionine, glycine, and arginine	Creatine
Aspartic acid and glutamine	Pyrimidines
Aspartic acid, glutamine, and glycine	Purines
Tyrosine or phenylalanine	Epinephrine, norepinephrine, thyroid hormone, dopamine

TABLE 6.3. Approximate Protein Content of Various Foods

Food	Protein (g)
Beef (3 oz)	22
Pork (3 oz)	21
Cod, poached (32 oz)	21
Oysters (32 oz)	14
Milk (1 cup)	8
Cheddar cheese (1 oz)	7
Egg (1 large)	6
Peanut butter (1 Tbsp)	5
Potato (1)	3
Bread (1 slice)	2
Banana (1 med)	1
Carrots, sliced (2 cups)	1
Apple (1)	2
Sugar, oil	0

when dough rises. Soy lacks these proteins, and ingredients need to be added to soy flour to make it rise to a light bread.

How are proteins digested and absorbed?

The goal of protein digestion is to disassemble proteins to their constituent amino acids. The liberated amino acids can then be absorbed across the wall of our small intestine into circulation. Unlike carbohydrates and fat, protein digestion does not begin in the mouth, as there is not a protein-digesting enzyme in our saliva. However, protein digestion does begin in our stomach as swallowed food is bathed in its acidic juice. The acid serves to straighten out the complex three-dimensional design characteristic of many proteins. This will make it easier for protein-digesting enzymes in the stomach and small intestine to do their job.

A protein-digesting enzyme called *pepsin* is an important component of stomach juice. Pepsin begins to break the bonds between amino acids. The impact of pepsin is significant yet incomplete, as most of the protein digestion to amino acids will ultimately take place in the small intestine. As partially digested proteins make their way into the small intestine, they are attacked and broken down to very small amino acid links and individual amino acids by a battery of protein-digesting enzymes, most of which come from our pancreas. Pancreatic protein-digesting enzymes include *trypsin, chymotrypsin, carboxypeptidase A and B, elastase,* and *collagenase.* These enzymes are actually made, packaged, and released by our pancreas in an inactive form. Upon reaching our small intestine they are activated by a process initiated by the small intestinal enzyme *enterokinase (enteropeptidase).* This process protects the pancreas and the connecting ducts from the protein-digesting activity of these enzymes.

While liberated amino acids are transported into small intestine wall cells, a fair amount of small peptides, consisting of just a few amino acids linked together, can also be transported into these cells. The final digestion of these small links of amino acids will then take place within those cells. Therefore, as a general rule, the absorbed form of protein will be individual amino acids.

The processes of digestion and absorption are by no means perfect. Occasionally, partially digested proteins are able to sneak between the cells that line the small intestine and get into the blood. These tiny peptides will either be digested by plasma enzymes or be recognized by immune factors. If the latter occurs, an allergic reaction may result. Food allergies will be addressed in Chapter 12.

What happens to amino acids once they are absorbed?

Amino acids make their way across the wall of the small intestine and enter the blood by way of the portal vein. The portal vein delivers the amino acids to our liver, which then removes a lot of them. In fact, it is typical for only about one-fourth of the absorbed amino acids to circulate because of the aggressive actions of our liver. Furthermore, much of the amino acids that survive the efforts of our liver are the so-called branch-chain amino acids (BCAA), which are the essential amino acids leucine, isoleucine, and valine. This is probably because these amino acids are needed by our skeletal muscle to replace what was used for energy during fasting or exercise.

The amino acids that enter our blood from our digestive tract evoke a release of insulin from our pancreas. However, the ability of elevated blood amino acid concentrations to cause the release of insulin is nowhere near as potent as elevated glucose. Regardless, the increased presence of circulating insulin will promote the uptake of amino acids in certain tissue, primarily muscle, as well as promote the building of new protein in muscle and tissue throughout our body. Interestingly, the increase in the level of circulating amino acids after a meal can slightly increase the level of glucagon as well. Considering this, aren't the actions of insulin and glucagon opposite, thus making this scenario counterproductive? Consider the following scenario. What if our only source of food was wild game (land or sea animals)? Having the effects of insulin and glucagon might allow the following to occur: Glucagon would promote the conversion of some amino acids to glucose in the liver while insulin would promote the formation of glycogen and muscle protein as well as promote the production and storage of fat. All of these efforts would leave that person in better shape for enduring an extended period of time before they ate again. This certainly may have been the case for our distant ancestors when enduring winters or prolonged dry seasons when vegetation might not have been available.

What happens to excess amino acids absorbed from the diet?

Diet-derived amino acids in excess of the needs of cells are not stored in the form of protein. Unlike fat, we do not store excessive diet protein as body protein. Therefore, our liver breaks down amino acids in excess of our needs and several of these amino acids can be used to make fatty acids, which then can be used to build fat. The hormone insulin promotes this process of making fatty acids from excessive amino acids. However, the conversion of excessive amino acids to fat is not as efficient as was once thought. Therefore, while some of the energy in excessive diet protein is stored as fat, our immediate use of amino acids to power our cell operations increases as well. So, if we eat a higher protein diet, more of our energy expenditure will be attributable to the breakdown of amino acids. This is similar to carbohydrates. When we eat more carbohydrates we tend to immediately use more carbohydrate for fuel. Later we will discuss how it can take several days to adapt to using more fat as an energy source if we eat a very high fat diet.

SOME AMINO ACIDS ARE ESSENTIAL COMPONENTS OF OUR DIET

What are essential and nonessential amino acids?

From a nutritional standpoint, only eight to ten of the twenty amino acids found in protein are actually dietarily *essential*. These amino acids present us with the same situation as do the other essential nutrients. We simply cannot make them or at least not in the amounts necessary to promote growth, development, and health. As a result, these amino acids must be provided by our diet. As listed in Table 6.1, arginine and histidine are noted as essential during periods of growth but not at other times.

The remaining amino acids, deemed dietarily *nonessential,* can be made in the body by using essential amino acids and/or other molecules. The easiest way to remember the essential amino acids is by the acronym TV-TILL-PM-AH! These are the first letters of the essential amino acids tryptophan, valine, threonine, isoleucine, leucine, lysine, phenylalanine, methionine, and the two semi-essential amino acids arginine and histidine.

Dietary essentiality or nonessentiality by no means is meant to imply biological essentiality or nonessentiality. All twenty amino acids must be present in cells to make the proteins needed to support the health of those cells and our body in general. Further, if a problem exists in making a nonessential amino acid, as is the case in some genetic anomalies, then that amino acid would also become a dietary essential as well. This is the case with some individuals who lack the ability to produce the appropriate enzyme to convert phenylalanine (essential amino acid) to tyrosine (nonessential amino acid). In these cases (i.e., phenylketonuria [PKU]), tyrosine becomes an essential amino acid.

Are there better food protein sources than others?

The goal of protein nutrition is fairly simple. We need to provide our body with food protein that closely resembles our own protein. This is to say that it is desirable for the protein within a particular food (or combinations of foods) to provide all of the essential amino acids, in proportion to human protein, while at the same time providing a respectable assortment of the nonessential amino acids. However, since the nonessential amino acids can be made in the body, we judge the ability of a food (or food combinations) to accomplish this task by focusing upon essential amino acid content.

All life-forms on this planet vary to some degree. Therefore, the protein nutrition goals stated may be met by eating foods derived from life-forms that are very similar to people—the idea being that closely related life-forms, such as other animals, will have much of the same proteins as we do, and in comparable amounts. Therefore, using the amino acids in that food to make proteins in our cells is a simple conversion because of the similarity in amino acid compositions. Protein sources such as beef, pork, fish, poultry, eggs, milk, and milk products are often called "higher-biological value" proteins because their relative essential amino acid concentrations more closely resemble our own protein. These protein sources are also called "complete" proteins because they will contain adequate amounts of all essential amino acids relative to our protein.

On the other hand, plants and foods derived from plants will provide "incomplete" or "lower-biological value" proteins. This is to say that their proteins' essential amino acid composition is less similar to our protein. Some of this is due to the immobility of plants. Meanwhile, animals contain muscle protein that is very similar from one animal to the next (including humans). Since a large proportion of the protein in animals (including us) is found in muscle, a strong foundation for protein/amino acid compatibility exists. Another reason for protein compatibility between animals is that most of the other cell proteins and other proteins (i.e., collagen) are highly similar as well. Plants, on the other hand, grow, survive, and reproduce by vastly different means than we do and, as a result, many of their proteins vary as well. When we compare the protein content endowed to a given plant food, we tend to find that one or more of the essential amino acids is in a limited quantity relative to our protein (see Figure 6.4). The amino acids in limited concentration are often referred to as "limiting amino acids."

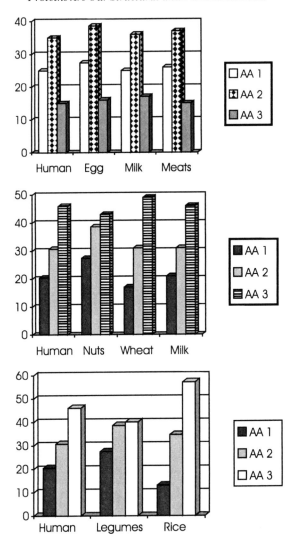

FIGURE 6.4. Hypothetical content of three essential amino acids (AA) in human protein and three high biological value protein sources (top). Comparison of two lower biological value protein sources (nuts and wheat) to human protein and milk (middle). Eating two lower biological value foods allows them to complement each other to make a higher biological value meal (bottom). Here, the limitations of legumes to provide AA 3 is compensated for by the abundance of AA 3 in rice. The opposite is true for rice and AA 1. (The three amino acids are not necessarily the same in the different graphics.)

Because adequate amounts of all essential amino acids are needed to make protein, strict vegetarians who eat only plants or plant-derived foods must consider this issue. However, less strict vegetarians who eat eggs and/or dairy products may be less concerned. Fortunately, the essential amino acids that are of limited quantity within plants can vary among plant sources. This allows us to combine different plant-derived food sources to acquire adequate quantities of all the essential amino acids. For example, we could combine cereals (i.e., oats, wheat, rice, rye) which are low in lysine but a good source of methionine, with legumes, which are low in methionine but a good source of lysine. This practice is called "complementing" proteins. Complementing incomplete proteins allows one plant-derived food source to pick up the essential amino acid slack for one another. The practice of complementing proteins may be best served within the same meal; however, many nutritionists feel that complementing within adjacent meals is acceptable as well. Examples of complementing proteins include a peanut butter sandwich or beans and rice.

Plant proteins are inferior to more complete animal protein sources only in their inability to supply us with all of the essential amino acids. However, with thoughtful planning we can easily meet the dietary requirements for all essential amino acids. Furthermore, obtaining protein from plant sources, such as vegetables and whole grain products, certainly has its advantages. Plants and plant products generally contain less fat and no cholesterol relative to animal products. Also plants and plant products are generally rich in many vitamins and minerals as well as water, fiber, and other phytochemicals.

BODY PROTEIN IS A FUEL RESERVE SIMILAR TO GLYCOGEN AND FAT, BUT NOT EXACTLY

What happens to body protein when we fast or exercise?

Situations can occur whereby the amount of body protein used for energy increases. Calorie dieting and exercise render our body more reliant upon body protein as an energy source. During periods of fasting or prolonged aerobic exercise, the concentrations of glucagon, cortisol, and epinephrine will be higher in our blood. All three of these hormones will promote the conversion of amino acids to glucose in our liver, while cortisol will promote the breakdown of our body proteins to amino acids to feed this operation. The amount of amino acids used to make glucose is related to the length of fasting or exercise. When our body glycogen stores become depleted, as in prolonged fasting and endurance exercise for several hours, the reliance upon amino acids to make glucose increases.

During a longer period of fasting, such as several weeks, our reliance upon amino acids lessens a bit as our brain adapts to utilize more ketone bodies. This is to say that the reliance upon amino acids during this adaptive fasting period is still greater than during more normal times; however, part of the metabolic adaptation to prolonged fasting is to try to conserve (slow the loss of) our body protein. Clearly the cause of death in most cases of starvation is related to protein malnutrition. For instance, if the cause of death is due to an infection, the true cause is probably a failure to maintain an optimal immune defense because of poor protein status.

If we use some body protein for energy on other things, how much do we need to eat?

During a single day about 300 to 400 g (about 4.6 g/kg body weight) of an adult man's body protein is "turned over." This is to say that on a daily basis, throughout our body a little less than one pound of protein is broken down to amino acids. Meanwhile, throughout that same day, a relative amount of protein is also made. Therefore, even though there is this seemingly significant quantity of protein turnover, we seem to be mostly the same from one day to the next.

Protein is either broken down or manufactured to allow us to adapt to the most current metabolic situation within cells, and also in our body. This process also allows us to maintain the integrity of proteins subjected to daily wear and tear. These activities allow cells to make or break down enzymes, which are either involved or not involved in different metabolic states such as fasting, feeding, and exercise. These processes also allow us to remodel tissue such as muscle and bone and to make and break down hormones and neurotransmitters. It is important to remember that our cells are constantly active. This allows us to grow, heal, remodel, and internally defend ourselves on a continual basis.

All proteins in our body have a certain life expectancy. For instance, when insulin and glucagon are released into our blood they may circulate only for about five to ten minutes before they are removed and broken down. Some enzymes within cells may exist only for a few minutes or so before they are replaced or not remade. This can allow cells to shift metabolic gears, so to speak, when going from a fasting to a fed state, resting to exercise state, and so on. Contractile proteins in muscle (e.g., myosin and actin) may last only a couple of days, while connective tissue proteins, such as collagen, may last weeks to months before they are broken down and replaced. The rate of turnover or remodeling of skeletal muscle contractile proteins and connective tissue proteins helps us understand why the human body seems to get bigger and stronger in just a couple of weeks or so when lifting weights regularly. Meanwhile, it seems to take months and years for scar tissue to change.

Most cells in the body have a small assortment of amino acids. Along with the small amount of amino acids circulating in the blood, scientists refer to this as the "amino acid pool." These amino acids are either derived from the breakdown of body proteins or from the diet. Whichever the case, these amino acids are available to cells to make new proteins or amino acid-derived substances. Over the course of the day some of these amino acids can also become involved in energy pathways. In fact, scientists estimate that about 20 to 40 g of body protein in the form of individual amino acids is utilized to make each day as energy. Therefore, if our diet failed to include amino acids (protein) we would lose a significant amount of body protein over time. To avoid this situation we must include at least 20 to 40 g of protein in our diet daily. The RDA for protein for adults is set at 0.8 g of protein per kg body weight. This works out to about 54 to 60 g for most men and about 44 to 50 g for most women. Thus, the RDA for protein provides a little cushioning for reasons that we will not go into at this time.

What happens if we do not eat enough protein?

Our diet needs to at least replace a quantity of protein equivalent to what is lost to energy pathways and processes that produce amino acid-derived molecules such as neurotransmitters, nucleic acids, and some hormones. More specifically, our diet needs to replace the essential amino acids that were lost. If one or more essential amino acids are in limited quantity in our cells, then protein synthesis is limited to that level. If this continues over time, there will be a decrease in total body protein content. This would be most obvious in reductions in skeletal muscle mass, and if the deficiency continues then the level of various proteins in blood would decrease and in addition our immune system could become compromised, leaving us more prone to infections.

There are two important factors to consider when evaluating a diet in its ability to meet our essential amino acid needs. The first is protein quality and the second is protein quantity. Protein quality becomes a factor only when protein quantity is lower. For instance, if a person derives all of their diet protein from one plant source whose limiting amino acid was, say, lysine, they could still meet their lysine needs by eating a lot of that plant source. However, this is not practical or nutritionally sound. Yet, this does make the point that protein quantity could potentially negate protein quality for strict vegetarians. What we do know is that vegetarians tend to eat less protein than nonvegetarians because plant foods tend to be less concentrated with protein than animal foods. So, the more strict the vegetarianism, the more effort these people should make to complement protein sources.

Several levels of vegetarianism exist. Among the most restrictive are the fruitarians, who mostly eat what certain plants bear (i.e., fruits, nuts) and not necessarily the foundational plant tissue. Vegans are also very restrictive in their dietary choices. Their diet will include only plant tissues and derivatives. Lactovegetarians will include milk and dairy products while ovovegetarians will include eggs. As you may have guessed, lactoovovegetarians will complement the plant-based foods in their diet with dairy, eggs, and recipe foods that include eggs and dairy products as ingredients. Again, the less restrictive one's diet tends to be, the higher the protein intake and the less need for concern about protein quality. For instance, the typical omnivorous (plant and animal eating) American adult will eat on average about 100 to 125 g of protein daily. This would provide a more than ample quantity of the essential amino acids.

Can our protein requirements be increased during certain times in our life?

At no time in our life are our protein requirements higher than during infancy. Furthermore, not only is the total protein need greater but so too are the requirements for the essential amino acids. For instance, the protein needs of an infant are more than double that of adults, 2 g versus 0.8 kg body weight. This is because of the extremely rapid growth that occurs during infancy. Also, during pregnancy and lactation a woman's protein requirements are raised as well to 1.2 and 1.0 kg body weight, respectively. In addition, protein needs are increased during resistance training (e.g., weight lifting) and endurance training. For individuals who train hard on a regular basis, their protein requirements may increase to 1.4-1.7 g/kg. This level of protein would support the development of muscle tissue for weight trainers or the maintenance of body protein in endurance athletes. We will discuss this further in Chapter 11.

What happens to the nitrogen when amino acids are used for energy purposes?

The composition of elements in amino acids differs from carbohydrate and fat, as they contain nitrogen (N). This creates a dilemma for the body if it wishes to use amino acids for energy or to make fat or glucose. Thus an important step in using amino acids for any of these purposes is to remove the nitrogen-containing portion of the molecule. Since the removed nitrogen portion of amino acids will become ammonia (NH_4^+), which is potentially toxic to the CNS, it must be removed from the body before it builds up in the blood. The most prevalent way to rid the body of the nitrogen removed from amino acids is to use it in the construction of a molecule called *urea* (Figure 6.5). Urea is made by the liver and released into the blood. Urea circulates to the kidneys and is subsequently lost from the body in urine. Each molecule of urea allows us to efficiently remove two nitrogen atoms from our body.

INTEREST IN SPECIFIC AMINO ACIDS IS GROWING

Can amino acids affect our mood, memory, and emotions?

As noted previously, certain amino acids are precursors for neurotransmitters and are therefore believed to have the ability to influence mood, memory, and emotions. For instance, the amino acids tryptophan and tyrosine are used by brain cells to make serotonin and catecholamines (norepinephrine and dopamine), respectively. Also, choline, which can be made from the amino acid serine, is a building block for the neurotransmitter acetylcholine.

Serotonin is a neurotransmitter mostly associated with a calming and sleepy feeling. In order for serotonin to be produced, tryptophan

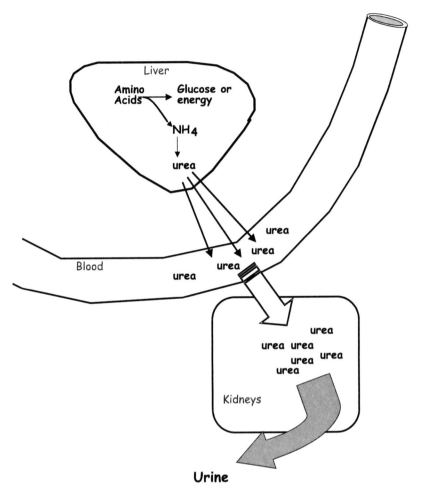

FIGURE 6.5. The nitrogen that is removed from amino acids is used to make urea in the liver. Urea then circulates to the kidneys and is released in the urine.

must exit the blood and enter our brain cells. The movement of tryptophan out of the blood requires a special transport system. However, tryptophan must compete with several other amino acids, namely valine, leucine, tyrosine, and phenylalanine, to do so. Traditionally, a glass of warm milk in the evening is believed to produce drowsiness. It was assumed that the tryptophan content of milk proteins increased the concentration of typtophan in our blood, which in turn resulted in more tryptophan entering our brain. However, the proteins in milk contain a lot more of the other amino acids that tryptophan must compete against in order to enter the brain, so scientists questioned this notion. It seems that the calming effect of milk is probably not directly related to its tryptophan content. It is more likely that the carbohydrate content of milk or other high carbohydrate foods (e.g., soda, candy, cake) increases the insulin content of our blood, which then promotes the uptake of amino acids in skeletal muscle. Unlike the amino acids that compete with tryptophan for entry into the brain, tryptophan is not removed from the blood by the actions of insulin. Therefore, the relative amount of tryptophan to the amino acids it competes with to enter the brain increases. More tryptophan is able to enter the brain and subsequently more serotonin can be made. This may also be true for turkey, another food that is believed to cause drowsiness. By and large, turkey is eaten on bread or with potatoes. Thus, again, the carbohydrate may be the real culprit that causes drowsiness by decreasing tryptophan's competitors for uptake into the brain.

Chapter 7

We Are All Wet

WATER IS THE BASIS OF OUR BODY

Water makes up about 60 percent of our total body weight, typically a little more for men and a little less for women. So then, for a 175-pound man more than 100 pounds of his weight would be water. Roughly two-thirds of our body water is found within our cells as intracellular fluid, while the remaining one-third is extracellular fluid found bathing our cells. As mentioned earlier, extracellular fluid includes both the fluid between our cells and also the plasma portion of our blood.

When looking at our body tissue, skeletal muscle is about 73 percent water by weight, while fat tissue is less than 10 percent water (see Figure 7.1). By and large, it is the ratio of skeletal muscle to fat tissue that dictates the amount of water in the body. Because men tend to have a slightly greater percentage of muscle and a slightly lower percentage of fat in comparison to women, they tend to have a slightly greater percentage of body water. However, regardless of gender, a lean muscular person will have a higher percentage of body water while a nonmuscular overweight person will have a lower percentage of body water. Interestingly, the ratio skeletal muscle to fat tissue not only influences our body water content but our buoyancy within a body of water as well. Having more skeletal muscle to fat tissue translates to a higher ratio of body protein to fat, thereby resulting in a more dense and less buoyant person.

What does water do for us?

Water provides the medium or environment for the body. This is to say that substances within the body are dissolved, suspended, and/or

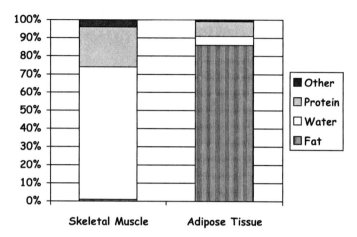

FIGURE 7.1. Composition difference between skeletal muscle and adipose (fat) tissue. Skeletal muscle is largely water and then protein, while adipose tissue is mostly fat and very little water, protein, and other material.

bathed within water. In accordance, the transport of lipid materials in our blood requires transporters such as proteins or lipoproteins. For instance, fat-soluble vitamin D hitches a ride upon a vitamin D binding protein (DBP), while sex hormones (i.e., estrogen, testosterone) can latch onto sex hormone binding protein (SHBP). In the meantime, fats and cholesterol are transported in lipoproteins, which are in essence submarines carrying lipid cargo.

Our body water is dynamic. Individual water molecules can move into and out of cells and travel throughout our body. So even if the distribution of your body water has not changed since yesterday, a water molecule that was in a skeletal muscle cell at 3:00 p.m. yesterday could possibly be found in a liver cell or a neuron in your brain twenty-four hours later.

One of the most interesting features of water is its capability to absorb heat to keep us from overheating (hyperthermia) and at times overcooling (hypothermia). In comparison to other materials, water can absorb a relatively high amount of heat before its own temperature changes. This allows our body water to absorb the heat generated during normal metabolism and during times when we engage in exercise. Water then facilitates the removal of extra heat from our body. Heat that is produced via the operations in our cells warms the water surrounding them, which in turn warms the water in the blood surging through that tissue. The blood then circulates the heat to the skin, where it can be released to the outside environment. This allows the body to cool down.

On the other hand, because we are water based this helps prevent our body temperature from dropping too fast in a cold environment. This is because water tends to hold onto heat energy longer than most other materials. This means that if you brought a cup of water, a copper penny, and an aluminum bat outside on a cold day, the latter two materials would become colder more quickly. The ability of water to absorb and hold onto heat helps us understand why cities located close to a large body of water tend to have more moderate temperature highs and lows during a twenty-four-hour period than those located away from bodies of water. It also helps us understand how the water temperature at beaches can be lower than the air temperature in the summer and higher than the air temperature in the winter.

Water also provides the basis for the lubricating substances found in our joints and for the amniotic fluid that cushions and protects a fetus during pregnancy. It is also the basis of our urine, bile, saliva, mucus, lacrimal fluid (tears), and digestive secretions.

OUR BODY LOSES WATER

What is sweat?

One way that we remove excess heat from the body is by sweating. Our brain prompts sweating when our internal body temperature increases. Scientists sometimes refer to the temperature in and around our vital organs (brain, heart, intestines, liver, etc.) as the "core" body temperature. The other ways that we lose heat from our body are by conduction, convection, and radiation (see Table 7.1). As the temperature around us increases, the potential to lose heat from our body via conduction, convection, and radiation decreases, thus rendering us more reliant upon sweating. Sweating is also stimulated by circulating epinephrine, which is released into the blood by our adrenal glands during exercise. This helps us understand why we sweat more when we exercise and why we sweat more when we exercise in warmer climates.

TABLE 7.1. How We Lose Heat from Our Body

Method	Mechanism	Factors
Evaporation	Transfer of our body heat to sweat water. This warms the water to its vapor point. Heat leaves the body in evaporated water.	Sweating is increased relative to the intensity of exercise and/or as temperature increases.
Convection	Transfer of our body heat into the surrounding air or water (e.g., swimming in a pool).	Convection increases as air or water temperature decreases, and vice versa.
Conduction	Transfer of our body heat to an object or surface. (This could be a chair, bed, bare feet on the floor, etc.)	The warmer the objects the less heat is transferred, and vice versa.
Radiation	Transfer of our body heat to other entities by radiating energy waves. This is similar to the energy waves from the sun warming our body on a sunny day.	The warmer the objects the less heat is transferred, and vice versa.

Sweat is mostly water with a varying amount of dissolved substances, such as sodium and chloride. It is released from skin glands into pores, which are in essence tubes leading to the surface of skin. Excessive body heat warms the sweat reaching our skin until the water reaches its vapor point. Sweat water changes from a liquid to a vapor and then lifts off into the air, thus taking heat with it. Each liter of sweat can remove 580 Cal of heat. However, when sweat evaporates, it leaves the once-dissolved substances caked on our skin.

The process of sweating is fascinating. As shown in Figure 7.2, our sweat glands are based pretty deep in our skin, probably deeper than many people realize. This is actually very important. When we sweat, the initial fluid oozing into the tubes leading to our skin surface is fairly concentrated with sodium and chloride. In fact, the concentration of these minerals in that fluid is similar to their concentration in our blood (plasma). However, as that initial sweat flows through the tube, sodium and chloride can be absorbed back into our body along with some of the water. What is most important in determining the final amount and composition of the sweat reaching our skin surface is how rapid the sweat flows through the tubes. The flow rate itself is related to the degree of stimulation. For instance, even if you are sitting

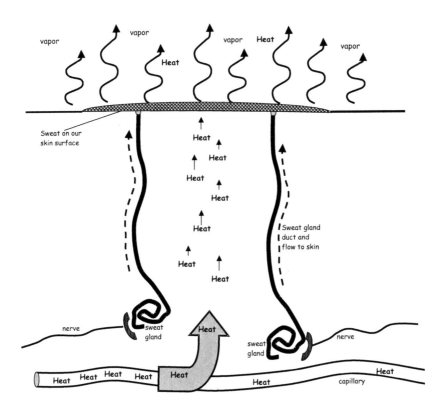

FIGURE 7.2. Our sweat glands begin deep in our skin and they ooze sweat when they are stimulated by our brain, when our body temperature rises, and by circulating epinephrine during exercise.

in your living room, the sweating process is only lightly stimulated. Therefore, as that produced sweat moves slowly through the tubes, practically all of the sodium and chloride are brought back into our body along with some water. This results in only tiny amounts of water reaching our skin. In fact, you probably do not even realize that you are sweating, but you are. Oppositely, in a warmer environment and/or during exercise, when sweating is more strongly stimulated, the flow of sweat through the tubes is much faster. In this situation less and less sodium, chloride, and water are removed, resulting in more sweat reaching the skin's surface. The sweat is also more concentrated with sodium and chloride, which can leave a salty residue on the skin and on clothing. Because sweating is such an important means of removing heat, distance runners and other endurance athletes become "better sweaters." This means that their sweat glands and tubes have adapted during the athlete's training to produce larger volumes of sweat but containing less sodium and chloride. This helps keep them from overheating but at the same time it keeps them from losing excessive amounts of the key electrolytes in sweat. A well-trained endurance athlete may sweat 2 to 3 L/h.

How do we lose water from our body and how much?

As suggested earlier we probably sweat throughout the day to help remove extra body heat produced by normal cell operations, but we probably do not even notice it because it is so minimal. For an adult this can add up to about .5 L (see Figure 7.3). However, when we exercise or find ourselves in a hot environment, sweating certainly becomes more obvious, especially if it is humid. Increased moisture in the air can hinder the evaporation process, allowing sweat to accumulate on our skin.

Water is also lost from our body through breathing. When we inhale, air moving through our air passageways (i.e., trachea and bronchi) becomes humidified. This means that we are adding moisture to

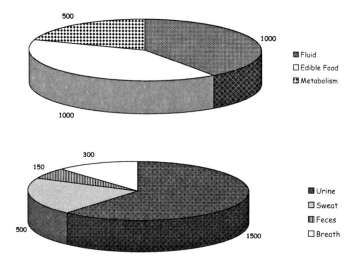

FIGURE 7.3. Water provision (top) and water losses (bottom) throughout the day. Approximate volumes (mL) are listed next to each factor.

it. Subsequently, when we exhale, much of the humidified air is lost to the outside environment. This is noticeable on a cold day as humidified exhaled air condenses to form little clouds. The amount of body water lost in this process is about 3 to 500 mL, depending on the humidity level of the air. For instance, in a dry environment, such as a desert climate or at higher altitudes, a little more of our body water is used to humidify the air we inhale. This in turn means that a little more water would be lost during exhalation. Conversely, breathing more humid air decreases the amount of water lost through our lungs.

Every day our kidneys process about 180 L (47.5 gals) of blood-derived fluid to regulate blood composition. Of the 180 L, more than 99 percent is returned to our blood, while the remaining 1 percent becomes urine. Dissolved in our urine will be waste products of our metabolism (e.g., urea) and other substances in excess of our needs (e.g., sodium, chloride). About 1 to 2 L of our body water is lost daily as urine. This quantity will change relative to our water consumption. For instance, people who ingest more water will tend to produce more urine daily. In addition, their urine will also be less concentrated with waste products and excess substances. Meanwhile, people who ingest less water will tend to produce less urine, which will be more concentrated. For these reasons people sometimes look at the color of their urine to gauge their body water or "hydration" status. However, while this can certainly provide insight, food factors, such as the vitamin riboflavin, can darken the color of urine and/or alter its odor, such as with coffee.

Last, water is also lost from our body in feces. Water helps moisten feces for easier transit through and out of the colon. We lose about 100 to 200 mL of water in this process daily. As you might expect, we would lose more water from our body via the feces during bouts of diarrhea. This also means that we need to drink more water as tolerated during, as well as after, these unpleasant episodes.

WATER IS AN ESSENTIAL NUTRIENT

How much water do we need and where do we get it?

If we combine these routes of water loss from our body, it totals about 2 to 3 L (2 to 3 quarts or 8 to 12 cups) per day. If the amount of water lost from the body is not at least matched by the amount of water provided to the body, then dehydration can occur. However, this does not necessarily mean that we need to drink eight to twelve cups of pure water every day because there is water in most of the foods we eat, including water-based fluids such as milk, juices, and drinks such as soda and Kool-Aid. In addition to the water we ingest, we can also count on normal metabolic reactions in our cells to generate some water as well. For instance, when our cells completely break down (combust) the glucose and the fatty acid, two of our most significant energy nutrients, water is created.

Glucose: $\quad C_6H_{12}O_6 + 6\,O_2 \quad \longrightarrow \quad 6\,CO_2 + 6\,H_2O$

Palmitic Acid: $\,C_{16}H_{32}O_2 + 23\,O_2 \quad \longrightarrow \quad 16\,CO_2 + 16\,H_2O$

On the average we drink about 1 L of water daily in the form of water or other fluids such as soft drinks. Also, we receive about 1 L of water in the foods we eat and generate about .5 L in our normal metabolic reactions. Foods such as fruits and vegetables will have a relatively high water content compared to meats, breads, and fats (see Table 7.2).

What is thirst?

When our body needs water, a region of our brain called the hypothalamus initiates *thirst*. Thirst is a symptom of dehydration and is a

TABLE 7.2. Water Content of Common Foods

Food	% Water
Collards, lettuce (iceberg)	96
Radishes, celery, cabbage (raw)	93-95
Watermelon, broccoli, beets	90-92
Snap beans, milk, carrots, orange	87-90
Apples, cereals (cooked)	83-85
Potatoes (boiled), banana, egg (raw), fish (baked flounder)	74-78
Corn, prunes	70
Chicken (roast)	67
Beef (lean sirloin)	59
Cheese (Swiss)	42
Bread (white)	37
Cake (devil's food)	24
Butter	16
Almonds, soda crackers (e.g., Saltines)	4
Sugar (white), oils	0-5

signal to replenish body water. However, this also means that by the time thirst occurs, our body water is already slightly depleted. This probably is not that big a deal for most of us; however, to an athlete engaged in competition, this can result in decreased performance and the difference between victory and defeat. Most athletes who compete in endurance sports will drink prior to and during an event. A common belief among endurance athletes is that we should drink before we are thirsty.

By the time we have lost about 2 percent of our body weight as water we will become thirsty and may experience a slight reduction in strength. By the time we are dehydrated by 4 percent of our body weight, muscular strength and endurance are significantly hindered, while a 10 percent reduction of our body weight as water is associated with heat intolerance and general weakness. If dehydration continues, life itself becomes threatened. If dehydration continues to a 20 percent loss in our body weight, we become susceptible to coma and death.

How does water compare to other essential nutrients?

Many people regard water as our most important essential nutrient. This is because of three principal concepts. First, when we do the math, our dietary need for water far exceeds any other essential nutrient. For instance, 1 mL of water weighs exactly 1 g, therefore daily need for water for an adult would be approximately 2,000 to 3,000 g (2 to 3 kg). This is about 30 to 60 times greater than our need for protein and millions of times greater than our need for different vitamins and minerals. Second, signs and symptoms of water deficiency begin to show much more rapidly than any other essential nutrient. If we abstain from all food and drink, we would develop signs of water deprivation by the end of the first day or two. Furthermore, we may die from severe dehydration by the week's end. Third, as water is the basis of the human body, water imbalance (dehydration or toxicity) could not occur without influencing the metabolism of all other nutrients in some way.

Chapter 8

Energy Metabolism
and Body Composition

HUMAN COMPOSITION

When I was a kid I was told that little girls were made of sugar and spice and everything nice and little boys were made of snakes and snails and puppy-dog tails. I was happy with that then, but as I got older it just did not seem possible! Well, what did you think when you were six?

What are we really made of?

When we step on a scale, it registers the total weight or mass of our body. However, this is just a general measurement and does not really provide us with an accurate assessment of the individual contributions made by the different types of substances to our body weight. Said another way, the scale is not sensitive to body composition. In the first chapter we recognized that the elements carbon, hydrogen, oxygen, and nitrogen make up greater than 90 percent of our body weight. We also acknowledged that these elements are components of the major types of molecules in our body. These molecules are water, protein, fat (triglycerides), carbohydrate, variations and combinations of the latter three molecule types, as well as other fascinating substances such as DNA. Minerals, which obviously are not molecules, make up most of our remaining body weight. Look at some examples of body compositions of what are deemed to be average adults in Table 8.1.

If we were able to remove the water from our body, we would find that we are then mostly made up of energy molecules such as protein, fat, and carbohydrate. In fact, greater than 80 percent of what would be left over are energy molecules in one form or another. So we are a

TABLE 8.1. Theoretical Contributors to Body Weight for a Lean Man and Woman

Component (Substance)	Lean Man (%)	Lean Woman (%)
Water	62	59
Fat	16	22
Protein	16	14
Minerals	5-6	4-5
Carbohydrate	< 1	< 1

container of energy similar to the foods we eat. This means that if we were the prey of another sophisticated animal who farmed people and then marketed them with food labels, our energy content could be listed on the label. This also means that when we do not externally eat energy, we must internally eat energy sources. Thus we must eat ourselves. Keep in mind that our cells are tireless in their operational efforts and must be fed twenty-four hours a day.

Why do we store excessive energy as fat?

Fat is how we store excessive energy; it is a matter of efficiency. More than double the amount of energy can be stored in a gram of fat than in carbohydrate and protein. Furthermore, carbohydrate and protein attract water, thus storing excessive energy exclusively as glycogen or protein would increase our body water tremendously. For instance, for each gram of glycogen there would be about 3 g of water hanging around it. Thus storing energy primarily as carbohydrate or protein would make people (and other animals) much heavier, larger, and somewhat waterlogged. This would be a huge disadvantage, as body weight would probably triple!

Do we "burn" fat and other energy nutrients?

From time to time someone will attempt to compare our metabolism to a furnace. Although both would expend energy as heat, this is about where the comparison should stop. For example, throwing more energy-endowed material (e.g., wood) into a furnace would increase the energy expenditure in a relative fashion. However, eating more energy-endowed material would have a comparative small impact on human energy expenditure. We would store the extra energy. On the other hand, when less wood is tossed into the furnace, the flame wanes and energy expenditure decreases and possibly ends, while our body can tap into stores and maintain a fairly constant energy expenditure.

SUPPLY AND DEMAND ECONOMICS
OF BODY WEIGHT

Weight loss and weight gain are not a matter of magic. There are no smoke and mirrors, sleight of hand, or rabbits pulled from a hat. Weight loss and weight gain are more of a simple model of balance—energy balance, that is. To an economist, it would be a simple model of supply and demand; for us, it allows us to use those algebra skills we developed in high school. If the energy contained in the food we eat (supply or positive) exceeds the energy needed or expended by our body (demand or negative), then we are destined to store the surplus.

Quantifying the energy content of foods is easy. We can simply read the food label or look at a Calorie chart. A food's energy content is the sum total of the energy contributions of its protein, carbohydrate, fat, and alcohol. However, quantifying the energy that we expend over the course of a single day and assessing how our energy expenditure may fluctuate over time with respect to different situations is a bit more complicated.

How do scientists know how much energy is in food?

When scientists want to know the energy content of a food, they can place the food item in an insulated chamber, called a *bomb calorimeter,* and "combust" it. Combustion is an O_2 requiring process and is often applied in the breakdown of nature's energy molecules. Combustion is how we completely break down energy nutrients in our body. Combustion is how the carbohydrate in paper and wood "burns" in our fireplace. Because of this, the term "burn" is often applied to the combustion of fuel sources in our cells.

The products of combusting foods in a bomb calorimeter include CO_2, H_2O, and heat. In addition, if the food contains protein or amino acids, some nitrogen-containing gases will also be produced. Since heat energy is typically measured as a unit called the kilocalorie (kcal) or Calorie (capital "C") this is how the energy content of the food is measured. All too often Calorie is used interchangeably with calorie (lower case "C"), but they are not the same. In fact, a calorie is 1/1000 of a Calorie or kilocalorie. However, because popular magazines and books often use calorie to mean Calorie, their interchangeable use has become acceptable. Food labels correctly use Calories.

In separate experiments, scientists can also determine the individual amounts of carbohydrate, protein, fat, and alcohol in a given food. The approximate energy equivalent of 1 g of these substances is as follows:

- 1 gram of carbohydrate = 4 Calories (kcals)
- 1 gram of protein = 4 Calories (kcals)
- 1 gram of alcohol = 7 Calories (kcals)
- 1 gram of fat = 9 Calories (kcals)

If we were to add up the energy contribution of the individual energy nutrients in a food, it should approximate the total Calories of heat measured by the bomb calorimeter.

Do we generate the same amount of energy when using energy nutrients in our body as generated in a bomb calorimeter?

We combust energy nutrients in our cells and in the process generate the same amount of energy as in the bomb calorimeter. In fact, the reason we bring O_2 into our body is so that it can be used in the combustion of energy nutrients within our cells. Furthermore, CO_2 is produced during the combustion of these energy nutrients in our cells and we must breathe it out.

Despite several similarities between the combustion of energy nutrients in a bomb calorimeter and in our cells there are a couple of fundamental differences. First, when amino acids and proteins are combusted in a bomb calorimeter, nitrogen-containing gases are produced. Contrarily, when amino acids are used for energy in our cells, most of the nitrogen is ultimately used to make urea. Second, the combustion of energy nutrients in a bomb calorimeter is for the most part an instantaneous process, while the combustion of energy nutrients occurring within our cells happens over a series of many chemical reactions (energy pathways). Last, unlike a bomb calorimeter, when we combust energy nutrients in our cells, we initially harness some (~40 percent) of the energy released in the form of ATP and to a lesser degree GTP (see Chapter 1). Meanwhile, the remainder of the energy released in the breakdown of energy nutrients is converted to heat.

The harnessed energy is stored in the bonds that link the phosphorus groups (phosphates) together as we discussed in one of the earliest chapters (see Figure 8.1). These links are referred to as "high-energy bonds." Cells can purposely break a phosphate bond when they need a burst of energy. The energy can be used to make molecules, contract muscle cells, or pump substances across membranes.

How are energy nutrients used by our cells?

Carbohydrates, amino acids, fat, and alcohol can all be used by our cells to make ATP. Although the specific energy pathways involved in the metabolism of these substances are somewhat unique, they are indeed interconnected at various points. This allows us to convert glucose and certain amino acids to fatty acids and also to convert amino acids, glycerol, and lactate to glucose. However, only cells of certain tissue will engage in these conversion activities.

Energy pathways in our cells occur in either the mitochondria or the intracellular fluid (cytoplasm). In the intracellular fluid, glucose becomes engaged in an energy pathway called *glycolysis*. This pathway converts glucose to two molecules of *pyruvate*. In this process, two ATP and heat energy will be generated (see Figure 8.2). Since these ATP will be generated without the need for O_2, glycolysis is often referred to as *anaerobic* energy metabolism.

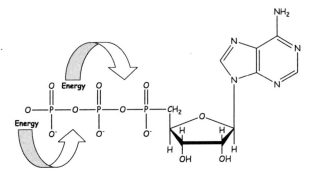

FIGURE 8.1. Adenosine triphosphate (ATP) molecule. Three phosphate groups (PO_4) are linked holding some of the energy released during the breakdown of energy nutrients.

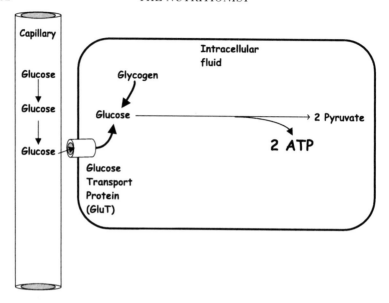

FIGURE 8.2. Inside all of the cells glucose is broken down into two molecules of pyruvate and in the process two ATP are formed. This operation does not require O_2 and is referred to as anaerobic ATP production or anaerobic energy metabolism. Glucose can be delivered by our blood, or depending on the type of cell, it can come from glycogen storage.

Pyruvate has several options, depending on the type of cell and what is going on inside of that cell (see Figure 8.3). If the cell lacks mitochondria, such as in RBCs, or if there is a shortage of oxygen in that cell, pyruvate can be converted to *lactic acid* (lactate). On the other hand, if the cell is endowed with mitochondria and has ample O_2, pyruvate will more likely enter the mitochondria for combustion. Once inside the mitochondria, pyruvate can be converted to another molecule called *acetyl CoA*. Acetyl CoA can then enter another energy pathway called the *Kreb's cycle* (see Figure 8.4).

During several of the chemical reactions that take place in our mitochondria, electrons are removed by carrier molecules and transported to special links of proteins embedded in the inner membrane of mitochondria. These special links of protein are called the *electron-transport chain* (see Figure 8.5). The electrons are passed from the carrier molecules to the electron-transport chain and then, like a

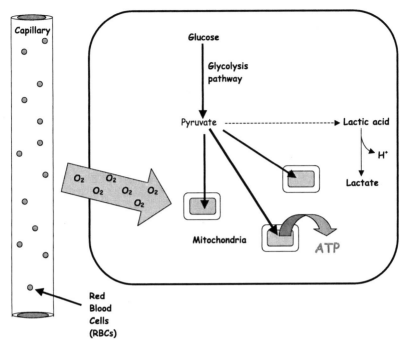

FIGURE 8.3. In our cells pyruvate can enter mitochondria where it is broken down further to produce ATP. Because O_2 is needed for our mitochondria to produce ATP the processes are called aerobic. If O_2 is not abundant in that cell or if the cell does not have mitochondria (i.e., RBCs) then pyruvate is converted to lactic acid.

bucket brigade, are passed along its length. As electrons are passed along the electron-transport chain, energy is released which drives the formation of ATP. Each of our mitochondria probably contains thousands of electron-transport chains.

Oxygen is needed to receive the electrons reaching the end of the electron-transport chain. Subsequently, the oxygen and electrons are coupled with hydrogen to make H_2O (see Box 8.1). This serves to generate water in our body on a daily basis. We use the term *aerobic* to describe the absolute need for O_2 in the formation of ATP via the electron-transport chain.

When energy nutrients are combusted completely by aerobic processes, the end products will be CO_2, H_2O, ATP, and heat. The CO_2 is

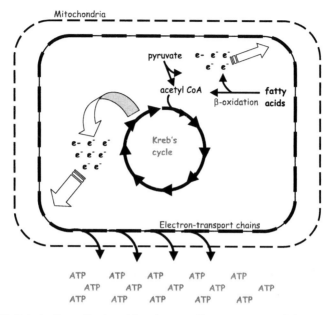

FIGURE 8.4. In the mitochondria of our cells, pyruvate and fatty acids are broken down to acetyl CoA, which then is broken down in a series of chemical reactions called the Kreb's cycle. During the breakdown of fatty acids, pyruvate, and acetyl CoA, electrons are removed and carried to the electron-transport chains that are stitched into the inner membrane. The electrons then become important in the making of ATP, which can be used by that cell to power an operation. These processes also produce CO_2 and H_2O.

actually a product of several reactions in our mitochondria. Since the need for CO_2 is somewhat limited in our body, it is considered a waste product and must be removed by our lungs. If O_2 is absent from a cell, the electron-transport chain will become jammed up with electrons and stop functioning. At this point that cell will have to rely more heavily upon anaerobic ATP generation. This is perhaps most obvious in skeletal muscle during heavy exercise. The increased reliance on anaerobic energy metabolism in skeletal muscle leads to the production of more and more lactic acid.

The lactate generated by RBCs and skeletal muscle can be used by other cells as an energy source. This is accomplished by first converting the lactate back to pyruvate, which can then enter mitochondria. Furthermore, the liver can use the lactate to make new glucose, which

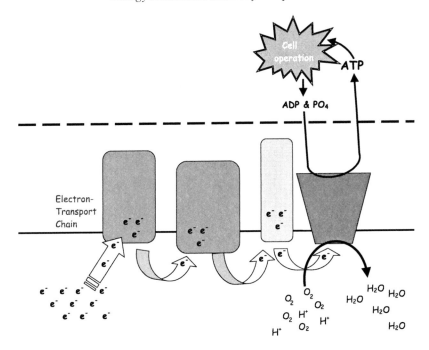

FIGURE 8.5. Electrons are moved down the electron-transport chain allowing the production of ATP. The electrons reaching the end of the chain are used to make H_2O from available O_2 and H^+.

BOX 8.1. Formation of Water in Our Cells	
$O_2 + 2\,H^+ \longrightarrow H_2O$	Electrons reaching the end of the transport chain are used, along with oxygen and hydrogen, to make water. Oxygen (O_2) in the atmosphere must be split into single atoms of oxygen.

can circulate to working muscles and help power muscle contractions. This occurs during exercise and between meals.

Do all energy nutrients use both aerobic and anaerobic processes?

When glucose is to be used in our cells for energy, it must first begin with glycolysis and anaerobic metabolism. Once it is converted to pyruvate, however, and if the conditions mentioned are met, pyruvate can enter mitochondria and become involved in aerobic energy metabolism. Like glucose, the monosaccharides fructose and galactose will also be used for energy by engaging in the glycolysis pathway. This happens mainly in the liver. So carbohydrates must use glycolysis to feed into the aerobic processes within the mitochondria.

When we use fat (triglyceride) for energy, both the fatty acid and glycerol can be used in energy pathways. Fatty acids enter an energy pathway called *beta-oxidation* (β-oxidation), which takes place within the mitochondria (see Figures 8.4 and 8.1). Beta-oxidation produces several molecules of acetyl CoA, which can then enter the Kreb's cycle. Also during β-oxidation electrons are removed and transported to the electron-transport chain by the special carriers mentioned previously and discussed in more detail in Chapter 9. Therefore, fatty acids require mitochondria and oxygen in order to be used for energy; they are completely aerobic.

Glycerol's importance, from an energy standpoint, lies mainly in its ability to be converted to glucose in the liver during fasting or exercise. Amino acids, on the other hand, can be used for ATP production in several ways. By consuming a lot of protein, excessive amino acids will be broken down in the liver. Once the nitrogen is removed from the amino acids, the remaining molecule can be converted to molecules in the energy pathways such as pyruvate, acetyl CoA, or those that are part of the Kreb's cycle. This makes amino acids aerobic. However, during fasting and endurance exercise some amino acids can be converted to glucose, which can then be used in glycolysis (anaerobic), and then the pyruvate can be used for energy in mitochondria (aerobic). In the meantime, some amino acids can be used during fasting to produce ketone bodies, whose subsequent use will be aerobic.

METABOLISM EQUALS ENERGY EXPENDITURE

What is our metabolic rate?

The chemical reactions that take place in our cells will release energy, and this energy is ultimately derived from the breakdown of energy nutrients. This energy is mostly lost from the body as heat. Therefore, our metabolic rate can be viewed as the amount of heat we produce within a specified period of time, such as over an hour or a day.

If energy expenditure is measured over an hour's time, it only estimates the expenditure during that hour and cannot be confidently extrapolated to longer periods of time. For instance, if energy expenditure is measured for one hour just after lunch during an afternoon, surely your energy expenditure would be greater than when you are sleeping. On the other hand, if energy expenditure is expressed over a day's time, it will not indicate periods within the day when the metabolic rate was greater, such as in more active times of the day, or lower, as in less active times of the day or when sleeping (see Figure 8.6).

How do we measure metabolic rate?

The human body works very hard to maintain its temperature at about 37°C (98.6°F). This means that excess heat generated by chemical reactions in cells must be dissipated. Because this dissipated heat is a direct indicator of our metabolism, we can use an insulated chamber sensitive to temperature change to determine how much heat we produce (energy expenditure). This method of estimating metabolic rate is often referred to as *direct calorimetry*. Calorimetry literally means "heat measurement." However, since the operational expense

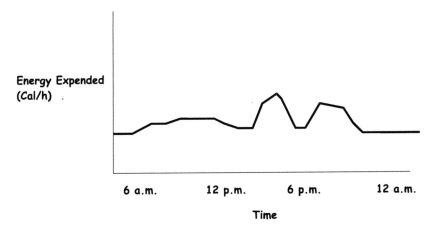

FIGURE 8.6. Hypothetical fluctuations in energy expenditure over a twenty-four-hour period. This would include periods of sleep, eating, and physical activity as well as the potential influence of the environmental

for this scientific tool is overwhelming, facilities designed to perform direct calorimetry may be found at only a handful of universities and research institutions.

An alternative method can be employed to assess metabolic rate called *indirect calorimetry*. Because ATP is generated from the combustion of energy molecules and because combustion requires O_2 and produces CO_2 it is possible to estimate energy expenditure based upon the exchange of these gases with the environment (see Photo 8.1). Representative chemical reactions for the combustion of carbohydrates, protein, and fat are shown below. You see that O_2 is used as a reactant for each reaction while CO_2 is a product. Utilizing mathematic equations we can estimate the amount of heat produced in a given period of time based upon the amount of O_2 inhaled or the amount of CO_2 expired. As it turns out, indirect calorimetry is not only a very accurate indicator of metabolism, but it also gives us an idea of the mixture of energy substances our body is using during that time.

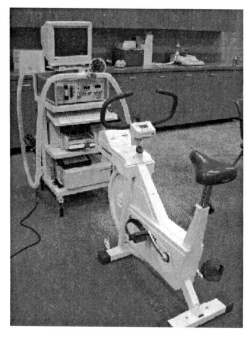

PHOTO 8.1. The metabolic cart can estimate energy expenditure and the contributions made by carbohydrate and fat by measuring O_2 and CO_2 produced by a person.

Carbohydrate
$$C_6H_{12}O_6 + 6\ O_2 \longrightarrow 6\ CO_2 + 6\ H_2O$$

Triglyceride (fat)
$$2\ C_{57}H_{110}O_6 + 163\ O_2 \longrightarrow 114\ CO_2 + 110\ H_2O$$

Protein
$$C_{72}H_{112}N_2O_{22}S + 77\ O_2 \longrightarrow 63\ CO_2 + 38\ H_2O + SO_3 + 9\ CO(NH_2)_2$$

From the chemical reactions shown, we can calculate the respiratory exchange ratio (RER) or respiratory quotient (RQ) for a given time period. RQ is equal to the amount of CO_2 exhaled divided by the amount of O_2 inhaled.

$$RQ = CO_2 / O_2$$

- RQ of glucose 6 CO_2 /6 O_2 = 1.0
- RQ for the triglyceride 114 CO_2 / 163 O_2 = 0.70
- RQ for the protein 63 CO_2 / 77 O_2 = 0.82

If we measure a person's gas exchange during a period of time we can calculate a few things. For example, say that during one hour a person consumed 15 L O_2 and expired 12 L of CO_2; we can first calculate their RQ for that hour:

$$RQ = 12/15 = 0.80$$

We can find the RQ 0.80 on Table 8.2 and follow it over to the Calorie source columns. At an RQ of 0.80 this individual would be using approximately 33 percent carbohydrates and 66 percent fat to fuel his or her metabolism. We will assume that the contribution from amino acids toward energy production during that time is minimal. This is a fair assumption for a healthy person not engaged in prolonged fasting or endurance exercise during this time. Furthermore, we can estimate metabolic rate by multiplying the amount of O_2 consumed (15 L) by the Caloric Value for 1 L O_2 for an RQ = 0.80. Their metabolic rate would be:

$$15 \times 4.801 = 72\ Cal/hour$$

What factors contribute to our metabolism or energy expenditure?

So far we have discussed metabolism as a single entity; however, there are four components to our metabolism or total energy expendi-

TABLE 8.2. Thermal Equivalent of O_2 and CO_2 for Nonprotein RQ

Nonprotein RQ	Caloric Value 1 L O_2	Caloric Value 1 L CO_2	Carbohydrate (%)	Fat (%)
0.707	4.686	6.629	0	100.0
0.71	4.690	6.606	1.1	98.9
0.72	4.702	6.531	4.76	95.2
0.73	4.714	6.458	8.4	91.6
0.74	4.727	6.388	12.0	88.0
0.75	4.739	6.319	15.6	84.4
0.76	4.751	6.253	19.2	80.8
0.77	4.640	6.187	22.8	77.2
0.78	4.776	6.123	26.3	73.7
0.79	4.788	6.062	29.9	70.1
0.80	4.801	6.001	33.4	66.6
0.81	4.813	5.942	36.9	63.1
0.82	4.825	5.884	40.3	59.7
0.83	4.838	5.829	43.8	56.2
0.84	4.850	5.774	47.2	52.8
0.85	4.862	5.721	50.7	49.3
0.86	4.875	5.669	54.1	45.9
0.87	4.887	5.617	57.5	42.5
0.88	4.899	5.568	60.8	39.2
0.89	4.911	5.519	64.2	35.8
0.90	4.924	5.471	67.5	32.5
0.91	4.936	5.424	70.8	29.2
0.92	4.948	5.378	74.1	25.9
0.93	4.961	5.333	77.4	22.6
0.94	4.973	5.290	80.7	19.3
0.95	4.985	5.247	84.0	16.0
0.96	4.998	5.205	87.2	12.8
0.97	5.010	5.165	90.4	9.58
0.98	5.022	5.124	93.6	6.37
0.99	5.035	5.085	96.8	3.18
100	5.047	5.047	100	0

ture (TEE). These are *basal metabolism* (BM), *thermal effect of activity* (TEA), *the thermal effect of food* (TEF), and *adaptive thermogenesis* (AT):

$$TEE = BM + TEA + TEF + AT$$

What is basal metabolism?

We will begin with the most basic or basal level of metabolism. *Basal metabolism* is the energy expended (heat) by chemical reactions during a period of complete rest (nonactive), when the body is not subjected to an unusually cold or warm environment and also at a time long after a meal, say, greater than ten to twelve hours.

The processes that occur as part of basal metabolism include those that fundamentally support life. Thus basal metabolism will include the energy expended for the beating of the heart, breathing, urine production, and the building of new cells. Surprisingly, the energy necessary to maintain tightly regulated electrolyte concentrations across cell membranes takes its place among the major contributors to basal metabolism. This occurs in all cells but is particularly significant in excitable tissue (nervous tissue and muscle). All of these activities release a substantial amount of energy as heat as they perform their duties.

Looking specifically at basal metabolism occurring within various tissue in the body we find that the most metabolically active tissue (Calories expended/gram tissue) are organs such as the heart, kidneys, lungs, pancreas, brain, and liver. These organs make up only about 10 percent of our total body weight, but the energy expended by these organs accounts for as much as 50 to 60 percent of our basal metabolism. Interestingly, the retina of the eye is the most metabolically active tissue (per gram of tissue) when we are engaged in visual processes. Skeletal muscle, which makes up about 40 percent of an adult's body weight, is not as metabolically active as the organs just mentioned. Skeletal muscle energy expenditure contributes about 25 percent to our basal metabolism. Keep in mind that this expenditure takes place when skeletal muscle is not working! Last, fat tissue contributes relatively little to our basal metabolism.

We can now see that the energy expended in basal metabolism is strongly related to the ratio of lean body tissue (organs, muscle, and bone) to fat tissue. For example, we would expect a 200-pound man

(91 kg) with 12 percent body fat to have a higher basal metabolism than a man who weighs the same but has 25 percent body fat. Basal metabolism on a per-weight basis is typically higher in males than in females because men tend to have a higher skeletal muscle to body fat ratio.

Basal metabolism is highest during infancy. At this stage basal metabolism not only reflects normal life-sustaining operations of the infant but also must power the building of new tissue. The same can be said for growth spurts in children and teens. Conversely, as we age, our basal metabolism seems to slow down. However, while researchers agree that some of this is related to declining hormones, much of it is related to changing body composition. As we age we become less active and thus lose muscle mass and gain fat mass.

How can we estimate basal metabolism?

The measurement of energy expended by basal metabolic processes over a given period of time is called basal metabolic rate (BMR). Scientists have devised a rule of thumb and more precise equations for estimating BMR for twenty-four hours. One limitation of these calculations is that they tend to overestimate basal metabolism in heavier individuals with a higher percentage of body fat.

- Rule of thumb:
  $$BMR = BW \times 24 \text{ hours}$$
- Body weight raised to the power of three-fourths:
  $$BMR = 70 \times BW^{.75}$$
- Harris and Benedict equation for men and women, respectively:
  $$BMR = 66 + (13.7 \times BW) + (5 \times Ht) - (6.8 \times age)$$
  $$BMR = 655 + (9.6 \times BW) + (1.8 \times Ht) - (4.7 \times age)$$
  (Wt [weight] = kg and Ht [height] = cm)

Calculate an estimated BMR for a thirty-five-year-old man who is 180 pounds (82 kg) and five feet eleven inches using the different equations.

- Rule of thumb: 1,963 Calories
- Body weight .75 × 70:   1,904 Calories
- Harris and Benedict: 1,853 Calories

What is the thermal effect of activity and how do we estimate it?

Skeletal muscular activity expends a lot of energy. Quite simply, the more we contract our skeletal muscle the more ATP is needed to power this activity. The thermal effect of activity (TEA) is the heat produced by skeletal muscle activity. We can use Table 8.3 to calculate a general estimation of the thermal effect of activity for various sports.

To use Table 8.4 we would need to keep an activity journal for a twenty-four-hour period. Then use the activity factors to calculate the amount of energy you expended while engaged in various activities

TABLE 8.3. Energy Expended During Various Sports

Activity	Approximate Energy Expended (Calories/pound of body weight)					
	100 lb (45.5 kg)	120 lg (54.5 kg)	140 lb (63.6 kg)	160 lb (72.7 kg)	180 lb (82 kg)	200 lb (90 kg)
Bicycling						
5 mph	1.9	2.3	2.7	3.1	3.5	3.9
10 mph	4.2	5.1	5.9	6.8	7.6	8.5
15 mph	7.3	8.7	10.0	11.6	13.1	14.5
20 mph	10.7	12.8	14.9	17.1	19.2	21.3
Running						
6 mph	7.2	8.7	10.2	11.7	13.1	14.6
7 mph	8.5	10.2	11.9	13.6	15.4	17.1
8 mph	9.7	11.6	13.6	15.6	17.6	19.5
9 mph	10.8	12.9	15.1	17.3	19.5	21.7
Skiing[1]	6.5	7.8	9.2	10.5	11.9	13.2
Skiing[2]						
2.5 mph	5.0	6.0	7.0	8.0	9.0	10.0
4.0 mph	6.5	7.8	9.2	10.5	11.9	13.2
5.0 mph	7.7	9.2	10.8	12.3	13.9	15.4
Soccer	5.9	7.2	8.4	9.6	10.8	12.0
Tennis	5.0	6.0	7.0	8.0	9.0	10.0
Walking						
3 mph	2.7	3.3	3.8	4.4	4.9	5.4
4 mph	4.2	5.1	5.9	6.8	7.6	8.5
5 mph	5.4	6.5	7.7	8.7	9.8	10.9
Weight lifting	5.2	6.0	7.3	8.3	9.4	10.5

[1]Downhill skiing
[2]Cross-country skiing

during that time. The activity factors are provided in ranges to allow for slight variations of effort. For example, if you walked two miles across town on two different days you would probably consider this light activity. However, if you noticed that on the second day that you reached your destination two minutes earlier than on the first day, then use the higher end of the range for the second day versus the first day.

What is the thermal effect of food?

Most people do not realize that their metabolic rate increases during the digesting and processing of a meal. It does. This extra heat produced is called the thermal effect of food (TEF). There are a couple a reasons for the extra heat production after a meal. Some heat is generated by the muscular activities of chewing and swallowing and the churning and propulsion of food in our stomach and intestines. The release of hormones and digestive enzymes associated with digestion as well as the activities associated with absorption will also have their input into the expenditure of energy during this time. However, most of the heat generated by a meal is generated by the processing of the absorbed nutrients once they reach our liver and other tissue. Depending

TABLE 8.4. Energy Expended for General Physical Activity

Type of Activity	Energy Expended (Calories/kg body weight/min)	
	Female	Male
Sleeping or lying still	0.00	0.00
Sitting or standing still (e.g., sewing, writing, eating)	0.001-0.007	0.003-0.012
Very light activity (e.g., driving, walking slowly)	0.009-0.016	0.014-0.022
Light activity (e.g., sweeping, walking moderately, carrying objects)	0.018-0.035	0.023-0.040
Moderate activity (e.g., fast walking, dancing, biking, cleaning vigorously)	0.036-0.053	0.042-0.060
Heavy activity (e.g., fast dancing, swimming, tennis, gymnastics, fast uphill walking)	0.055	0.062

upon the size of a meal and its composition, the thermal effect of food can endure for several hours after you finish eating. Perhaps the most common estimate of energy expended by the thermal effect of food is 10 percent of energy intake. For example, if you ate 2,500 Calories during a one-day period, the energy expended attributable to the thermal effect of food would be about 250 Calories. The TEF will tend to be a little higher for higher protein meals in comparison to higher fat.

What is adaptive thermogenesis?

Changes in environmental temperature can influence metabolic rate. Because body temperature is tightly regulated, the body will either try to increase or decrease metabolism in an effort to adapt to environmental conditions. Located throughout the body are sensors that alert the CNS when body and/or environmental temperature is changing. If body temperature begins to fall in a cooler environment, specific chemical reactions in certain cells increase in an effort to release extra heat. Also, the body begins to shiver. Shivering is tiny contractions within muscle cells that are not significant enough to cause a whole muscle to contract. However, the small contraction efforts of those muscle cells will generate some heat that can help warm the body. On the other hand, if the body temperature increases, aspects of cell metabolism will slow a bit in an effort to produce less heat.

Adaptive thermogenesis (AT) is of minor consequence for many of us who reside, work, and drive in climate-controlled environments. But for many people who work outside on cold winter days or blistering hot summer days, adaptive thermogenesis becomes a more influential part of their daily metabolism.

OBESITY HAS BECOME A MODERN-DAY NUTRITION EPIDEMIC IN SOME COUNTRIES

In Chapters 9 and 10 we will discuss vitamins and minerals. In doing so our discussion will include symptoms related to deficiencies of these substances. Many of these deficiency disorders, such as goiter, were fairly common in the United States as the twentieth century began, and these deficiency diseases are still a concern in many underdeveloped countries. However, embracing the twenty-first century, the greatest nutritional concern in the United States is not one of deficiency but toxicity. Obesity is a disorder resulting from chronic excessive energy consumption whose signs and symptoms include high blood pressure, high blood lipids, glucose intolerance, and often complaints of lethargy. Thus obesity can be viewed as energy toxicity syndrome.

What does it mean to be overweight?

The term *overweight* is used to describe an individual's body weight relative to a reference or what has been deemed a more ideal body weight (IBW). Several decades ago, the Metropolitan Life Insurance Company developed the Height-Weight Table for adults (see Table 8.5 a and b). The weights listed on this table are based upon the statistical association between the occurrence of various diseases and body weight. This table lists body weight ranges for men and women of different heights and body frame sizes. The IBW range is then understood to be the weight whereby the association with various diseases is the lowest. Since diseases can influence longevity, the Metropolitan Life Insurance Company used this table as a tool to adjust life insurance premiums.

Body frame size can be estimated by dividing our height (Ht) by our wrist circumference (WC), as per this formula:

$$r \;=\; \frac{Ht \text{ (cm)}}{WC \text{ (cm)}}$$

Wrist circumference is measured at the point where the wrist meets our hand. Other methods of estimating body frame size are available, including measuring the breadth of the elbow. However, wrist circumference is probably the easiest and most popular method used to estimate frame size (see Table 8.6). You can use a measuring tape or a piece of string. The measuring tape will need to include metric measurements or you will need to do a conversion (1 in = 2.54 cm). If you use a string it can then be laid out and measured against a ruler. Remember to take up the slack but do not compress the skin when making your measurements with either the tape or string.

Another method of estimating IBW for adults applies a rule of thumb (ROT) formula based on height (± 10 percent for range of frame size):

- Women: 100 pounds for the first 60 inches and then 5 pounds for each inch beyond
- Men: 106 pounds for the first 60 inches and then 6 pounds for each inch beyond

To gauge a person's body weight status health professionals commonly use the Metropolitan Life Insurance Company's table and the Rule of Thumb. They are also used to help set goals for better health. Having a body weight that is 10 to 20 percent greater than a person's IBW is identified as being overweight. Having a body weight that is

TABLE 8.5a. Height & Weight Table for Men

Height Feet Inches	Small Frame	Medium Frame	Large Frame
5'2"	128-134	131-141	138-150
5'3"	130-136	133-143	140-153
5'4"	132-138	135-145	142-156
5'5"	134-140	137-148	144-160
5'6"	136-142	139-151	146-164
5'7"	138-145	145-154	149-168
5'8"	140-148	145-157	152-172
5'9"	142-151	148-160	155-176
5'10"	144-154	151-163	158-180
5'11"	146-157	154-166	161-184
6'0"	149-160	157-170	164-188
6'1"	152-164	160-174	168-192
6'2"	155-168	164-178	172-197
6'3"	158-172	167-182	176-202
6'4"	162-176	171-187	181-207

Weights at ages 25-59 based on lowest mortality. Weight in pounds according to frame (in indoor clothing weighing 5 lbs.; shoes with 1" heels)

MetLife®

Copyright 1996, 1999 Metropolitan Life Insurance Company
One Madison Avenue, New York, NY 10010
All Rights Reserved

TABLE 8.5b. Height & Weight Table for Women

Height Feet Inches	Small Frame	Medium Frame	Large Frame
4'10"	102-111	109-121	118-131
4'11"	101-113	111-123	120-134
5'0"	104-115	113-126	122-137
5'1"	106-118	115-129	115-140
5'2"	108-121	118-132	128-143
5'3"	111-124	121-135	131-147
5'4"	114-127	124-138	134-151
5'5"	117-130	127-141	137-155
5'6"	120-133	130-144	140-159
5'7"	123-136	133-147	143-163
5'8"	126-139	136-150	146-167
5'9"	129-142	139-153	149-170
5'10"	132-145	142-156	152-173
5'11"	135-148	145-159	155-176
6'0"	138-151	148-162	158-179

Weights at ages 25-59 based on lowest mortality. Weight in pounds according to frame (in indoor clothing weighing 3 lbs.; shoes with 1" heels)

MetLife®

20 to 40 percent greater that a person's IBW is recognized as mild obesity; 41 to 99 percent greater than IBW is recognized as moderate obesity; and a body weight 100 percent or more greater than IBW is defined as morbid obesity.

What exactly is obesity?

Simply stated, obesity is a state of excessive body fat. However, since the equipment and trained personnel needed to precisely determine body fat percentage are generally not available to the majority

TABLE 8.6. r Value Application for Body Frame Size

Frame Size	Men	Women
Small	> 10.4	> 10.9
Medium	10.4-9.6	10.9-9.9
Large	< 9.6	< 9.9

of people, we turn to the scale as an alternative method of determining obesity. Recent reports estimate that roughly 60 million Americans are obese as defined as a body weight in excess of IBW by 20 percent or more.

One potential downfall to relating our actual weight to IBW is that our body weight may not be sensitive to body composition. Remember, obesity refers to excessive contribution of fat to an individual's body weight, not necessarily total body weight. However, more times than not, the two go hand in hand. One exception is in the case of heavier yet more muscular people. These people would include bodybuilders and other strength athletes who train with weights or other resistance tools. The training leads to the development of greater than typical amounts of muscle tissue. Thus, if we merely use body weight to determine the status of a five-feet, ten-inch 220-pound man with 12 percent body fat, he would be considered mildly obese. This is because his body weight is more than 20 percent greater than his IBW. Consequently, to accurately identify obesity, we must measure body fatness, not just body weight. A body fat percentage greater than 25 percent for men and 33 percent for women is generally considered obese.

What health concerns are associated with obesity?

Time and time again researchers have reported that strong associations exist between obesity and a greater occurrence of various diseases. These diseases include hypertension (high blood pressure), type 2 diabetes mellitus, arthritis, gallstones, heart disease, and various forms of cancer. Also, a greater risk exists of complications during pregnancy and surgery and, sadly, obese people tend to live relatively shorter lives. Furthermore, it seems that the greater the obesity, the greater the risk. The risk for type 2 diabetes mellitus is particularly disturbing. Roughly 90 percent of the people diagnosed with type 2 diabetes mellitus are obese. What has also become clear is that when these people reduce their body fat, this disease lessens in severity. Whether obesity is a direct cause of type 2 diabetes mellitus remains unclear, but scientists have determined that as fat cells swell during the accumulation of more fat, they release factors that probably make the disease worse.

Is obesity due to genetics?

This is a difficult question to answer in the manner in which we would like it to be answered. Quite simply, obesity results from an energy imbalance whereby more energy is brought into our body than is expended. As fat is how we store the excessive energy, we thus accumulate more body fat. Certainly that seems simple enough. However, identifying the reason for the imbalance is a bit more complicated. Is it merely a matter of excessive energy intake, meager energy expenditure, or a combination of both?

An argument can easily be made that nearly all aspects of our being have a genetic basis. Thus genetic disposition might certainly be involved in determining body weight and composition. But how? Although "faulty genes" can certainly play a role in establishing a sluggish metabolism in some people, scientists estimate that this may account for only a small percentage of obese individuals. The problem may lie in hormonal imbalances, such as lowered thyroid hormone. Scientists also believe that some people are genetically inclined to store body fat and hold on to it once it is stored. In this situation the cause is not hormonal but more related to increased activity of the enzymes involved in storing fat.

Whether a genetic basis is evident for the remaining obesity is matter for an interesting debate. Can genetics pattern an individual's behavior thereby rendering him or her more inclined to develop obesity? For example, people who prefer to be less active or favor energy-dense foods are likely candidates for an energy imbalance. If we apply genetics to the incidence of obesity in this manner, we can certainly attribute obesity in many people to a genetic origin of some form. For others, excessive energy consumption may be a manifestation of psychological disturbances. Here, food may serve more as an instrument of comfort or as a way to cope.

Regardless of the exact causes for obesity, one thing is certain: the incidence of obesity in America has increased dramatically within the past few decades. In fact, modern-day America appears to nurture the development of obesity. In no other country is food so readily available, especially energy-dense high-fat foods. Almost everywhere we turn in America we can find soda and vending machines. It also seems that most of the commercials on television are for chips, soda, candy, and other energy-dense foods. Interestingly, a fair portion of the other commercials market athletic apparel and gear. Yet, when was the last time you saw a commercial for broccoli or apples or heard a radio jingle for carrots? Furthermore, we seem to take great pride in developing ways to reduce our activity level. Escalators grace every mall; airports have moving sidewalks; and everywhere you go, you can sit down. All too often roads are constructed without sidewalks or bicycle lanes.

Long ago, even eating itself involved significant energy expenditure. As hunters and gatherers, our ancestors had to spear their fish, hunt and scavenge animals, dig up roots, climb trees for leaves, and pick fruits and vegetables. Today, one simple trip to the convenience store or dialing a phone number yields a bounty of food. Even the act of preparing food, which could take hours even a generation ago has been greatly simplified and requires less expenditure of energy.

What is the ob *protein, and what potential applications might it have for humans?*

In 1995, scientists detailed a genetically obese breed of mice *(ob)* that have a defective gene that codes for the protein leptin. As you may have already realized, *ob* is an abbreviation of obesity. Therefore, these mice develop·obesity because they cannot make this particular protein. It seems that leptin, which is made and released into the blood by fat tissue, signals the brain as to the status of fat stores. As fat stores swell, more leptin is released into the blood, telling the brain to slow down energy consumption. This is "satiety." Over time, then, the animal should expend more energy than it eats and the body fat level is reduced. In essence, fat tissue serves to gauge energy storage levels and leptin is a message that is sent to the brain to update the brain on the status of these levels.

Interestingly, those mice that had a faulty *ob* gene not only overate but were also less active and had a sluggish metabolism. In the reported studies, the scientists gave daily injections of leptin to the *ob/ob* mice. The scientists reported that the injected obese mice not only lost weight but also showed an increase in their activity and metabolism levels. In essence, their obesity seemed to be reversed. Furthermore, one study also reported that injections of leptin in normal mice caused them to become leaner as well.

The potential for leptin therapy in treating human obesity is somewhat confusing at this time. It seems that most obese humans already have normal levels of leptin. However, it does increase our understanding of the complexity of human obesity. Leptin is now added to a growing list of hormones and neurotransmitters that seem to be involved. This growing list includes neuropeptide Y, cholecystokinin (CCK), galalin, serotonin, gastrin, and insulin. Abnormal levels of these and potentially other factors may invoke continuous hunger despite increasing energy storage. Many drugs attempt to inhibit or increase the influence of these factors, as will be discussed shortly.

Are there different kinds of obesity?

Visually it may indeed seem as if there are different types of obesity. Some people, particularly men, seem to store more fat above the waist in the abdominal region. Meanwhile, some people, particularly women, seem to have increased storage below the waist localized in the buttocks and thighs. If the majority of body fat has accumulated above the waist, we refer to this type as upper-body obesity. Often this body shaping is described as "applelike." On the other hand, if the majority of body fat has accumulated below the waist, we refer to this situation as lower-body obesity. This type of body design has been described as "pear shaped."

Those of us who exhibit the upper-body obesity pattern seem to be at a higher risk for heart disease, stroke, diabetes mellitus, and some types of cancers. There also may be some fundamental differences between the functions of fat cells in the abdomen in comparison to those found below the waist. While the reasons for preferential storage of fat in specific sites are still unclear, hormone levels (e.g., estrogen) and different levels of activity of fat-storing enzymes in different parts of our body probably play the biggest roles. These enzymes are called lipoprotein lipase (LPL) and hormone-sensitive lipase (HSL).

PINCHING, DUNKING, AND ELECTRICITY
ARE ALL USED TO ASSESS BODY FAT

How is body fat assessed?

Some of the more common methods used to estimate body fat percentage include skinfold measurements, underwater weighing, and bioelectrical impedance. Underwater weighing is the most accurate of these methods, as body fat content is determined by comparing body weight on land versus body weight when submerged in water. Since our body is about 60 percent water, this weight would be negated when we are submerged in a tank of water (see Photo 8.2). After removing as much air from the lungs as possible, the remaining body weight underwater is largely attributed to the relative amounts of body fat and nonfat or lean body mass (LBM). A person with a

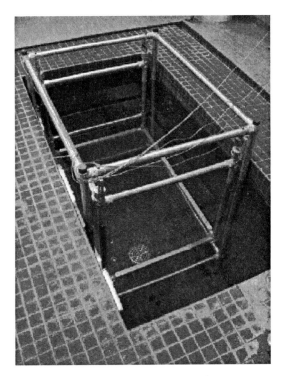

PHOTO 8.2. An underwater weighing tank can provide an accurate estimation of body fat levels.

higher percentage of body fat will be less dense and thus a little more buoyant than a leaner person who weighs the same. Thus the person with the higher body fat level would actually weigh less underwater than a leaner individual of the same body weight. Underwater weighing tanks are found at many universities; if the assessment is performed correctly, they are extremely accurate.

Skin-fold or fat-fold measurements rely on the premise that the layer of fat found beneath the skin, called subcutaneous fat, is a reliable indicator of total body fat. Skinfolds are pinched and measured with calipers from regions of the body such as the back of the arm (tricep), midback (subscapular), above the hip (suprailiac), abdomen, and thigh. Care must be taken to pinch only the skin and the underlying layer of fat, not the skeletal muscle beneath. The measurements can then be used in an equation to determine body fat percentage. These equations were mostly generated from underwater weighing studies within specific groups of people, such as female college students, male swimmers, women or men ages thirty to fifty, and so forth. Therefore, to be accurate, we need to use the equation most applicable to the person being assessed.

The accuracy of skin-fold assessment in estimating body fat percentage depends largely on the person doing the assessment. The average of multiple measures should be applied and equations using multiple skin-fold sites should be applied. A minute or more to allow compressed tissue to recover should separate the multiple measurements at the same site. Also, a pinch should not be held for more than 4 to 5 seconds before taking a measurement. If performed correctly, skin-fold measurements can be accurate ±5 percent.

Another tool for estimating body fat is the bioelectrical impedance assessment or BIA. Here, electrodes would be put in contact with two of our limbs and a tiny electric current is passed from one electrode to the other using our body as a conductor (see Photo 8.3). Our body fat will act as an insulating material, while our lean tissue, such as muscle, will serve as a conducting material. This is because muscle contains a lot of water and electrolytes while fat tissue contains relatively little water and electrolytes. Therefore, the amount of body fat relative to leaner tissue in the body will determine the speed of conduction of the electric current. This is measured and body fat is estimated.

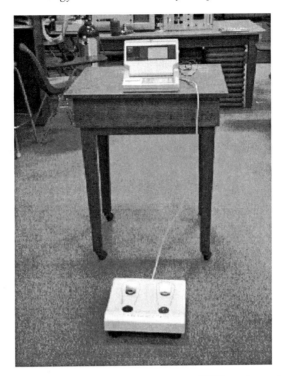

PHOTO 8.3. Bioelectrical impedance assessment (BIA) equipment. This device would pass a small electric current from one foot to the other and estimate body composition based upon the transit time.

Recently, some bathroom scales contain the components necessary to assess BIA. The accuracy of these scales has not been thoroughly tested by professionals. Other methods used by scientists to estimate body fat include infrared detection, total body potassium, total body water, and magnetic resonance imaging (MRI).

FOOD AND ACTIVITY ARE THE SCULPTORS OF OUR BODY COMPOSITION

What causes changes in body weight and composition?

Very rapid changes in body weight are usually caused by fluctuations in body water status. For instance, water losses via sweating and/or poor fluid consumption can reduce body weight by a little over 2 lb/L (1 kg/L) for each lost liter. Also, understand that the diuretic effects of caffeine and related substances in coffee, tea, and soft drinks may lead to a loss of body water. Keep in mind that you may not perceive thirst until you have reduced your body weight by about 1 percent as water. So you may actually reduce your body weight by a pound or so prior to feeling thirsty. Even if a person does not eat for one day, more than one-half of the weight loss experienced may be attributable to water loss. On the contrary, there are certainly times when we may hold a little extra water in our tissue. Women certainly know this to be true at certain points in their menstrual cycles.

However, changes in body weight and composition over time are more attributable to chronic overeating, undereating, the type of diet we eat, and exercise training. In general, the effects of these factors are relegated to specific hormones. The handling of energy nutrients being absorbed from the digestive tract is primarily influenced by insulin. In contrast, glucagon, cortisol, and epinephrine largely control the handling of stored body nutrients during fasting or exercise.

Are energy nutrient ratios important?

Over the past couple of decades several popular diet programs were founded on energy nutrient ratios. At the present time, very low carbohydrate diets enjoy the greatest popularity. For instance, *Dr. Atkins' Diet Revolution* and *Sugar Busters!* enjoyed several months on *The New York Times* bestseller lists and still may be in the top 100. The Atkins diet was first introduced in the late 1960s and was met by international criticism in the decade that followed. The late 1980s and early 1990s seemed to belong to Dr. Barry Sears and *The Zone*. But what do we really know about energy nutrient ratios and their influence on weight loss, weight gain, and body composition?

It does seem that when we eat carbohydrates and protein they are used for energy before fat; there may be a hierarchy of fuel utilization. This is probably due in part to the ability of insulin to promote the use of glucose for energy. Thus, it seems that if we eat 70 percent carbohydrate, then roughly 70 percent of our energy expenditure will be carbohydrate. If we eat 50 percent protein, then roughly that amount of our energy expenditure will be protein.

How would weight gain from overeating affect body composition?

When we eat more energy than we use (expend), much of it will be stored and we will gain weight. Remember, our ability to store carbohydrate (as glycogen) is limited to about 400 to 500 g, and body protein content is based upon the protein needs of our body, not how much protein we eat. This means that the more carbohydrate and protein we eat, the more we will use for energy during the hours that follow, as mentioned previously. This will decrease our use of fat as a fuel source. In addition, some of the energy in the carbohydrate and protein we ate will be used to make fat. So when we eat energy in excess of our expenditure, less body and food fat is used for energy and a little fat is made as well. Subsequently, more and more body fat will accumulate over time.

For the most part, fat will be stored in fat cells (adipose tissue). By virtue of expanding fat cells and of simply being a larger person, the absolute amount of body protein, mineral, and water also must increase. In fact, these substances may account for as much as 20 percent of our weight gain from chronic overeating. However, since the increase of these nonfat substances is small relative to the increase in fat, their percentage of our total body weight will ultimately decrease. For example, if a person's body weight increases by 10 pounds (~ 4.5 kilograms) due to overeating, the amount of protein in the body may increase by .25 to .5 lb (~ .5 to 1 kg). However, the protein percentage of their total body weight will actually decrease a little. A body fat percentage of about 14 to 18 percent for men and 15 to 25 percent for women is considered typical (see Table 8.1); however, body fat percentage can climb upward of 70 percent of total body weight in morbidly obese people. This latter situation would leave only about 30 percent for all other body components.

Will different types of diets evoke the same weight gain?

The conversion of excess glucose and amino acids to fat is not a simple process. These substances must engage in chemical reaction pathways, which will require some energy to power. Therefore, we must actually expend a little energy to make fat. This means that a person eating a higher-carbohydrate/protein diet in excess of energy needs will not store quite as much energy in the form of fat in comparison to an individual who eats a high fat diet in excess of energy needs. So, to address the notion that higher-carbohydrate diets make us "fat," the answer is clearly yes! But only when we eat more energy than we expend. However, if we eat the same amount of energy (in excess of expenditure) with a higher amount of fat, we may probably gain even more body fat.

In addition, the type of fat we eat may also influence our ability to make fat from excessive diet-derived carbohydrate and amino acids. Some studies have shown that eating a diet which derives more of its fat from good food sources of omega-3 PUFAs (e.g., fish) may actually decrease our ability to make fat from excessive diet-derived carbohydrate and amino acids—perhaps another good reason to eat more fish.

What happens to our body composition during complete fasting?

Over time, when our energy intake does not meet energy expenditure, we should lose weight. However, the nature of the weight loss depends largely upon how much energy we eat and whether we are exercising during that time. For instance, if we completely fast for a day or two, weight loss would certainly be rapid and this fact is encouraging for "crash dieters." However, the composition of the weight loss may not be as expected. As much as 60 to 70 percent of that weight loss might be attributable to water loss. Meanwhile, much of the remaining weight loss would be carbohydrate, and to a lesser degree, fat and protein. Keep in mind that glycogen is stored in association with water. As mentioned earlier, scientists estimate that every gram of glycogen sponges about three grams of water. So during that fasting period when glucagon levels are elevated and liver glycogen is broken down for energy, water will move out of liver cells into our blood, circulate to our kidneys, and be urinated out.

As the fast continues beyond a day or two, liver glycogen is no longer a major energy resource. Body fat breakdown is in high gear and becomes the major fuel source. Keep in mind that because all cells in the body have at least a minimal need for glucose at all times, our liver will need to generate some glucose. Amino acids become the major resource for this process. Most of the amino acids will be derived from skeletal muscle protein at first. Thus, with severe energy restriction you can certainly count on burning body fat, but you will also lose body protein (i.e., muscle mass). This is usually not what we want.

Even though your body would be fueled mostly by fat during prolonged fasting, protein would still make a remarkable contribution to your weight loss. The reason lies in the energy density differences between fat and protein. Consider this example: if a man has been fasting for five days, on the fifth day he might be deriving about 75 percent of his energy from body fat and the remainder from protein. If he expended 2,400 Calories that day, then 1,800 Calories would have come from fat and 600 Calories from body protein. If we calculate the mass equivalent of the fat and protein utilized we would cipher roughly 200 grams of fat and 125 grams of protein. That's nearly .5 lb of fat and a little more than .25 lb of protein. Some weight loss from water would be expected due to its association to lost protein.

If starvation were to endure for even longer, less body protein would be broken down on a daily basis and used as energy. This happens for a couple of reasons. First, our brain would require lesser amounts of glucose as it adapts to using more ketone bodies. Remember, ketone bodies are made in our liver during periods of high fat utilization. This is a survival mechanism serving to reduce the rate of loss of body protein. During prolonged starvation, the cause of death is usually related to body protein loss. Amazingly, our brain can replace about half of its glucose requirement with ketone bodies after a week or so of complete starvation. Second, during prolonged energy restriction the thyroid gland may release less and less thyroid hormone. This slows our TEE and thus decreases the requirement for protein breakdown. TEE is also reduced as less protein is made in the body over the course of the day and muscle tissue is lost.

What happens to our body composition during semi-starvation?

During extended periods when our energy intake is mildly to moderately restricted and most of the diet energy is derived from carbohydrate and protein, the composition of the weight loss would be different than during complete starvation. Since glycogen stores would be partially restored in response to the carbohydrate-containing meals, this would lead to less reliance upon the breakdown of our body protein. Furthermore, our diet will also provide protein to replace some of the amino acids used for energy. Insulin would promote the rebuilding of body protein, especially muscle, as well as liver and muscle glycogen. Contrary to the complete fast (zero energy) there would not be the early rapid weight loss that is attributable mostly to water. The weight loss experienced during extended periods of a mild to moderate energy restriction will largely be a mixture of fat, some protein, and a little water. However, the relative fat to protein contribution to energy expenditure would be much more favorable versus complete fasting. In addition, resistance training will also help minimize body protein loss as will be discussed.

Some moderate energy-restricted diet plans (1,000 to 1,200 Calories) include protein levels that well exceed the RDA. This design is believed to help spare body protein during weight loss. The reason is that the diet protein-derived amino acids can be used for glucose production, thus sparing some body protein. Furthermore, if the energy restriction is also limited in carbohydrate (as popular today), amino acids can also stimulate the release of insulin, although to a much lesser degree than carbohydrate. Insulin will help move amino acids into skeletal muscle and promote the rebuilding of some of the protein that is being lost.

The energy nutrient ratio may have an impact on the rate of weight loss. If the energy restriction includes a very low carbohydrate protocol, some of the weight loss is probably related to water. For instance, if you expend 2,500 Calories and your diet provides 1,500 Calories, there is a 1,000 Calorie imbalance. In the first day or two, much of the energy will come from waning glycogen stores. So, during the first day, if 60 percent of the energy imbalance is covered by carbohydrate, this translates to 150 g of carbohydrate ($^1/_3$ lb), which will be associated with roughly 450 g of water (another 1 lb). Meanwhile, if fat accounted for most of the other 40 percent of the energy imbalance (400 Calories), then about 45 g of fat would have been lost (about 1/10 or .1 lb). As the energy restriction continues and fat becomes the primary fuel covering the imbalance, weight loss will slow. Meanwhile, if the energy-restricted diet contained mostly a mixture of carbohydrate and protein, more of the energy imbalance would be covered by fat. This would result in a slower and more consistent rate of weight loss.

Because the very low carbohydrate diet tends to yield a greater weight loss in the first week or so, it is often deemed more effective. But is it really? The bottom line is that any time you use more body carbohydrate and protein to fuel cells, the associated weight loss will be more significant. Again, this is because of the energy density differences between carbohydrate and protein in comparison to fat as well as losses of water associated with body carbohydrate and fat. This is why changes in body composition must be assessed in relation to changes in body weight.

If a person strays from the very low carbohydrate protocol and eats a carbohydrate-containing meal or two, he or she may experience a weight gain, even if the person consumed less energy than he or she expended that day. Again, this is because of the water associating with partially replenished glycogen stores, not necessarily fat. Recently the USDA reported that very low carbohydrate diets were not more effective than higher carbohydrate diets in reducing body weight and fat. Furthermore, very low carbohydrate diets tend to be restrictive in fruits and some vegetables and whole grain products. These are major contributors of nutraceuticals, which promote general health.

In some circumstances a lower carbohydrate diet may be helpful. For many obese people, blood insulin levels are elevated. The health risks associated with hyperinsulinemia (chronic elevated blood insulin) include elevated blood cholesterol, triglycerides, and elevated blood pressure. Thus, a very low carbohydrate intake may lead to improved insulin levels. Furthermore, some people may be able to more successfully adhere to an energy-restricted protocol that is very low in carbohydrates. Some people claim that their appetite is suppressed as the higher level of ketone bodies is produced. For a long time researchers have speculated that ketone bodies may decrease appetite, but this has been difficult to prove in studies.

Can we lose only fat during weight loss?

When body weight is reduced, we must expect some obligatory loss in protein, water, and minerals. This only makes sense because these nutrients were important to a person before the weight loss. Even though fat tissue is composed of about 86 percent fat, when fat cells expand more of the other nutrients are needed to support the new size and metabolism of the larger cells and tissue. For instance, plasma membranes of fat cells must expand and more enzymes may be needed. Furthermore, new fat cells may have been made during the accumulation of body fat. On the contrary, when fat is mobilized from fat cells, these cells shrink, thereby decreasing the need for the extra supporting nutrients. Also, when the body was heavier, the amount of skeletal muscle and density of the bones may have been a little greater to support and move the larger body. Researchers usually find that heavier people have denser bones. Thus, as body weight decreases, it is only reasonable that these areas will decrease as well. Excessive skin and some connective tissue would be broken down during weight loss as well; both of these tissues are protein rich.

If you incorporate resistance training in your efforts to change your body composition, it certainly is possible to lose primarily body fat. Here, the maintenance of body protein, minerals, and water may be necessary as you enhance your muscle mass. In fact, it is possible that you might not even lose weight as you lose body fat. This might be indicative for people who are slightly overweight compared to those who are obese.

SMART WEIGHT LOSS EMPLOYS
SMART PLANNING AND EXECUTION

How can we plan for weight loss?

Traditionally, weight loss programs were limited to reducing energy intake. We have to look back only a few decades to recall the popularity of various formula diets, such as the Cambridge diet, which were very low calorie diets (VLCD). These diets provided as little as 400 to 600 Calories per day. Today, most health professionals recommend a much less drastic energy reduction coupled with exercise for weight reduction. Rarely are energy levels restricted below 1,000 to 1,200 Calories.

Before engaging in any type of weight loss program, some things must be understood and considered. First, begin by assessing the current situation. Keep a journal. What is your current body weight and what makes up this body weight? It is a good idea to have your body-fat percentage determined by an individual trained to do so. This should be someone you can go to again and again in the future, especially if the individual is using skin-fold measurements. Your goal should be focused upon the reduction of your body-fat percentage rather than simply reducing your body weight. However, your goals must be realistic and healthy. Note in your journal body weight, composition, and tape measurements. Also, note how your clothes fit and keep a recent picture if possible. The sample clothes should be set aside or worn less frequently, while the photo should display your appearance in a reproducible manner for later comparison.

Also, realize that the rate of weight loss may not be consistent throughout your efforts. Weight loss rate may be greater earlier on and taper off as the regimen continues. Periods of plateau can represent your body's adaptation to the energy restriction by slowing down a bit. This phenomenon is called the set-point regulation. As a survival mechanism, your metabolism can slow down and speed up to a degree to accommodate imbalances in energy intake. Patience is important. Keep in mind that changes in body weight do not always reflect changes in body composition. This is why it is important to monitor body composition with body weight. Also, make note of changes in "fatty" regions of the body such as the waist, face, and chin. Your clothes may begin to fit differently and you may feel less jiggling when climbing stairs.

Aerobic or cardiovascular training will increase daily energy expenditure not only by increasing the TEA but also BMR as muscle tissue recovers and repairs itself over the ensuing hours. Resistance training (e.g., weight training) will also help maintain or even increase muscle tissue. Increasing muscle mass will positively influence energy expenditure. Remember, skeletal muscle has a moderately high metabolic rate, meaning that it will expend a great deal of energy even when it is resting.

How much energy should be eaten during weight loss?

Before planning an energy level to allow for weight loss, we must first determine how much energy is being expended. Because most of us do not have access to direct or indirect calorimetry, we can use mathematical methods for estimating the components of TEE.

Once TEE is known, we can establish an energy level that will allow for a more desirable weight loss. A good recommendation for overweight and mildly obese individuals is to plan for a weight loss of about .5 to 1.5 lb per week. Again, it is important to focus upon a reduction in body-fat rather than body weight. A slow, thoughtfully planned weight loss will allow for a higher percentage of the weight loss to come from fat.

The golden rule of dieting states that to theoretically lose one pound of body-fat tissue, you need to create an energy imbalance of

3,500 Calories in the favor of weight loss. Since 1 lb of fat weighs 454 g and because fat cells are roughly 86 percent fat, to lose 1 lb of fat it would require about 3,500 Cal.

$$454 \text{ g} \times .86 = 390 \text{ g of fat} \times 9 \text{ Cal} = 3,510 \text{ Cal}$$

Therefore to reduce body weight by 1 lb of fat per week an individual would need to create an energy imbalance of 3,500 Cal per week favoring weight loss. Dividing 3,500 Cal by seven days, one would need to create an average energy deficit of 500 Cal per day. You can do this by increasing your activity and/or restricting your energy intake. However, as mentioned above, not all of the weight that is lost during an energy imbalance is fat.

Increasing activity in the form of exercise can account for most, if not all, of the energy imbalance. Table 8.4 provides the approximate number of Calories expended during various exercises. For example, a 185-lb man walking at a 5 mph pace for sixty minutes would expend about 600 Calories of energy. It is also important to remember that if skeletal muscle mass is increased via resistance training BMR energy expenditure increases as well.

Can drugs help people lose weight?

The short answer is possibly or more than likely. There are two primary ways for substances such as these to work. They can decrease a person's appetite, increase one's energy expenditure, or both. However, keep in mind that these benefits can come with side effects and risks of toxicity.

Drugs such as fenfluramine (Pondimin) and dexfenfluramine (Redux) were extremely popular in the early 1990s, especially in the United States. The combination of fenfluramine and phentermine was commonly called "fen-phen." These drugs worked by increasing the influence of serotonin in the brain, thereby suppressing appetite. However, these drugs were pulled from the market in the latter part of the 1990s as mounting evidence suggested that these drugs promoted the development of cardiovascular problems in some people. Today, other similar substances are available as appetite suppressants, such as simetidine. However, as with their predecessors, these substances could carry the risk of side effects.

Can nutrition supplements help us lose weight and body fat?

Ma huang (ephedra) is a Chinese herb that has been used for thousands of years to treat asthma and other conditions. "Herbal fen-phen," a combination of ephredrine (ma huang) and St. John's Wort, was popularized after pharmaceutical fen-phen was pulled from the market. Ephedrine is the potent chemical found in the ephedra plant. It seems to work by acting as a stimulant, much in the same way that the neurotransmitter norepinephrine and the hormone epinephrine work. So, ephedrine can stimulate our heart, increase our blood pressure, dilate our airways, and increase our alertness. The pharmacological properties of ma huang's ephedrine alkaloids are undetermined at this time. Meanwhile, the FDA has recommended that daily doses not exceed 24 mg and the length of use not exceed seven days.

Caffeine can be found in some plant leafs, nuts, and seeds, such as the coffee bean, tea leaf, kola nut, and cacao seed. An average cup of coffee may contain 50 to 150 mg of caffeine, while a cup of tea may contain 50 mg. A 12 oz (355 mL) can of soda can contain about 35 mg. Although chocolate contains some caffeine, most of its caffeine-like potency comes from a similar substance called theobromine, while tea contains some theophylline.

Caffeine can promote wakefulness and alertness. Caffeine seems to do this by competing with the neurotransmitter adenosine in the brain. Adenosine seems to be more of a relaxing substance, as it appears to decrease the activity of the brain. However, to counter the effects of caffeine competition, the brain adapts by producing more and more receptors for adenosine. So adenosine can overcome the presence of caffeine. This means that we will begin to need to ingest more caffeine to feel the same stimulating effects. This also explains why we feel especially groggy and "washed out" when we do not have the usual morning coffee. Some people call this feeling "caffeine withdrawal." Here, the influence of adenosine goes unchallenged, and because of the increased number of adenosine receptors, the withdrawal symptoms are very strong. However, over the next couple of days without caffeine, the brain would produce less and less adenosine receptors and the symptoms of caffeine withdrawal would in turn subside.

So caffeine may enhance energy expenditure by increasing wakefulness and alertness, which can promote more activity. Caffeine also can have cardiovascular stimulatory effects and possibly increase the use of fat as an energy source in the body. One of the major differences between caffeine and ephedrine is that caffeine tends to be ingested as part of foods while ephedrine is consumed more often in supplement form. Thus any additional energy in caffeine-endowed foods can negate the influence of caffeine to increase energy expenditure. For instance, the carbohydrates in chocolate candies and soda can lead to an increase in serotonin levels. Serotonin tends to make us feel tired, thereby counteracting the stimulation of caffeine. Sugar is often added to coffee and tea along with milk. Because coffee is such a strong source of caffeine, its effects tend to prevail despite the presence of sugar.

Ephedrine is often the most active ingredient in supplements marketed as metabolism enhancers. Supplements such as Ripped Fuel and Metabolift by Twinlabs also contain guarana (root) extract, which contains caffeinelike substances. These supplements should be used very cautiously as several deaths have been attributed to toxicity of ephedrine, which is attracting the attention of physicians and the Food and Drug Administration (FDA).

Can frequent dieting have derogatory effects?

Many people are on a dieting roller coaster. Some starve or semi-starve themselves for several days to weeks and then eat excessively for a period of time. This is sometimes called *yo-yo dieting.* During the period of drastic energy restriction, the body will deplete its glycogen stores and rely heavily upon stored fat and protein to power metabolic activities. Since protein is largely derived from lean body tissue, such as skeletal muscle, this practice tends to reduce muscle mass and in turn decrease basal metabolism. This can result in a decrease in TEE and a greater likelihood of gaining weight when we return to eating an unrestricted amount of energy. Furthermore, it may be that the activity of some of the enzymes involved in making fat from excessive carbohydrates and amino acids may be slightly higher once we begin to eat again. Therefore, we have ultimately set ourselves up for a potentially quick return of body weight, especially body fat.

Is it possible to be too lean?

Contrary to what some people believe, it is not healthy to be excessively lean. Excessively lean people are at greater risk for various diseases as well as malnutrition. Furthermore, excessively lean girls often fail to produce adequate sex hormones (e.g., estrogens), a condition which is associated with irregular or halted menstrual cycles as well as bone mineral losses. An excessively lean male would have less than 5 percent body fat, while an excessively lean female would have less than 10 percent body fat. Do not forget that 0 percent body fat cannot be a goal, as not all body fat is stored in adipose tissue, which is classically called "fat." Some fat is stored in bone marrow and other vital places.

Today, an excessively skinny appearance does not seem to be as in vogue as it was in the 1970s and 1980s. With the exception of some supermodels, many magazine covers are graced with photos of teens and adults with more muscle tissue than in years gone by. However, many of these models and celebrities strive for an excessively lean, yet muscular, appearance. This can be a driving force for experimentation with supplements or even drugs.

Chapter 9

We Need Vitamins for Vitality

VITAMINS ARE VITAL MOLECULES IN OUR FOOD

Almost a century ago a scientist coined the term *vitamine* when describing a vital nitrogen (amine)-containing component of food. Vitamine was a condensed word for a *vital amine*-containing substance. However, as more and more vitamines were discovered, scientists observed that many did not contain nitrogen, so eventually the "e" was dropped from vitamine, converting it to the more familiar term *vitamin*.

What are vitamins?

For a substance to be added to the exalted list of vitamins, it must be recognized as an essential player in at least one necessary chemical reaction or process in the body. Also, a vitamin is a substance that is made in the body either not at all or in sufficient quantities to meet our needs. We will discuss two vitamins, niacin and vitamin D, that can be made in the body, and two others, vitamin K and biotin, that are made by the bacteria inhabiting the large intestine. However, they are still considered vitamins, which will be explained shortly. In addition, vitamins are non-Caloric substances and are required in very small amounts, typically micrograms (µg) to milligram (mg) quantities. A microgram and a milligram are one-millionth and one-thousandth of a gram, respectively.

What is the difference between fat-soluble and water-soluble vitamins?

Because the basis of the body is water, it only makes sense that vitamins are grouped together based upon their ability to dissolve in water. There are nine water-soluble and four fat-soluble vitamins (see Table 9.1). Some general assumptions regarding the two different classes of vitamins can be made. For instance, water-soluble vitamins generally have limited storage ability in the body, with the exception of vitamin B_{12}. Therefore, it is logical to think that signs of a deficiency of a water-soluble vitamin may appear more rapidly than would fat-soluble vitamins' symptoms when they are lacking from the diet. One reason is that water-soluble vitamins are more susceptible to removal from the body in the urine, which is water based. Again, the major exception is vitamin B_{12}.

On the other hand, fat-soluble vitamins are very dependent upon the processes of normal lipid digestion and absorption, such as the presence of bile and the construction of chylomicrons in the cells lining our small intestine. Any situation in which there is decreased bile production and/or delivery to our small intestine would greatly decrease fat-soluble vitamin absorption into our body. Because the presence of fat in the diet is the most powerful stimulus for bile delivery to the small intestine, it only makes sense that a nutrition supplement containing fat-soluble vitamins should be taken with a fat-containing food or meal. Fat-soluble vitamins are less likely to be removed from our body in the urine and, as mentioned previously, relatively longer periods of time would be required to bring about deficiency. However, there is an exception here as well, which is vitamin K.

We will begin our discussion with the water-soluble vitamins and then move to the fat-soluble vitamins.

TABLE 9.1. Vitamins

Water-Soluble		Fat-Soluble
Vitamin C	Vitamin B_{12}	Vitamin A
Thiamin (B_1)	Folate	Vitamin D
Riboflavin (B_2)	Pantothenic acid	Vitamin E
Niacin (B_3)	Biotin	Vitamin K
Vitamin B_6	Choline*	

*Not recognized as essential at this time, but many nutritionists think it should be.

WATER-SOLUBLE VITAMINS ARE VITAMIN C
AND THE B-COMPLEX VITAMINS

Vitamin C

What is vitamin C and where do we get it?

Vitamin C is the common name for ascorbic acid. People, along with other primates, guinea pigs, and birds, are unable to make vitamin C. Other animals and plants can make their own vitamin C from glucose. When we think of good sources of vitamin C, citrus fruits instantly come to mind. However, other fruits and some vegetables can make a significant contribution to our vitamin C intake (see Table 9.2). The vitamin C RDA for adults is 75 mg.

Vitamin C is susceptible to breakdown during certain cooking, processing, and storage procedures (i.e., heat or cooking in neutral or basic medium). For instance, potatoes can lose nearly half of their vitamin C by boiling. Spinach can lose nearly all its vitamin C if stored for two to three days at room temperature. Thus, for practical purposes, citrus fruits and other vitamin C-containing fruits and vegetables usually are better dietary sources of vitamin C as they are generally eaten uncooked and shortly after harvest.

Vitamin C is fairly well absorbed from our digestive tract when consumed in typical dietary amounts. However, as the amount of vitamin C increases in our diet its absorption efficiency decreases. For example, a vitamin C intake of 180 mg (three times the RDA for an adult) is about 80 to 90 percent absorbed, while an intake approximating 5 g is only about 24 percent absorbed. However, 24 percent absorption of 5 g is still about 1.2 g of vitamin C. Much of this excessive vitamin C will be quickly removed from the body as part of urine.

What does vitamin C do in our body?

Vitamin C is found in most of the tissue throughout the body. Greater concentrations of vitamin C can be found in the heart, brain, pancreas, adrenal glands, thymus, and lungs, and two of the most vitamin C-dense regions in the body are the pituitary gland and the lens of the eye. As vitamin C circulates in the blood it is vulnerable to kidney filtration and subsequent loss in the urine. Vitamin C is lost in the urine either as ascorbic acid or derivatives (metabolites) of vitamin C,

TABLE 9.2. Vitamin C Content of Select Foods

FOOD	VITAMIN C (mg)
Fruits*	
Orange juice (1 c)	124
Kiwi (1)	108
Grapefruit juice (1 c)	94
Cranberry juice cocktail (1 c)	90
Orange (1)	85
Strawberries (1 c)	84
Cantaloupe (1/4)	63
Grapefruit (1)	51
Raspberries (1 c)	31
Watermelon (1 c)	15
Vegetables*	
Green peppers (½ c)	95
Cauliflower, raw (½ c)	75
Broccoli (½ c)	70
Brussels sprouts (½ c)	65
Collard greens (½ c)	48
Cauliflower, cooked (½ c)	30
Potato (1)	29
Tomato (1)	23

*All fruits and vegetables and juices are fresh.

such as oxalates, which will become more important later on in our discussion.

The activity of vitamin C is realized in its ability to either donate or accept electrons. In doing so it participates in many metabolic processes. Perhaps its most famous role is its involvement in the production of collagen. Collagen is a connective tissue protein, which is a protein that tends to have structural or physical significance. This makes it different from more functional proteins such as transporters, enzymes, protein hormones, and so on. Connective tissue proteins can be found holding cells together and are very concentrated in very strong tissue such as teeth, bone, tendons, ligaments, cartilage, and arteries.

Collagen is the most abundant protein in the body, representing one-fourth of our total protein mass. It is found in teeth, bone, ligaments, cartilage, tendons, and in the space between the cells. Without question, proper collagen production (quantity and quality) is vital to existence. Vitamin C is fundamentally involved in modifying specific amino acids in the collagen protein. These modified amino acids will ultimately affect collagen's structure and function. Without this processing, the collagen that is made is relatively worthless.

Vitamin C is also involved in the production of norepinephrine and carnitine. Norepinephrine functions mostly as a neurotransmitter in the body and is made from the amino acid tyrosine. The making of carnitine in the liver requires vitamin C among other substances. Carnitine is needed to use longer chain length fatty acids for energy, as it basically chaperones these fatty acids into the mitochondria of our cells where they can be broken down for ATP production.

Other functions of vitamin C appear to include the enhancement of iron absorption from our digestive tract. This means that both iron and vitamin C would need to be part of the same meal for this to occur. Vitamin C is also an antihistamine factor and an immune function potentiator, and is involved in the making of thyroid hormone, serotonin, bile acids, and steroid hormones.

Another role of vitamin C, which is receiving more and more attention today, is that of antioxidant. Antioxidants serve as lines of protection against free radicals, as discussed previously. Antioxidants provide protection against free-radical activity that can lead to heart disease, cancers, and other medical concerns, so this role of vitamin C is more of a nutraceutical role.

As an antioxidant and also an immune function potentiator vitamin C has been suggested for use in decreasing the incidence and severity of the common cold. However, the benefit of a greater intake of vitamin C in regard to the common cold remains debatable. Yet most scientists will not deny that those of us not receiving adequate vitamin C in our diet are at greater risk of catching the common cold and may have a more difficult time recovering.

What happens if too little vitamin C is consumed?

The classical vitamin C deficiency syndrome is referred to as *scurvy*. For adults, scurvy will appear approximately one to three months after discontinuing vitamin C consumption. Medical signs and symptoms include impaired wound healing, fluid buildup in ankles and wrists (edema), swollen bleeding gums with tooth loss, fatigue, lethargy, and joint pain. In infants who are not breast-fed, deficiency can be recognized at around six months of age when the vitamin C stores transferred from the mother during pregnancy have been exhausted. Medical signs of this syndrome (Moeller-Barlow disease) include abnormal bone character and development, severe joint pain, anemia, and fever. The abnormalities in bone are directly related to vitamin C's involvement in the proper manufacturing of collagen.

What happens if too much vitamin C is consumed?

If you set out to increase your vitamin C intake through the use of supplements, a couple of possible side effects and a practical issue should be considered. First, as discussed, as vitamin C intake increases, the efficiency of absorption decreases. This still leads to more vitamin C absorbed per day, but a proportionate increase in urinary loss of vitamin C and its metabolites also occurs. Perhaps one of the biggest concerns associated with consuming gram-size doses ("gram dosing") over time is that it may increase the production of oxalates, a principal type of metabolite of vitamin C. Oxalates are a primary component of the most prevalent type of kidney stones (i.e., calcium oxalates). Therefore, those with a medical history of kidney stones may be placing themselves at risk and they should discuss this with a physician. Although the research in this area is also debatable, most health practitioners do agree that people prone to forming kidney stones should avoid gram doses of vitamin C.

Thiamin (vitamin B_1)

What is thiamin and where do we get it?

Classically known as vitamin B_1, thiamin is found widely distributed in foods, although most contain low concentrations. Brewer's yeast, pork, and whole grain and enriched grain products are better sources of thiamin (see Table 9.3). The RDA for adults is 1 to 1.2 mg of thiamin.

Similar to vitamin C, thiamin is not very stable during cooking processes. Convection cooking of meat may result in destruction of roughly half of its thiamin content. The baking of breads and the pas-

TABLE 9.3. Thiamin Content of Select Foods

Food	Thiamin (mg)
Meats	
Pork roast (3 oz)	0.8
Beef (3 oz)	0.4
Ham (3 oz)	0.4
Liver (3 oz)	0.2
Nuts and seeds	
Sunflower seeds (1/4 c)	0.7
Peanuts (1/4 c)	0.1
Almonds (1/4 c)	0.1
Fruits	
Orange juice (1 c)	0.2
Orange (1)	0.1
Avocado (1/2)	0.1
Grains	
Bran flakes (1 c)	0.6
Macaroni (1/2 c)	0.1
Rice (1/2 c)	0.1
Bread (1 slice)	0.1
Vegetables	
Peas (1/2 c)	0.3
Lima beans (1/2 c)	0.2
Corn (1/2 c)	0.1
Broccoli (1/2 c)	0.1
Potato (1)	0.1

teurization of milk may result in destruction of approximately 25 percent and 15 percent of thiamin content, respectively. Certain fish and shellfish contain natural *thiaminases,* which are enzymes that specifically break down thiamin. Fortunately, cooking inactivates these enzymes. In light of its water-soluble nature, some thiamin may also be washed away in the thaw drip. The thaw drip is the watery fluid that drains from thawing meats.

What does thiamin do in our body?

Much of the thiamin that we eat is absorbed in the small intestine. Once inside the body, thiamin circulates around primarily aboard red blood cells (RBCs). Thiamin does not seem to have a primary organ of storage. However, the brain, kidneys, liver, and skeletal muscle seem to have higher concentrations, with the latter accounting for as much as one-half of the total thiamin in the body. Thiamin and its metabolites are subject to removal from the body in urine.

Thiamin serves as a *coenzyme* in many key reactions in the cells. A coenzyme is a substance that will interact directly with an enzyme; together the two allow a chemical reaction to proceed. The enzyme will not function optimally without the presence of the coenzyme. Many water-soluble vitamins function as coenzymes.

Thiamin is active in the form of *thiamin pyrophosphate* (TPP) and TPP is a coenzyme for a couple of enzymes involved in energy pathways. TPP as a coenzyme is necessary in the mitochondria to convert pyruvate to acetyl CoA and also in one reaction within the Kreb's cycle (see Figure 9.1).

Because of the need for thiamin at these two vital points in our energy pathways it is easy to understand why thiamin is most often associated with energy metabolism. In fact, many scientists have stated that the RDA for thiamin might be more appropriately expressed in terms of energy intake, whereby 0.5 mg of thiamin would be recommended per 1,000 Calories, with a lower limit of 1 mg per day.

Thiamin is also involved in converting glucose to ribose in the cells. Ribose, and a slightly modified form, deoxyribose, are key components of deoxyribonucleic acids (DNA) and ribonucleic acids (RNA). You will remember that DNA provides the instructions or blueprints for making cells, while RNA is involved in reading the blueprints and constructing proteins.

Scientists have also concluded that thiamin is crucial to the proper functioning of the brain and nerves. However, the exact involvement of thiamin may not be easily explained within the confines of thiamin's classic functions. Researchers have shown that when thiamin is deficient in the diet the brain tends to hold on to its thiamin more vigorously than other tissues do. This suggests that a very special relationship exists between the brain and thiamin.

Is thiamin a B-complex vitamin?

Along with the other water-soluble vitamins (except vitamin C), thiamin is considered a B-complex vitamin. Decades ago scientists knew there was a complex of factors involved in proper energy me-

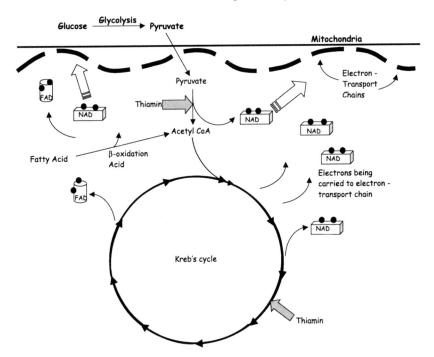

FIGURE 9.1. Chemical reaction pathways in the mitochondria allow for electrons to be removed from involved molecules and carried to electron-transport chains found in the mitochondria membrane (inner). The carriers are niacin (NAD) and riboflavin (FAD) based.

tabolism in the cells. They called this the B complex. As scientific instruments were modernized, scientists were able to identify the specific individual factors involved in the B complex. Hence, the classification of vitamins B_1, B_2, B_3, B_6, and B_{12}. Folate, biotin, and pantothenic acid are also involved in the processing of energy nutrients and are thus included in the B-complex family. Vitamin C is not included in the B-complex family with its water-soluble brethren because it is not directly involved in the chemical reaction pathways that either break down or build energy nutrients.

What happens if too little thiamin is consumed?

If thiamin is deficient from our diet for several weeks, symptoms will begin to appear. Classic thiamin deficiency has been termed *beri-*

beri, which is often separated into two types. *Wet* and *dry* beriberi describe the effects of thiamin deficiency with special reference to the presence of fluid buildup in tissue (edema). Enlargement of the heart sometimes occurs and appears to be more prevalent in those individuals with the fluid buildup (wet beriberi). Muscular weakness, loss of appetite, and atrophy of legs are also characteristic symptoms of thiamin deficiency. Beriberi is said to mean "I can't, I can't," which probably refers to the deficits in voluntary movement that accompany thiamin deficiency.

An infant who is breast-fed by a thiamin-deficient mother is also at risk of thiamin deficiency. This situation, called infantile beriberi, typically occurs between two and six months of age, and these infants may lose their desire to eat, may regurgitate milk, and may also experience vomiting and diarrhea. A rapid heart rate and a bluish tint to the skin may also develop.

Alcoholics are also at risk for thiamin deficiency. An alcoholic's diet is typically low in thiamin along with other essential nutrients. Furthermore, there appears to be a reduced ability to absorb thiamin in the digestive tract of alcoholics with an accompanying increase in metabolic need for this vitamin.

Can too much thiamin be consumed?

Because much of excessive thiamin will be rapidly removed from the body in the urine, excessive consumption of thiamin appears relatively safe. However, long-term thiamin intake of greater than 100 times the RDA has been associated with headaches, convulsions, weakness, allergic reactions, and irregular heart rhythms.

Riboflavin (vitamin B₂)

What is riboflavin and what foods provide riboflavin?

Riboflavin is a B-complex vitamin and has long been called vitamin B_2. The name riboflavin refers both to a component of its molecular structure and also its yellow color: *ribo-* with respect to the ribose portion of the molecule and *flavin* from the Latin word for yellow, *flavus.*

Better sources of riboflavin include rapidly growing, green leafy vegetables, beef liver, beef, and dairy products (see Table 9.4). About one-fourth to one-half of the riboflavin Americans consume is pro-

TABLE 9.4. Riboflavin Content of Select Foods

Food	Riboflavin (mg)
Milk and milk products	
Milk, whole (1 c)	0.5
Milk, 2% (1 c)	0.5
Yogurt, low fat (1 c)	0.5
Milk, skim (1 c)	0.4
Yogurt (1 c)	0.1
Cheese, American (1 oz)	0.1
Cheese, cheddar (1 oz)	0.1
Grains	
Macaroni (1/2 c)	0.1
Bread (1 slice)	0.1
Meats	
Liver (3 oz)	3.6
Pork chop (3 oz)	0.3
Beef (3 oz)	0.2
Tuna (3 oz)	0.1
Vegetables	
Collard greens (1/2 c)	0.3
Broccoli (1/2 c)	0.2
Spinach, cooked (1/2 c)	0.1
Eggs	
Egg (1)	0.2

vided by milk and milk products. Meats are also a primary supplier of dietary riboflavin along with fortified and enriched foods (breads, breakfast cereals). The RDA for adults is 1.1 to 1.3 mg of riboflavin.

Riboflavin appears to be more stable than vitamin C and thiamin with regard to cooking and storage. However, significant riboflavin losses in foods are experienced when foods are exposed directly to light (e.g., sunlight). This was a bigger concern back when milk was packaged in clear glass bottles and delivered to your doorstep usually before people got out of bed. The milk would then be exposed to the morning sunlight until it was brought in the house. Fortunately, most milk producers no longer package their product in clear containers such as glass bottles. This helps milk retain most of its riboflavin. Sun drying and cooking foods in an open pot can lead to significant ribo-flavin losses as well. Also, like other water-soluble vitamins, ribofla-vin can be washed away during boiling and thawing (thaw drip).

What does riboflavin do in the body?

Riboflavin in foods is well absorbed from our digestive tract. Al-though riboflavin is found in most cells in the body, higher concentra-tions will be found in very active tissue, such as the heart, liver, and kidneys. This makes sense due to riboflavin's heavy involvement with aerobic energy metabolism. Also, because of its water solubility, riboflavin is lost from the body in urine.

Riboflavin functions in the cells as an essential component of two coenzymes, *FAD* and *FMN*. With regard to energy metabolism, FAD (flavin adenine dinucleotide) serves as one of the electron carriers men-tioned in our discussion of aerobic energy metabolism in Chapter 8. FAD transfers electrons from reactions in the Kreb's cycle and also the breakdown of fatty acids, a pathway that scientists call β-oxida-tion (see Figure 9.1).

FMN (flavin mononucleotide), on the other hand, also functions in electron transfer as a key component of the electron-transport chain in the mitochondria in our cells. Beyond energy metabolism FAD and FMN are used in many of our cell systems such as amino acid and ste-roid hormone metabolism. As you might have guessed, these and other riboflavin-requiring cell activities involve the transfer of elec-trons from one molecule to another. That is what riboflavin-based co-enzymes do: they transfer electrons.

What happens if too little or too much riboflavin is consumed?

Deficiency of riboflavin rarely occurs by itself. However, if a diet contains very little riboflavin, a person would begin to show defi-ciency signs after a couple of months, such as inflammation of the mouth and tongue. Other signs of riboflavin deficiency include dry-ness and cracking at the corners of the mouth, lesions on the lips, ac-cumulation of fluid in tissue (edema), anemia, and neurological dis-orders, as well as mental confusion.

There does not appear to be great concern regarding riboflavin tox-icity. Much of the excessive riboflavin present in the human body is rapidly voided in the urine. However, unlike the removal of most other substances in our urine, riboflavin removal is visually obvious as urine turns a bright yellow. This effect is noticeable even with smaller doses of riboflavin.

Niacin (vitamin B₃)

What is niacin and what foods contribute niacin to our diet?

Niacin is more commonly recognized as vitamin B_3 and is part of the B-complex vitamins. Niacin in its two forms, nicotinic acid and nicotinamide, is found well distributed throughout most foods. Brewer's yeast and most fish, pork, beef, poultry, mushrooms, and potatoes offer higher niacin content (see Table 9.5). Niacin in foods appears to be stable in most forms of cooking and storage while some losses may occur during the boiling of foods and during the thaw drip. In these cases some niacin can dissolve into the water that becomes separated from the food. The adult RDA is 14 to 16 niacin equivalents (NE).

What does niacin do in the body?

Niacin is well absorbed from our small intestine and is found in all of our cells. Like riboflavin we can expect to find higher concentrations of niacin in more metabolically active tissue, or those tissues with higher energy demands such as the heart, brain, liver, and skeletal muscle. Niacin will be lost from the body mostly as part of our urine.

Like riboflavin, niacin imparts coenzyme activity to our cells. In fact, hundreds of chemical reactions depend upon niacin to proceed. Like riboflavin in the form of FAD, niacin in the form of *NAD* (nicotinamide dinucleotide) is a carrier of electrons from energy pathways to the electron-transport chain during aerobic energy metabolism (see Figure 9.1). Niacin is also part of another electron-transferring molecule called *NADP* (nicotinamide dinucleotide phosphate). NADP also transfers electrons between molecules and is vitally important in making cholesterol and fatty acids.

Can we make niacin in our body?

Earlier it was mentioned that a vitamin is a substance that cannot be made in the body in adequate quantity to meet our needs. Niacin offers the first potential contradiction to this rule as it can be made in the body starting with the essential amino acid tryptophan. However,

TABLE 9.5. Niacin Content of Select Foods

Food	Niacin (NE*)
Meats	
Liver (3 oz)	14.0
Tuna (3 oz)	10.3
Turkey (3 oz)	9.5
Chicken (3 oz)	7.9
Salmon (3 oz)	6.9
Veal (3 oz)	5.2
Beef, round steak (3 oz)	5.1
Pork (3 oz)	4.5
Haddock (3 oz)	2.7
Scallops (3 oz)	1.1
Nuts and Seeds	
Peanuts (1 oz)	4.9
Vegetables	
Asparagus (1/2 c)	1.5
Grains	
Wheat germ (1 oz)	1.5
Rice, brown (1/2 c)	1.2
Noodles, enriched (1/2 c)	1.0
Rice, white, enriched (1/2 c)	1.0
Bread, enriched (1 slice)	0.7
Milk and milk products	
Milk (1 c)	1.9
Cheese, cottage (1/2 c)	2.6

*1 NE = 1 mg niacin and 60 mg tryptophan

the conversion is very inefficient. It requires about 60 mg of tryptophan to produce 1 mg of niacin. Since daily niacin needs are 13 to 20 mg for adults, it is unrealistic to rely upon the conversion of tryptophan to niacin, especially since tryptophan is not one of the most abundant amino acids humans eat. Nevertheless, since some niacin can be made from tryptophan, the RDA is stated as niacin equivalents (NE) where 1 NE is equal to 1 mg of niacin or 60 mg of tryptophan.

What happens if too much niacin is consumed?

Those of us who have ingested more than 100 mg of niacin as nicotinic acid may recall quite clearly the uncomfortable feeling that resulted. Headache and itching were probably accompanied by an increased blood flow to our skin ("flushing"). On the other hand, physicians often prescribe niacin (2 to 5 g/day) as a means of reducing blood cholesterol. Because gram doses of niacin can have a pharmaceutical effect, this practice is not suggested unless under medical supervision.

What happens in niacin deficiency?

Niacin deficiency can result in a severe disease syndrome called *pellagra* which is characterized by the three "D's" (dermatitis, diarrhea, dementia) possibly leading to the fourth "D" (death). Some of the earlier symptoms of a niacin deficiency include a decreased appetite, weight loss, and a general feeling of weakness. Aerobic ATP production suffers tremendously when our niacin status is compromised.

Biotin

What sources help us meet our biotin needs?

Biotin is widely dispersed throughout the foods we eat, although its concentration is somewhat limited. Liver, oatmeal, almonds, roasted peanuts, wheat bran, brewer's yeast, and molasses are better sources. While milk and milk products contain only mediocre amounts of biotin they actually are some of the best providers of biotin in our diet because of their popularity. Eggs offer a respectable amount of biotin, but there is one concern regarding biotin availability and the consumption of raw eggs or whites. Egg whites contain a protein called *avidin* that will bind to biotin in our digestive tract and decrease its absorption. People who eat a lot of raw eggs or just the whites must be aware that this will reduce the absorption of biotin derived from all foods consumed at the same time. In the past, bodybuilders and other individuals seeking higher protein intakes often included egg whites with meals or as a component within high-protein shakes. If this practice takes place daily, over time the body's biotin status can become compromised. Fortunately, the practice of consuming raw eggs or egg white is not very popular today. Also, fortunately, avidin's ability to bind biotin is diminished when eggs, or their whites, are cooked. There are other reasons to avoid consuming raw eggs or egg whites, such as lowering the risk of bacteria infection. Cooking eggs will also kill the harmful bacteria.

The bacteria living in the colon also produce biotin, and some of this biotin can be absorbed. This seems to make a respectable contribution toward meeting our biotin needs, but it is not enough to be relied upon exclusively. Furthermore, as it is actually bacterial cells and not our own cells making the biotin, biotin should not really be viewed as a vitamin that the human body can make. Therefore, biotin indisputably maintains its place on the list of vitamins. The RDA for adults is 30 μg of biotin daily.

What does biotin do in our body?

Similar to thiamin, riboflavin, and niacin, biotin also provides vital assistance to energy operations in its function as a coenzyme. First, biotin is pivotal in making glucose from other substances such as amino acids and lactate. You will recall that this process (gluconeogenesis) takes place in the liver and the glucose generated can be released into the blood to maintain glucose levels during periods of fasting or exercise. Biotin is also necessary in the chemical reaction pathway that makes fatty acids from excessive glucose and certain amino acids. Last, biotin is necessary for the pathways that help break down odd-chain-length fatty acids and certain amino acids for energy. By and large, most of the fatty acids in foods and in the body have an even number of carbons, but some do indeed have an uneven number of carbon atoms (e.g., 3:0). To completely break down those fatty acids to make ATP, biotin is needed in a special chemical reaction. Because of its involvement in the breakdown of energy nutrients as well as converting energy nutrients, biotin is vital in all aspects of energy nutrient metabolism (i.e., fed, fasting, exercising).

Can too much or too little biotin be consumed?

Because biotin is widely available in foods and is also derived from the bacteria in our intestinal tract, deficiency is very uncommon. However, some of the documented cases of biotin deficiency include hospital patients fed a biotin-deficient solution intravenously (IV) or in infants fed a lot of egg whites as a protein supplement. Conversely, biotin seems to be relatively nontoxic.

Pantothenic acid

What foods contribute pantothenic acid to the human diet?

The term *pantothenic acid* is derived from the Greek word *pantothen* which means "from every side." This name was given to imply pantothenic acid's widespread availability in foods. Good sources of pantothenic acid include egg yolk, animal tissue, whole grain products, legumes, broccoli, milk, sweet potatoes, and molasses. Some losses of pantothenic acid can be expected in cooking and during the thawing of foods. Americans probably eat between 5 and 20 mg of pantothenic acid daily, which at least equals the RDA for adults.

What does pantothenic acid do in the body?

Pantothenic acid's claim to nutritional fame lies in its incorporation into two very special molecules that impact carbohydrate, protein, and fat metabolism. These molecules are called *coenzyme A* (CoA) and *acyl carrier protein* (ACP). We have mentioned CoA a few times already in regard to acetyl CoA, the "dump-in" molecule for the Kreb's cycle. Furthermore, CoA is also utilized in a chemical reaction in the Kreb's cycle as well as during the breakdown of fatty acids for ATP production. In these situations, CoA is attached to specific molecules and enhances their metabolism tremendously.

ACP is also indispensable but for different reasons than CoA. Where CoA is fundamental in the processes that help generate ATP from energy molecules, ACP is fundamental in a preliminary step whereby fatty acids are made from excessive carbohydrates and amino acids. Here pantothenic acid, as part of ACP, is essential for storing energy in the form of fat in our body.

Can too little or too much pantothenic acid be consumed?

Even though foods will experience some loss of pantothenic acid during cooking and thawing, a deficiency is still unlikely. In fact, a case of true nonexperimental pantothenic acid deficiency in humans has yet to be reported. Just as a pantothenic acid deficiency has not been documented, neither has a toxicity of pantothenic acid. However, there have been reports that large doses of pantothenic acid do cause diarrhea.

Vitamin B_6

What is vitamin B_6 and where do we get it?

Vitamin B_6 is the general name for five compounds in food with similar structures that provide vitamin B_6 activity in our cells. One form of vitamin B_6 is pyridoxine, which is mostly found in plant foods, with better sources being bananas, navy beans, and walnuts. The remaining four forms of vitamin B_6 are found mostly in animal foods with good sources being meats, fish, and poultry (see Table 9.6). Vitamin B_6 is fairly stable in cooking processes; however, some losses are experienced with prolonged exposure to heat, light, or alkaline conditions. The RDA for adults is 1.3 to 1.7 mg of vitamin B_6 daily.

What does vitamin B_6 do in the body?

Vitamin B_6 is fairly well absorbed from the small intestine. However, evidence suggests that vitamin B_6 from animal sources may be better absorbed than B_6 from plant sources. Vitamin B_6 can be found in nearly if not all cells throughout the body with higher concentrations found in muscle and liver tissue. Similar to most of its water-soluble vitamin siblings, vitamin B_6 is primarily lost from the body in urine.

Once inside the cells, vitamin B_6 forms can be converted to the active forms of vitamin B_6, *PLP* (pyridoxal phosphate) and *PMP* (pyridoxamine phosphate). PLP and PMP are key participants in many cell reactions committed to the metabolism of amino acids. For instance, it was mentioned that the nonessential amino acids are made from other amino acids. During this process, the nitrogen-containing *amine* portion of an amino acid is transferred to a specific molecule (see Figure 9.2), which creates a nonessential amino acid. In fact, if an individual developed a vitamin B_6 deficiency, most of the nonessential amino acids would actually become dietary essentials.

The bottom line is that the metabolism of every amino acid at some point or another will encounter a chemical reaction requiring vitamin B_6 as a coenzyme. In fact, vitamin B_6 is so deeply rooted in the metabolism of amino acids that the RDA is based on the typical protein content of the American diet. Approximately 0.016 mg of vitamin B_6 is apportioned per gram of protein in our diet. Therefore, since the typical daily protein intake of an American adult is approximately

TABLE 9.6. Vitamin B$_6$ Content of Select Foods

Food	Vitamin B$_6$ (mg)
Meats	
Liver (3 oz)	0.8
Salmon (3 oz)	0.7
Chicken (3 oz)	0.4
Ham (3 oz)	0.4
Hamburger (3 oz)	0.4
Veal (3 oz)	0.4
Pork (3 oz)	0.3
Beef (3 oz)	0.2
Eggs	
Egg (1)	0.3
Legumes	
Split peas (1/2 c)	0.6
Beans, cooked (1/2 c)	0.4
Fruits	
Banana (1)	0.6
Avocado (1/2)	0.4
Watermelon (1 c)	0.3
Vegetables	
Brussels sprouts (1/2 c)	0.4
Potato (1)	0.2
Sweet potato (1/2 c)	0.2
Carrots (1/2 c)	0.2
Peas (1/2 c)	0.1

100 to 125 g of protein, this translates to about 1.6 to 2 mg of vitamin B$_6$.

Vitamin B$_6$ is also necessary to convert certain amino acids into important body compounds, such as the neurotransmitters gama-amino-butyric acid (GABA) and serotonin. In addition, vitamin B$_6$ is essential in the formation of hemoglobin and white blood cells. Finally, vitamin B$_6$ also seems to be necessary to break down glycogen stores during exercise and fasting.

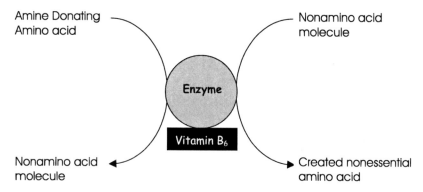

FIGURE 9.2. Some nonessential amino acids can be made by transferring the nitrogen-containing amine group from an existing amino acid to another molecule, thereby creating a nonessential amino acid.

What happens if too little vitamin B_6 is consumed?

Deficiency of vitamin B_6 is unlikely due to the popularity of meat, fish, and poultry as components of the American diet. However, if a deficiency occurred, amino acid metabolism would be greatly restrained, leading to poor protein synthesis. The production of hemoglobin, white blood cells, and many neurotransmitters would also be greatly hindered. Therefore the signs of a vitamin B_6 deficiency would significantly affect human body functions at many levels, including growth, immunity, and reproduction.

Can vitamin B_6 be toxic?

If vitamin B_6 is consumed in gram doses (2 to 6 g) over many months, it can affect nervous function and possibly lead to irreversible damage to nervous tissue. At one time, vitamin B_6 was considered a possible treatment for premenstrual syndrome (PMS), but this concept has since been abandoned and should not be pursued due to lack of promising supportive research and the potential for toxicity.

Folate (Folic Acid)

What foods in the diet contribute folate?

The name *folate,* as well as the other names associated with this vitamin (folacin and folic acid), suggests its food sources. *Folium* is

Latin for foliage or forage. Better food sources of folate include green leafy vegetables such as spinach, turnip greens, and asparagus (Table 9.7). Other vegetables and many fruits, juices, and organ meats also are good contributors of folate. Folate's molecular structure is somewhat unstable when it is heated, making fresh, uncooked fruits and vegetables better sources than cooked foods. The RDA for adults is 400 µg of folate daily.

What does folate do in the body?

Earlier we mentioned that when most molecules are made in the body they are constructed from smaller molecules or parts of other molecules. Folate, functioning as a coenzyme, is dedicated to transferring small, single carbon atom-containing molecules to the processes involved in making some pretty special molecules (see Figure 9.3). These molecules include a key component of DNA. Folate is also involved in transferring single-carbon molecules in the metabo-

TABLE 9.7. Folate Content of Select Foods

Food	Folate (µg)
Vegetables	
Asparagus (1/2 c)	120
Brussels sprouts (1/2 c)	116
Black-eyed peas (1/2 c)	102
Spinach, cooked (1/2 c)	99
Lettuce, Romaine (1 c)	86
Lima beans (1/2 c)	71
Peas (1/2 c)	70
Sweet potato (1/2 c)	43
Broccoli (1/2 c)	43
Fruits	
Cantaloupe (1/4)	100
Orange juice (1 c)	87
Orange (1)	59
Grains	
Oatmeal (1/2 c)	97
Wild rice (1/2 c)	37
Wheat germ (1 T)	20

lism of certain amino acids as well. Recently a link has been made between homocysteine levels and heart disease. When folate transfers a carbon molecule to homocysteine it is converted to methionine (see Figure 9.3). The conversion requires the help of vitamin B_{12} as well. Therefore, a deficiency of folate and/or vitamin B_{12} can allow for homocysteine levels to become elevated. Vitamin B_6 is also important because it helps folate pick up the carbon unit that will be added to homocysteine to form methionine.

The necessity of folate is particularly realized in cells that rapidly reproduce. This includes cells associated with the body surfaces (i.e., skin, hair, and digestive, urinary, and reproductive tracts) as well as blood cells and certain liver cells. Cells of these tissues must constantly be replaced or turned over to guarantee proper function and

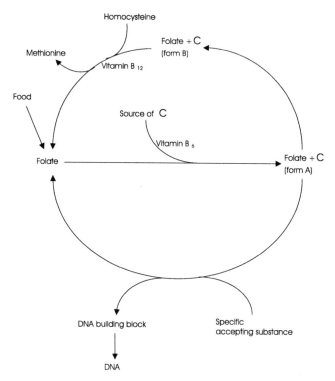

FIGURE 9.3. Folate passes a single carbon building block to the construction of various molecules, such as nucleic acids. In the process, folate is converted to a nonreusable form. Vitamin B_{12} can convert folate back to an active form.

integrity. However, in order for these cells to reproduce they must first make a duplicate copy of their DNA so that when the cell divides into two cells, both will get a complete set of DNA. Because folate is fundamentally involved in DNA production and thus the reproduction of cells, periods of life when rapid growth occurs demand a higher folate intake. During pregnancy a woman's diet must include extra folate to assist in the rapid reproduction of cells of the unborn infant and herself (e.g., blood cells, placenta). Most prenatal vitamin supplements include folate to help meet a pregnant woman's increased needs.

What happens if too little folate is consumed?

Red blood cells (RBCs) have a life span of about four months. They are constantly reproducing to compensate for their normal destruction. In fact, during the time it takes to finish this sentence, your bone marrow should have produced a few million new RBCs. Although an RBC will not contain a nucleus (with its DNA), there was a time in its development when it was created from the division of another cell. Before that cell divided into two new cells, it needed to copy its DNA. Normally, a RBC will lose its nucleus just prior to being released into circulation. During a folate deficiency, the original cell cannot properly copy its DNA because folate is not present to help construct the building blocks of DNA. This results in the development of large and immature RBCs, which then enter the blood and are readily noticeable with a microscope. Furthermore, less and less normal RBCs are produced, resulting in anemia. Anemia is a significant reduction in the level of hemoglobin in the blood. Remember: hemoglobin is found in RBCs, so a reduction in RBC concentration in our blood results in less hemoglobin. The anemia that results from folate deficiency is clinically referred to as *macrocytic megaloblastic anemia. Macrocytic* means big cell and *megaloblast* is the name for the pre-RBC form, which still has its nucleus. These changes in RBCs can be observed as early as a few months after consuming a folate-deficient diet.

Can folate be toxic?

Folate toxicity is rare for two principal reasons. First, it is difficult to consume too much folate through normal consumption of foods. Second, the folate content of nutrition supplements is limited by the government. The limitation in supplements is due to to an overlap between folate metabolism and vitamin B_{12} function. Vitamin B_{12} is fundamentally involved in folate metabolism in cells as it keeps folate in a form that can be used over and over again in cells (folate recycling). This means that a deficiency in vitamin B_{12} can in turn decrease folate recycling, resulting in the development of the anemia mentioned previously. Therefore, signs of a folate deficiency can actually help physicians identify a vitamin B_{12} deficiency. By taking higher dosages of folate (supplements) we can overcome the need for vitamin B_{12} in the recycling of existing folate in the cells. This is good for folate, but the vitamin B_{12} deficiency still remains and may go undetected. Thus, folate supplementation has eliminated an early warning sign (anemia) of vitamin B_{12} deficiency. If the vitamin B_{12} deficiency progresses it can lead to paralysis and death.

Vitamin B_{12}

What is vitamin B_{12} and what foods provide this vitamin?

Tucked away in the central part of the vitamin B_{12} molecule is an atom of cobalt. Therefore molecules that have vitamin B_{12} activity have been named the *cobalamins*. In the human diet, vitamin B_{12} is only found in foods of animal origin. Unlike animals, plants do not have a functional role for vitamin B_{12} and therefore do not make it. Interestingly, animals do not seem to make vitamin B_{12} either and rely instead upon their intestinal bacteria to make it. Vitamin B_{12} is then absorbed into that animal's body from its digestive tract.

The best sources of vitamin B_{12} are meats, fish, poultry, shellfish, eggs, milk, and milk products (see Table 9.8). The vitamin B_{12} content in these foods is modest but compatible with our needs. The RDA for adults is 2.4 µg, while the typical diet contains approximately 8 µg daily.

How is vitamin B_{12} absorbed and how is it lost
from the body?

First, with regard to absorption, vitamin B_{12} in foods needs a little help. Special proteins released by the stomach must interact with vitamin B_{12} both in the stomach and small intestine and facilitate its absorption. These proteins are called *R proteins* and *intrinsic factor*. A lack of these proteins can reduce vitamin B_{12} absorption dramati-

TABLE 9.8. Vitamin B_{12} Content of Select Foods

Food	Vitamin B_{12} (μg)
Meats	
Liver (3 oz)	6.8
Trout (3 oz)	3.6
Beef (3 oz)	2.2
Clams (3 oz)	2.0
Crab (3 oz)	1.8
Lamb (3 oz)	1.8
Tuna (3 oz)	1.8
Veal (3 oz)	1.7
Hamburger (3 oz)	1.5
Eggs	
Egg (1)	0.6
Milk and milk products	
Milk, skim (1 c)	1.0
Milk, whole (1 c)	0.9
Yogurt (1 c)	0.8
Cottage cheese (1/2 c)	0.7
Cheese, American (1 oz)	0.2
Cheese, cheddar (1 oz)	0.2

cally. This might be a concern for people who lack a properly functioning stomach, such as people who have had their stomach stapled or part (or all) of the stomach removed.

Once vitamin B_{12} is in the body it stays there for a while. Very little amounts of this vitamin are actually lost from the body on a daily basis, barring abnormalities. Contrary to the other water-soluble vitamins, the primary route of vitamin B_{12} loss from the body is not by way of the urine but rather in feces. The liver mixes a little vitamin B_{12} in with bile, which carries it to the digestive tract. A small portion of this vitamin B_{12} is not reabsorbed and becomes part of feces.

What does vitamin B_{12} do in the body?

Vitamin B_{12} is directly involved in the proper metabolism of folate. In fact, as discussed, a deficiency of vitamin B_{12} can impact folate metabolism to the point that signs of a folate deficiency appear. When folate is used to make molecules it is rendered "unusable," for lack of a better word. Vitamin B_{12} is involved in converting folate back to a usable form. Said another way, vitamin B_{12} is involved in folate recycling. This dramatically reduces the amount of folate we need to eat daily to have optimal levels of usable folate in our cells.

Vitamin B_{12} is also required for the breakdown of certain amino acids and fatty acids that have an odd chain length for ATP production. Finally, vitamin B_{12} appears vital in maintaining the special insulating wrapping around nerve cells called *myelin*. Myelin serves as insulation, which increases the velocity of a nerve impulse traveling from one part of the body to another.

What happens if too little vitamin B_{12} is consumed?

Contrary to other water-soluble vitamins, vitamin B_{12} losses from the body are small and occur primarily through the feces. Small quantities of vitamin B_{12} enter the digestive tract daily as part of bile released during meals. Most of this vitamin B_{12} is reabsorbed from the digestive tract while some is lost through feces. It has been estimated that we lose only about 0.1 percent of vitamin B_{12} stores daily through this process. Therefore, provided that there is optimal vitamin B_{12} reabsorption from the digestive tract, a person with good vitamin B_{12} stores could eat a diet lacking vitamin B_{12} for years before showing signs of deficiency—at least in theory. This also means that a strict vegetarian eating only plant-derived foods (vegan) and who became a vegetarian later in life may not show signs of a vitamin B_{12} deficiency for a very long time. The time period before signs and symptoms develop is directly related to how much vitamin B_{12} was stored in the body prior to becoming vegetarian. People who become vegetarians later in life and who continue to eat eggs and/or drink milk or eat some dairy products may never develop vitamin B_{12} deficiency. However, it should be understood that if children are raised vegetarian the need for a vitamin B_{12} supplement should be discussed with their pediatrician. The time frame for the onset of deficiency will be much shorter.

Factors that affect vitamin B_{12} digestion and absorption are more likely to cause vitamin B_{12} deficiency than insufficient dietary intake. Diseases and surgical manipulation of the stomach (i.e., removal and stapling) can affect its ability to make and release adequate intrinsic factor and R proteins. This can result in a dramatic decrease in vitamin B_{12} absorption. These proteins are very important in absorbing vitamin B_{12} in food and also reabsorbing the vitamin B_{12} entering the small intestine as part of bile.

Deficiency of vitamin B_{12} will result in a form of anemia in which red blood cells appear large and immature (macrocytic megaloblastic anemia). About 150 years ago, English physicians recognized that people with this type of anemia often died. They called this illness *pernicious anemia,* as pernicious means "leading to death." This anemia is usually related to the involvement of vitamin B_{12} in folate metabolism and DNA production. People who are vitamin B_{12} deficient also show destruction of nerve myelin, which can lead to nerve impulse conduction disturbances, paralysis, and ultimately death.

Older people are at increased risk of a vitamin B_{12} deficiency as their stomachs lose the ability to make sufficient acid with age. Stomach acid helps liberate the vitamin B_{12} in food so that it can interact with R proteins and intrinsic factor. Beyond anemia, other signs of a vitamin B_{12} deficiency include weakness, back pain, apathy, and a tingling in the extremities. These signs and symptoms usually appear before significant nerve damage occurs.

Some evidence suggests that excessive doses of vitamin C, such as ten times the RDA or greater, can render vitamin B_{12} inactive. Thus, if you choose to take large doses of vitamin C, you may wish to ask your physician to check your blood for indications of a vitamin B_{12} deficiency.

VITAMINS A, D, E, AND K ARE VITAL LIPIDS

Vitamin A

What is vitamin A and what foods contribute vitamin A?

Vitamin A in foods includes members of two chemical families, the *retinoids* such as retinol, retinal, and retinoic acid, and the *carotenoids* such as α-carotene, β-carotene, and other carotenes. However, in order for a carotenoid to have vitamin A activity it must first be converted to a retinoid in the body. Therefore, carotenoids are often referred to as provitamin A. Although there are hundreds of carotenoids found in nature, only about 50 may be converted to vitamin A. Furthermore, only about a half dozen of those carotenoids are found in the human diet in appreciable amounts. Because of its availability in the diet and relatively efficient conversion to a vitamin A, β-carotene may be the most significant carotenoid with regard to conversion to vitamin A.

Not all of the β-carotene eaten will be converted to vitamin A. Much of it, along with other carotenoids, will go unchanged and have different functions in the body. For instance, β-carotene and other carotenoids such as lutein and lycopene can function as antioxidants. In this capacity, the carotenoids function more as nutraceuticals helping to protect the body's cells against free radicals.

Vitamin A in the retinoid form is found in animal products with better sources being liver, fish oils, eggs, and vitamin A-fortified milk and milk products (see Table 9.9). Meanwhile, carotenoids are found in plant sources—mainly in orange and dark green vegetables and some fruits (squash, carrots, spinach, broccoli, papaya, sweet potatoes, pumpkin, cantaloupe, and apricots). In fact, the term *carotenoid* is derived from the species name for carrots. Thus, eating a diet rich in fruits and vegetables will not only support vitamin A intake but also provide carotenoids that help protect us from disease.

In Table 9.9 you will see that the vitamin A content of foods is listed as *retinol equivalents* (RE). This is because we derive vitamin A from two sources: retinoids and carotenoids. However, the question is whether these different sources provide the same quantity of vitamin A activity. For instance, carotenoids are absorbed from the digestive tract with about half the efficiency of the retinoids. Also, once inside the body, they must be converted to a retinoid, a process that varies in efficiency from one carotenoid to another. In order to account for the inherent differences in obtaining vitamin A activity from retinoids versus the carotenoids, vitamin A is listed in REs. One microgram of retinol equals 1 RE, whereas it takes 12 µg of β-carotene to equal 1 RE and 24 µg of other carotenes to equal 1 RE. The RDA for adults is 700 to 900 RE.

What does vitamin A do in the body?

Within the human eye lies a complex mechanism that registers the energy of light and couples it with the neural/sensory processes that allow us to perceive sight. Sight is really a perception or a mental vision of the world around us. We often use phrases such as "looking out over the area" or "I can see for miles." This implies that sight is

TABLE 9.9. Vitamin A Content of Select Foods

Food	Vitamin A (RE)
Vegetables	
Pumpkin, canned (1/2 c)	1350
Sweet potato, baked (1/2 c)	1000
Carrots, raw (1/2 c)	1913
Spinach, cooked (1/2 c)	739
Broccoli, cooked (1/2 c)	109
Winter squash (1/2 c)	53
Green peppers (1/2 c)	40
Fruits	
Cantaloupe (1/4)	430
Apricots, canned (1/2 c)	210
Nectarine (1)	101
Watermelon (1 c)	59
Peaches, canned (1/2 c)	47
Papaya (1/2 c)	20
Meats	
Liver (1 oz)	3045
Salmon (3 oz)	53
Tuna (3 oz)	14
Eggs	
Egg (1)	84
Milk and milk products*	
Milk, skim (1 c)	149
Milk, 2% (1 c)	139
Cheese, American (1 oz)	82
Cheese, Swiss (1 oz)	65
Fats	
Margarine* (1 tsp)	46
Butter (1 tsp)	38

RE - Retinol Equivalents; 1 RE = 1 μg Retinol or 12 μg β-carotene or 24 μg of α-carotene or β-carotene or β-cryptoxanthin
*Fortified

reaching out when in fact the opposite is true. Our eyes are being struck by waves of energy being emitted by entities around us.

Vitamin A is fundamentally involved in this process and is also involved in maintaining the health of the cornea, which is the clear outer window of the eye. Because of this relationship, poor vitamin A status in the human body is often recognized by changes in vision, as will be discussed.

Vitamin A is also indispensable for the maintenance and regulation of growth of many types of cells in the body. Cells that produce mucus, a lubricating and protecting substance, are particularly sensitive to vitamin A status. These types of cells are found lining the digestive tract and lungs and also in the eye's cornea. Vitamin A is also essential for normal growth and development of the human body as a whole. It is now clear that vitamin A acts in certain cells throughout the body at the genetic level. This means that some of the function of vitamin A is related to its ability to interact with DNA and affect the manufacture of certain proteins. This seems to be very important in the proper development and maintenance of various tissues throughout the body.

Vitamin A may play a pivotal role in the prevention of certain types of cancers and also in the proper activity of a class of white blood cells called T lymphocytes. Because vitamin A plays a role in regulating the growth and reproduction rate of many types of cells in the body, it may be involved in preventing or slowing the progression rate of certain cancers. Beyond vitamin A activity, the carotenoids may also present assistance in cancer prevention. As mentioned, carotenoids such as β-carotene appear to provide antioxidant protection. However, their role as supplements in the prevention of cancer and heart disease is not entirely clear at the present time and will be discussed in Chapter 13.

What happens if too little vitamin A is consumed?

When vitamin A is deficient from the diet for many months the body's internal stores are decreased, and proper vision and the health of the corneas of the eyes become compromised. *Night blindness* results from vitamin A deficiency. Night blindness is an inability to adapt to dim lighting and is usually accompanied by a prolonged transition from dim to bright light.

Vitamin A deficiency is one of the more recognized nutrient deficiencies worldwide, as roughly 2 million children in developing countries go blind each year as a result of vitamin A deficiency. International relief efforts to improve health conditions in these countries are attempting to correct this deficiency by giving children large amounts of vitamin A a couple of times per year. Hopefully, the doses are large enough to provide adequate vitamin A storage to last until the next treatment.

In vitamin A deficiency the mucus-producing cells of the cornea deteriorate and no longer produce mucus; a hard protein called keratin is produced instead. Keratin in combination with a decreased presence of mucus will dry out and harden the cornea of the eye. This condition is called *xerophthalmia,* which means dry, hard eyes. Inadequate mucus secretion of cells lining the respiratory, digestive, urinary, and reproductive tracts will greatly affect the function and health of these tissues as well. They are subject to drying and infection. Dry, hard skin is an observable sign of a vitamin A deficiency.

Can vitamin A become toxic?

Toxicity of vitamin A is seemingly just as severe as a deficiency. If a person consumes as little as ten times the RDA for vitamin A for several months, signs and symptoms such as bone pain, hair loss, dryness of the skin, and liver complications may develop. If toxicity persists it can eventually result in death. However, the risk of vitamin A toxicity from eating a balanced diet is low. Even those of us eating very large amounts of carotenoid-containing fruits and vegetables are not at significant risk of toxicity. This is due to the much lower rate of digestive absorption and conversion of carotenoids to vitamin A. Most people who develop vitamin A toxicity seem to do so through use of supplements. Furthermore, vitamin A toxicity during pregnancy can result in birth defects. We will look more closely at this situation in Chapter 12.

Vitamin D

Where do we get vitamin D?

Vitamin D is somewhat unique in relation to the other vitamins because the body can produce it in adequate amounts with the assistance of the sun. This is to say that there are two possible ways of supplying the body with vitamin D: through diet and exposure to the sunlight. Many scientists feel that since certain cells can produce vitamin D and because it then circulates and affects tissue throughout the body, it might be better classified as a hormone than a vitamin. However, as mentioned, the body's ability to make vitamin D relies upon exposure to sunlight (ultraviolet radiation), and not everyone receives adequate exposure. Furthermore, direct exposure to sunlight is not recommended due to the increased risk of skin cancers. For this reason, vitamin D will maintain its position as a vitamin. In the human diet, the richest sources of vitamin D are vitamin D-fortified milk and milk products, tuna, salmon, margarine (vitamin D fortified), herring, and vitamin D-fortified cereals (see Table 9.10). Vitamin D in foods appears fairly stable in various cooking and storing procedures. The RDA for adults is 5 to 10 µg vitamin D daily.

How do we make vitamin D in our body?

People with lighter skin color require only about 15 to 30 min of sun exposure to make adequate amounts of vitamin D while the necessary exposure time for people with darker skin color seems to increase relative to the degree of darkness. This also means that a person will make less and less vitamin D as they tan longer or over several days, as in a vacation at the beach. In addition, the ability to

TABLE 9.10. Vitamin D Content of Select Foods

Food	Vitamin D (µg)
Milk	
Milk (1 c)	2.5
Meats	
Beef liver (3 oz)	1.0
Eggs	
Egg (1)	0.7
Fish and seafood	
Salmon (3 oz)	8.5
Tuna (3 oz)	3.7
Shrimp (3 oz)	3.1

Note: 1 µg vitamin D = 40 IU

make vitamin D appears to be stronger during youth and decreases as humans get older. For this reason, scientists are debating whether to increase the RDA for vitamin D for older people.

The process of making vitamin D can be simplified to three primary locations within the body. First, within the skin a derivative of cholesterol called 7-dehydrocholesterol is converted to another substance called *cholecalciferol*. In order for this to occur, 7-dehydrocholesterol must be exposed to ultraviolet (UV) radiation from the sun or other UV sources (e.g., tanning beds). As mentioned, the efficiency of this conversion appears to decrease as UV exposure time increases. This helps to protect people from potentially making too much vitamin D.

Once cholecalciferol has been produced it leaves the skin region and circulates in the blood with the help of a transport protein called vitamin D binding protein (DBP). In the cholecalciferol form, vitamin D is only minimally active in the body. The activity of vitamin D depends on its ability to be recognized by vitamin D receptors in specific cells. In order for cholecalciferol to become more attractive to the vitamin D receptor, it must undergo more changes in its molecular design. The first change takes place in the liver as circulating cholecalciferol is removed and modified to become 25-hydroxycholecalciferol. This form of vitamin D is released by the liver and reenters the blood. This form of vitamin D is a little more attractive to vitamin D receptors and some of the effects of vitamin D are realized. 25-dihydroxycholecalciferol can circulate to the kidneys and be modified further to the most potent form of vitamin D—1,25-dihydroxycholecalciferol or calcitriol, which is released back into circulation (see Figure 9.4). In this form, vitamin D is exceptionally attractive to vitamin D receptors strategically located within certain cells in the body.

Does the vitamin D in foods need to be processed in the body?

The vitamin D in foods is fairly well absorbed across the wall of the small intestine. Because this form of vitamin D is fat soluble (water insoluble), it will require the same digestive and absorptive considerations as other lipid substances. This includes the presence of bile and the incorporation into chylomicrons. This vitamin D will eventually make it to the liver and must also undergo the same modifications in the liver and kidney as did the vitamin D made from cholesterol in the skin.

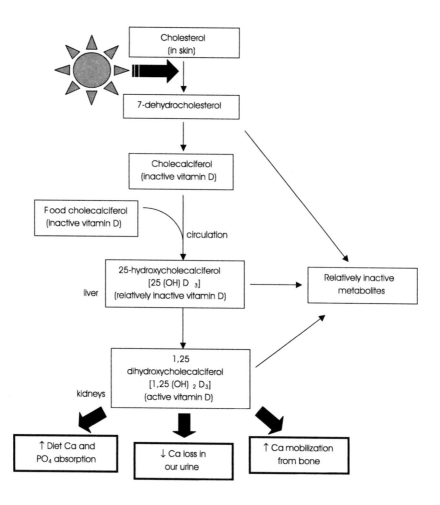

FIGURE 9.4. Sunlight (ultraviolet light) can convert a cholesterol derivative (7-dehydrocholesterol) to cholecalciferol. Cholecalciferol (from food or sunlight exposure) can be converted to active vitamin D by conversion in the liver and then kidneys. Vitamin D will increase available calcium in the body by increasing absorption from our diet and decreasing urine losses. Also, vitamin D can promote the mobilization of calcium from bone, which can become significant when dietary calcium is lacking.

What does vitamin D do in the body?

In order for a cell to be influenced by vitamin D it must possess vitamin D receptors. This further strengthens the argument that vitamin D is more like a hormone than a vitamin. Remember that a hormone must bind with a specific receptor in order to be active. While scientists continue to discover vitamin D receptors in various tissues throughout the body, most of the attention has centered around the bone, kidneys, and intestines. Vitamin D is classically recognized as being principally involved in bone and calcium metabolism although newer functions of vitamin D may be added to the list in the near future.

Vitamin D is principally involved in maintaining blood calcium levels. Since about 99 percent of the body's calcium is found in bone, it serves as a reservoir for blood calcium. The concentration of calcium in the blood is tightly regulated. When blood calcium levels begin to fall below normal levels, the parathyroid gland releases *parathyroid hormone* (PTH) into circulation. PTH is dedicated to reestablishing normal blood calcium levels. One of its activities is to increase the conversion of vitamin D in the kidneys to its most active form. Vitamin D can then work to promote an increase in calcium absorption from the digestive tract and to also decrease the amount of calcium lost from the body in urine. Scientists believe that vitamin D promotes the production and activity of proteins that help transport calcium across the wall of the small intestine.

Vitamin D also seems to be fundamentally involved in the remodeling of bone. Bone tissue is slowly but perpetually being broken down and remade. This means that bone is able to adapt according to the needs and demands of the body, such as growth or strengthening. Recently, some new roles of vitamin D have been suggested. These include the regulation of growth and maturation of certain normal cells, such as intestine, immune, and bone cells, and maybe cancer cells, such as skin and bone cancer cells. As advancements in laboratory techniques have allowed scientists to delve deeper into cell function, scientific understanding of other possible roles of vitamin D independent of calcium metabolism has increased.

What happens if too little vitamin D is consumed?

Deficiency of vitamin D can occur when a combination of factors is present. If vitamin D intake and/or absorption is low and an individual does not receive adequate exposure to sunlight, the potential for a vitamin D deficiency is present. In children, vitamin D deficiency results in *rickets,* a condition wherein bones are not properly formed and mineralized. Thin, pliable bones of the legs bow under the weight of a child's body. Bowed legs are often accompanied by an enlarged head, rib cage, and joints, which are considered the classic signs of rickets. It is important to remember that milk, whether it is from a human or from another mammal (e.g., cow, goat), is not a naturally rich source of vitamin D. However, most milk bought in a store is fortified with vitamin D thereby making it a good food source. Infants will be at greater risk of developing vitamin D deficiency if they do not receive periodical exposure to the sun and/or infant foods or a supplement containing vitamin D.

The adult form of rickets is medically referred to as *osteomalacia.* This name literally means "bad bones." In osteomalcia bones gradually lose their mineral content, become less dense and physically weaker, and are more susceptible to fracture. The underlying cause of osteomalacia may be related directly to a lack of dietary vitamin D as well as a lack of exposure to sunlight. Or it may be related to internal disease in a vitamin D-metabolizing organ, such as the liver and/or kidneys, or organs involved in digestion and absorption of vitamin D, such as the pancreas, gallbladder, liver, and small intestine. Osteomalacia and a seemingly similar disorder (osteoporosis) are discussed in Chapter 12.

Can too much vitamin D be consumed?

We may be more sensitive to vitamin D toxicity than other vitamins when looking at the intake level associated with signs and symptoms. Toxicity signs and symptoms can appear after several months of receiving as little as five times the RDA. Many of the manifestations appear to be related to vitamin D's increasing calcium absorption, which in turn results in too much calcium in the blood. Prolonged hypercalcemia (elevated blood calcium) can affect muscle cell activity, which includes the heart, and can induce nausea, vomiting, mental confusion, and lead to calcium deposition in various tissues throughout the body.

Luckily, as exposure to sunlight increases the body's ability to make vitamin D decreases. Also, as the level of active vitamin D increases, kidney cells produce less and less of the converting enzyme needed to make more active vitamin D. These mechanisms attempt to decrease the potential for toxicity.

Vitamin E

What is vitamin E and what foods provide vitamin E?

Similar to many other vitamins, vitamin E is not necessarily a single molecule but a class of similar molecules accomplishing related activities. There are about eight or so vitamin E molecules that can be subdivided into two major classes, *tocopherols* and *tocotrienols,* which themselves can be subdivided and given Greek descriptors (i.e., α, β, δ, γ). Good food sources of vitamin E include plant oils, margarine, and some fruits and vegetables, such as peaches and asparagus (see Table 9.11). The average adult intake of vitamin E approximates the RDA, which is 15 α-TE daily.

Among the vitamin E molecules, α-tocopherol is the most prevalent, popular, and probably potent in the body. For this reason the RDA for vitamin E is provided in α-tocopherol equivalents (α-TE). Here, 1 α-TE unit has the activity of 1 mg of α-tocopherol. Since other forms of vitamin E are not as potent, the α-TE unit amount bestowed to a food is based on the amount of α-tocopherol as well as the potential vitamin E activity contributions made by the other forms. For example, if a food contained 25 mg of α-tocopherol and 50 mg of another form of vitamin E which is only 50 percent as potent as α-tocopherol, the food is said to contain 50 α-TE (25 mg of α-tocopherol + 25 mg [50 percent of 50 mg] of other vitamin E form).

What does vitamin E do in the body?

Vitamin E shows a fair absorption (25 to 50 percent) from the small intestine. Factors such as an increased need or low stores of vitamin E may certainly increase the absorption percentage. Like other fat-soluble vitamins, vitamin E needs the assistance of lipid digestive and absorptive processes (e.g., chylomicrons). Much of the absorbed vitamin E will end up in the liver as chylomicron remnants are removed from the blood. The liver can then add vitamin E to VLDLs,

TABLE 9.11. Vitamin E (α-TE) Content of Select Foods

Food	Vitamin E (α-TE)
Oils/fats	
Oil (1 T)	6.7
Mayonnaise (1 T)	3.4
Margarine (1 T)	2.7
Nuts and seeds	
Sunflower seeds (1/4 c)	27.1
Almonds (1/4 c)	12.7
Peanuts (1/4 c)	4.9
Cashews (1/4 c)	0.7
Seafood	
Crab (3 oz)	4.5
Shrimp (3 oz)	3.7
Fish (3 oz)	2.4
Vegetables	
Sweet potato (1/2 c)	6.9
Collard greens (1/2 c)	3.1
Asparagus (1/2 c)	2.1
Spinach, raw (1 c)	1.5
Grains	
Wheat germ (1 T)	2.1
Bread, whole wheat (1 slice)	2.4
Bread, white (1 slice)	1.2

α-TE = α-tocopherol equivalents = 1 mg

which are then released into circulation where they can be delivered to most cells.

Because vitamin E is not very water soluble, very little is lost in urine; however, large intakes of vitamin E will result in a proportionate increase in urinary losses. The primary means for vitamin E loss from the body appears to be through the feces. The liver incorporates vitamin E into bile, which is dumped into the digestive tract. Some of this vitamin E, along with vitamin E from dietary sources, is not absorbed and becomes part of feces.

By and large, vitamin E functions as an antioxidant, protecting cells from free radicals. As vitamin E is a lipid-soluble molecule it is logical to think that vitamin E would be most active in lipid-rich areas of our cells. This appears to be the case, as vitamin E's antioxidant activities are recognized mostly in regard to protecting the lipid-rich cell membranes. Cell membranes contain a tremendous amount of phospholipids, each of which contain two fatty acids. Furthermore, double bonds within some of these fatty acids appear to be very vulnerable to free-radical attack. Vitamin E appears to protect fatty acids by donating one of its own electrons to a free radical. This pacifies the free radical and also spares the fatty acids in cell membranes.

Since lipoproteins provide a primary means of shuttling vitamin E throughout the body, scientists have speculated that vitamin E may be involved in the prevention of heart disease. Some evidence suggests that vitamin E helps protect LDL from oxidation. Oxidized LDL is believed to be a strong risk factor for atherosclerosis. This is discussed in more detail in Chapter 13.

As unsaturated fatty acids are more prone to free-radical attack, many scientists contend that diets containing more unsaturated fatty acids will increase the need for vitamin E. One fate of diet-derived fatty acids is to become part of phospholipids in cell membranes. In fact, the more unsaturated fatty acids found in the diet, the more unsaturated fatty acids found in cell membrane phospholipids. They argue that as we shift our fatty acid intake to more unsaturated fatty acids, such as the polyunsaturated ω-3 and ω-6 fatty acids, we may need to provide these fatty acids with adequate antioxidant escorts (e.g., vitamin E). Other antioxidants such as vitamin C are not as impressive in directly protecting unsaturated fatty acids. This is because their water solubility keeps them more involved in the watery intracellular fluid rather than the lipid portion of cell membranes.

The choice of unsaturated fatty acid sources, such as plant oils or fish (oil in fish), differs in regard to vitamin E contribution. Plant oils contain vitamin E while fish oils do not. Some scientists believe that if we derive most of our unsaturated fatty acids from fish sources those foods should be complemented with foods higher in vitamin E or a supplement containing vitamin E. The idea seems logical and awaits further study.

Can other antioxidants work together with vitamin E?

It should be recognized that other antioxidant-like compounds such as vitamin C and selenium can support vitamin E's efforts. After vitamin E concedes an electron to a free radical it can be restocked with another electron from vitamin C. Thus vitamin C helps keep vitamin E equipped in its battle against free radicals. This helps to recycle vitamin E. The mineral selenium, as part of the enzyme glutathione peroxidase, seems to have a beneficial effect upon vitamin E status. It has been suggested that like vitamin C, glutathione peroxidase also helps to recycle vitamin E by restocking it with an electron. Also, glutathione peroxidase helps inactivate free radicals such as peroxides, which ultimately reduces the workload of vitamin E.

What happens if too little vitamin E is consumed?

Vitamin E deficiency is somewhat rare in adults with the exception of those who have medical problems that impact the normal digestion of lipids. Any situation in which normal fat digestion and absorption are hindered can ultimately reduce the amount of vitamin E absorbed from the digestive tract. A deficiency may take many months or years to show itself through medical symptoms such as red blood cell fragility and neurological abnormalities. Usually the medical problem is treated long before vitamin E deficiency signs are recognized. However, children with cystic fibrosis are a special concern, as the pancreas produces inadequate amounts of digestive enzymes in those with this disease.

Can vitamin E become toxic?

Compared to the fat-soluble vitamins discussed so far, vitamin E is relatively nontoxic. However, studies on people eating fifty to one hundred times the RDA have demonstrated that these amounts can result in nausea, diarrhea, and headaches, while some individuals complained of general weakness and fatigue. It should be recognized that excessive vitamin E supplementation may interfere with vitamin K's activity in blood clotting.

Vitamin K

What is vitamin K and where do we get it?

Vitamin K is a general name for a few related compounds that possess vitamin K activity. *Phylloquinone* is the form of vitamin K found naturally in plants; *menaquinones* are the form of vitamin K derived from bacteria; and *menadione,* which is not natural, is the synthetic (laboratory derived) form of vitamin K.

Humans receive vitamin K not only from various foods but also from bacteria in the colon. Good sources of vitamin K include broccoli, spinach, cabbage, Brussels sprouts, turnip greens, cauliflower, beef liver, and asparagus. Foods lower in vitamin K such as cheeses, eggs, corn oil, sunflower oil, and butter also make a respectable contribution to our vitamin K intake because of their frequency of consumption. The RDA for adults is 90 to 120 µg of vitamin K.

It has been estimated that as much as one-half of the vitamin K absorbed from the digestive tract was originally made by intestinal bacteria. Being a fat-soluble substance, vitamin K relies somewhat upon the activities of normal lipid digestion for optimal absorption. Vitamin K must also be transported from the intestines by way of chylomicrons, which ultimately reach the liver. Once in the liver, vitamin K can be packaged into VLDL and carried throughout the body.

What does vitamin K do in the body?

For years the only recognized activity of vitamin K was its involvement in proper normal blood clotting. In fact, rumor has it that vitamin K was so named by Danish researchers with respect to blood *coagulation,* a word spelled with a "K" in Danish. The liver is responsible for making the proteins, or *clotting factors,* that circulate in the blood. These proteins are activated when there is a hemorrhage and allow blood to clot at that site.

When clotting factors are initially made by liver cells, but before they are released into circulation, several of these proteins are modified by vitamin K. The modification occurs only in few amino acids; however, it changes the design and function of the proteins significantly. With this slightly modified design, these and other clotting factors are released into circulation. Once in circulation, these proteins await the signal to initiate clot formation. The signal is a tear in a blood vessel wall producing a hemorrhage. In light of vitamin K's involvement with blood clotting, the vitamin K status of a patient is typically determined prior to any surgical procedure.

Vitamin K also seems to be active in other tissue besides the liver. In bone, muscles, and kidneys, vitamin K appears to be necessary for activities similar to those in the liver. At least two proteins in bone and one in the kidneys have been identified as needing modification by vitamin K to function properly.

Can too little or too much vitamin K be consumed?

Unlike other fat-soluble vitamins, vitamin K is not stored very well in the body and appreciable amounts are lost in urine and feces every day. This certainly presents the opportunity for a more rapid onset to deficiency. However, since vitamin K is abundant in the human diet and vitamin K is produced by bacteria in the digestive tract, vitamin K deficiency is uncommon in adults. The typical American adult may eat five to six times the RDA daily.

Opportunities for vitamin K deficiency do arise during infancy. There does not seem to be an appreciable transfer of vitamin K from the mother to the infant prior to birth. Thus newborns enter the world with very limited stores of vitamin K. Also, a newborn's digestive tract is sterile and will not develop a mature bacterial population for a couple months. Further, maternal breast milk is not a good source of vitamin K. All of these factors place infants at greater risk for developing vitamin K deficiency, which can lead to poor blood clotting and hemorrhage, among other considerations. With these concerns in mind, newborns are commonly provided with vitamin K shortly after birth.

One other situation may raise concern regarding the development of a vitamin K deficiency. People using antibiotics for long periods of time are at a greater risk for vitamin K deficiency. Certain antibiotics can reduce the number of vitamin K-producing bacteria from our colon which puts us at a greater risk of deficiency, especially if a person eats a low vitamin K diet and/or is experiencing problems with lipid digestion. But the combination of these factors is indeed rare.

Vitamin K is relatively nontoxic in natural forms; however, there have been situations of toxicity from chronic use of excessive vitamin K in the synthetic menadione form.

Chapter 10

The Minerals of Our Body

Minerals contribute about 5 to 6 percent to total body weight in humans and function in many different ways. Some minerals such as sodium, potassium, and chloride function as electrolytes, while other minerals, such as copper, zinc, iron, chromium, selenium, and manganese can be incorporated into enzyme molecules. Also, some minerals such as calcium, phosphorus, and fluoride can play a vital structural role in strengthening bones and teeth. After water, minerals are the primary inorganic component of the body; by and large they are what is left over (ash) after cremation of a body, as they will not combust like most organic molecules or evaporate like water.

Minerals can be broken into two broad groups based on their contribution to body weight (see Table 10.1). If a mineral accounts for more than one-thousandth of human body weight it is considered a *major mineral.* When a mineral accounts for less than one-thousandth of body weight it is called a *minor mineral* or *trace mineral.* Another way to designate the difference between major and minor minerals is through dietary need. The recommended dietary intake for major minerals is greater than 100 mg, while the recommendations for minor minerals are less than 100 mg. The term *mineral* is often used interchangeably with *element,* thereby indicating that all minerals are elements.

THE MAJOR MINERALS INCLUDE CALCIUM, PHOSPHORUS, AND ELECTROLYTES

Calcium (Ca)

Without question calcium is one of the most recognizable and popular minerals. Perhaps this is well deserved, as calcium is about 40 percent of total body mineral weight and about 1.5 percent of total

TABLE 10.1. The Minerals of Our Body

Major Minerals	Minor or Trace Minerals	
Calcium	Iron	Copper
Phosphorus	Chromium	Boron
Sulfur	Selenium	Manganese
Potassium	Zinc	Molybdenum
Sodium	Iodine	Fluoride
Chloride	Nickel	Vanadium
Magnesium	Arsenic	Silicon
	Cobalt*	Cadmium*
	Lithium*	Tin*

*Dietary essentiality is questionable despite presence in the body.

body weight. Furthermore, calcium tends to be portrayed as a hero for protecting the human body from osteoporosis. However, most people really do not understand how calcium functions. Calcium is found in foods and the body as an atom with a +2 charge (Ca^{++} or Ca^{2+}). Calcium atoms, therefore, are most stable after they have given up two electrons (see Chapter 1). Because of this heavy positive charge, calcium strongly interacts with substances bearing a negative charge.

What foods contribute to calcium intake?

Without question, dairy products are the greatest contributors of calcium to the diet. Perhaps more than 55 percent of the calcium in the American diet comes from dairy products. For instance, a glass of milk supplies about 300 mg of calcium (see Table 10.2). Other good sources of calcium include sardines, oysters, clams, tofu, molasses, almonds, calcium-fortified foods, and dark green leafy vegetables such as broccoli, kale, collards, mustard greens, and turnip greens. Other vegetables such as spinach, rhubarb, chard, and beet greens contain respectable amounts of calcium. However, other substances in plants, such as oxalates and phytate, can bind to calcium in the digestive tract and decrease its absorption (see Box 10.1). For example, as little as 5 percent of the calcium in spinach is actually absorbed due to the presence of inhibiting substances in the digestive tract.

TABLE 10.2. Calcium Content of Select Foods

Food	Calcium (mg)
Milk and Milk Products	
Yogurt, low-fat (1 c)	448
Milk, skim (1 c)	301
Cheese, Swiss (1 oz)	272
Ice cream (1 c)	180
Ice milk (1 c)	180
Custard (1/2 c)	150
Cottage cheese (1/2 c)	70
Vegetables	
Collard greens (1/2 c)	110
Spinach (1/2 c)	90
Broccoli (1/2 c)	70
Legumes and Products	
Tofu (1/2 c)	155
Dried beans (1/2 c)	50
Lima beans (1/2 c)	40

BOX 10.1. Influence of Various Factors Upon Calcium Absorption

↑ **Calcium Absorption**
- ↑ vitamin D and PTH
- lactose during same meal
- ↑ need (growth, pregnancy, lactation)

↓ **Calcium Absorption**
- ↓ vitamin D and PTH
- phytate, fiber, and oxalates during same meal
- ↓ need

PTH = Parathyroid Hormone

Factors such as normal stomach acidity and the presence of certain amino acids in the small intestine seem to increase the efficiency of calcium absorption. Therefore, many nutritionists recommend eating calcium-rich foods or taking a supplement with a meal. Some nutritionists also believe that a diet having a higher phosphorus-to-calcium ratio may reduce calcium absorption. They contend that the ratio of phosphorus to calcium in the diet should not exceed 2:1.

The RDA for calcium is the highest among the non-energy providing essential nutrients with the only exceptions being phosphorus and water, the latter of which does not have a RDA. The RDA for adults is 1000-1200 mg of calcium daily, depending on age and condition (e.g., pregnancy). The RDA for calcium takes into consideration daily losses of calcium from the body by way of urine, skin, and feces along with an absorption rate of about 20 to 40 percent for adults and up to 75 percent for children and during pregnancy.

The average calcium intake for American men seems to meet the RDA for all ages except for those over fifty-five years. Contrarily, the calcium intake for American women is significantly below the RDA for all age groups. Some nutritionists attribute the lower intake of calcium in women to weight-control efforts and the substitution of diet soft drinks for milk.

What does calcium do in the body?

About 99 percent of the calcium in the body can be found in the bones and teeth. The remaining 1 percent of calcium circulates in the blood and is distributed in tissue throughout the body such as muscle, glands, and nerves. Without question the most recognizable function of calcium is to make the bones and teeth hard. The two major calcium-containing complexes in these tissues are calcium phosphate $[Ca_3(PO_4)_2]$ and hydroxyapatite $[Ca_{10}(PO_4)_6OH_2]$ with the latter being the most abundant. Hydroxyapatite crystals have a structure somewhat similar to flagstone: they are basically long and flat. This design allows hydroxyapatite to lie on top of collagen fibers in bones and teeth, thereby complementing the strength of collagen with hardness and rigidity (see Figure 10.1). Calcium phosphate is a little different from hydroxyapatite in that it is broken down more readily than hydroxyapatite, which allows it to serve as a resource of both calcium and phosphate to help maintain blood levels of these minerals. Furthermore, calcium phosphate can be used to make hydroxyapatite in bones and teeth.

As mentioned, only a small portion of the body's calcium is found outside bone and teeth. This calcium is found in the blood as well as distributed in other tissues throughout the body including muscles, nerves, and glands. However, despite the relatively smaller quantity, it is this portion of calcium that is more important to human existence on a millisecond-to-millisecond, second-to-second, minute-to-minute ba-

Collagen fibers

Hydroxyapatite
containing calcium
and phosphate

FIGURE 10.1. Sheets of hydroxyapatite (calcium and phosphate crystals) coating collagen fibers in bone.

sis. For instance, calcium is involved in the function of excitable tissue (muscle and nerves). Before the heart can "beat," special cells in a region of the heart called the sinoatrial node (SA node) must spontaneously initiate an electrical impulse. This impulse then stimulates the rest of the heart to contract. Calcium is fundamentally involved in initiating that impulse in the SA node. Calcium is also involved in the contraction of heart muscle, as well as contraction of skeletal muscle.

Neurotransmitters and hormones are the means by which cells in the body can communicate with each other. However, in order for these substances to provide this service efficiently, they must be released from glands and nerve cells at appropriate times. Calcium is involved in the release of several of these substances. Furthermore, calcium is essential for certain hormones to have an impact upon certain cells. This means that when some hormones interact with their receptors, the result is an increase in the calcium concentration in that cell. As the level of calcium increases in these cells it will then interact with specific proteins and evoke the desired effect in that cell. Calcium sometimes can act as a middleman or intermediate factor as hormones cause things to happen. Scientists sometimes call this a "second messenger" role, whereby the first messenger was the hormone itself.

Calcium is also involved in proper blood clotting. When a hemorrhage occurs, clotting factors in the blood become activated and ultimately a clot is formed at the site of the hemorrhage. A clot is somewhat analogous to a bicycle tire patch that is placed specifically to seal off a hole. The clotting process consists of many steps, some which require calcium to proceed. Calcium binds to the clotting factors and allows them to become more active. Therefore, with a less than optimal amount of calcium in the blood, it might take longer to stop a hemorrhage.

How is the level of calcium in the blood regulated?

One thing is for certain: calcium is very busy in the body. Again, on an instant-to-instant basis, the calcium found in the blood and other tissues is more vital than the calcium complexes in bones and teeth. As we alluded to, bones serve as a reservoir for calcium to safeguard against falling blood calcium levels. Blood calcium levels are very tightly regulated; two hormones and one vitamin are directly involved in blood calcium status. Parathyroid hormone (PTH), calcitonin, and vitamin D all function with blood calcium levels in mind.

PTH is released into circulation from the parathyroid gland when blood calcium levels begin to decline. PTH increases the activation of vitamin D in the kidneys and, along with vitamin D, PTH decreases the loss of calcium in urine. Vitamin D and PTH also increase the release of calcium from bone into the blood as well as increase the efficiency of calcium absorption from the small intestine. The net result is an increase in the level of calcium in the blood, thus returning it to normal (8.8 to 10.8 mg/100 mL of blood). On the contrary, the level of the hormone calcitonin in the blood increases when calcium levels increase above the normal range. Calcitonin is made by the thyroid gland and generally works opposite to PTH and vitamin D. Calcitonin decreases bone release of calcium and with the help of urinary loss of calcium promotes a reduction in blood calcium, thus returning it to the more optimal range.

What contributes to a calcium deficiency
and what are its manifestations?

A deficiency of calcium results in bone abnormalities. If the deficiency occurs during growing years, poor bone mineralization will occur. Bones become soft and pliable due to a lack of mineralization. As bowed legs are often seen as a result of calcium deficiency during childhood, this disorder seems similar to rickets, which results from a vitamin D deficiency. If a calcium deficiency develops later in life, the result is a loss of mineral that renders bone less dense and more susceptible to fracture. This process is referred to as osteomalacia, which is often confused with osteoporosis. The differences will be explored in Chapter 12.

It is important to keep in mind that poor calcium intake may not be reflected by reductions in blood calcium. This is because the level of calcium in the blood is more influenced by the hormones mentioned previously in the short run (over a period of days and weeks). However, if calcium intake remains poor for longer periods of time, such as months, blood calcium levels can indeed begin to decrease. Therefore, an assessment of blood calcium levels is somewhat incomplete without an assessment of the hormones that regulate blood calcium levels. For instance, a person diagnosed with hypoparathyroidism may have reduced levels of calcium in his or her blood despite following a diet that might otherwise be rich in calcium. The same can be said for people who have impaired liver or kidney functions as these organs are responsible for the activation of vitamin D. Whatever the case may be, a reduced level of calcium in the blood may affect the calcium concentration found in tissues such as nerve, muscle, and glands. Low blood calcium levels are associated with irritability of nervous tissue, including the CNS as well as skeletal muscle cramping. Normal function of the SA node can be disrupted as well as influence the rhythm of the heart.

Is calcium toxic in large amounts?

Today, it is fairly common for people to ingest large supplemental amounts of calcium. Sometimes their intake can climb above five to ten times their RDA. Although the efficiency of calcium absorption decreases as more is ingested and body calcium status is optimal, this can still lead to increased entry of calcium into the body. Also, as mentioned previously, gram doses of vitamin C may increase calcium absorption to perhaps undesirable levels. Further still, excessive vitamin D intake may also increase body calcium by increasing its absorption and decreasing urinary losses. Whatever the case may be, excessive calcium in the body, over time, can lead to increased calcium content in tissues such as muscle (including our heart), blood vessels, and lungs. This will affect the activity of the tissues by making them more rigid.

In an effort to rid the body of excessive calcium, the kidneys will be forced to filter and void more calcium than normal. This situation may promote the formation of kidney stones. In addition, excessive calcium consumption may hinder iron absorption. Supplementing gram doses of calcium, therefore, is generally not recommended unless warranted for medical reasons.

What are calcium supplements?

Calcium supplements are necessary for those whose diets fail to provide ideal amounts of calcium. Most calcium supplements are in the form of calcium carbonate or calcium citrate. Calcium supplements should be taken with a meal unless the meal contains fiber-rich foods which often contain phytate and oxalates. Calcium carbonate is the form found in many antacids. Meanwhile, calcium citrate is itself an acid and therefore may be better suited for people lacking the ability to produce adequate stomach acid. Other forms of common calcium supplements include calcium gluconate, calcium acetate, and calcium lactate. Of all of the forms of calcium supplements, calcium carbonate supplies the most calcium (by weight); this form also possesses a slightly greater efficiency of absorption.

Some food manufacturers (e.g., orange juice manufacturers) use calcium citrate malate (CCM) to fortify their juices. Calcium has also become a popular nutrient for fortification in foods such as bread. Recently, supplements containing hydroxyapatite have also begun to appear on the shelves.

Phosphorus (P)

Phosphorus in food or in the body is usually in the form of phosphate (PO_4). Thus, phosphorus and phosphate are often used interchangeably. After calcium, phosphate is the most abundant mineral in our body. Similar to calcium, phosphate bears a strong charge, only in this case it is negative. Calcium and phosphate therefore interact with each other nicely in bone and teeth due to their strong, opposite charges.

What foods provide phosphorus, and can other substances influence absorption?

Those foods with a higher content of phosphorus include meat, poultry, fish, eggs, milk and milk products, cereals, legumes, grains, and chocolate (see Table 10.3). Many soft drinks contain phosphorus in the form of phosphoric acid. Go ahead and check the ingredients if

TABLE 10.3. Phosphorus Content of Select Foods

Food	Phosphorus (mg)
Milk and milk products	
Yogurt (1 c)	327
Milk (1 c)	250
Cheese, American (1 oz)	130
Meats and alternatives	
Pork (3 oz)	275
Hamburger (3 oz)	165
Tuna (3 oz)	162
Lobster (3 oz)	125
Chicken (3 oz)	120
Nuts and seeds	
Sunflower seeds (1/4 c)	319
Peanuts (1/4 c)	141
Peanut butter (1 T)	61
Grains	
Bran flakes (1 c)	180
Bread, whole wheat (1 slice)	52
Noodles, cooked (1/2 c)	47
Rice, cooked (1/2 c)	29
Bread, white (1 slice)	24
Vegetables	
Potato (1)	101
Corn (1/2 c)	73
Peas (1/2 c)	70
Broccoli (1/2 c)	54
Other	
Milk chocolate (1 oz)	66
Cola (12 oz)	51
Diet cola (12 oz)	45

you are drinking a soda right now. The recommended phosphorus intake for adults is below calcium recommendations at 700 mg daily for adults.

A meal containing a considerable quantity of magnesium can decrease phosphorus absorption; conversely, a meal low in magnesium might enhance phosphorus absorption. Also, aluminum-containing substances ingested with a meal can decrease phosphorus absorption. Aluminum hydroxide and magnesium hydroxide are common ingredients in antacids. As mentioned in the discussion on calcium, some scientists have speculated that diets containing higher phosphorus-to-calcium ratios may decrease calcium absorption and lead to greater calcium loss in the urine. Although this theory is still debatable, some nutritionists contend that choosing soft drinks over milk may significantly impact calcium status. They recommend that the phosphorus-to-calcium ratio should not exceed 2:1 and people should strive for a better balance between these two minerals.

What does phosphorus (phosphate) do in the body?

Approximately 85 percent of the phosphorus found in the body is in the skeleton and teeth as a component of calcium phosphate and hydroxyapatite. As mentioned previously, these complexes function to make bone and teeth hard. In addition, the phosphate found in bone can serve as a resource of this mineral to help maintain adequate amounts of phosphate in other tissues.

Phosphate is also vital to the processes that allow our cells to capture the energy released in the breakdown of carbohydrates, protein, fat, and alcohol. As mentioned several times, when energy is released from carbohydrates, protein, fat and alcohol some of it is trapped in chemical bonds involving phosphate of special molecules such as ATP (adenosine triphosphate). Other phosphate-containing energy molecules are creatine phosphate (CP) and guanosine triphosphate (GTP). It is important to keep in mind that while carbohydrates, protein, fat, and alcohol are endowed with energy, the body's cells cannot directly use that energy. Thus, these substances are broken down as needed to produce ATP and GTP, which then can be used to power cell operations.

In addition to the energy molecules, phosphate is used by the cells to help regulate the activity of key enzymes. For instance, a key enzyme involved in the breakdown of glycogen stores is activated when a phosphate is attached to it. It is like an on/off switch for that enzyme. In addition, phosphate is a vital component of phospholipids in cell membranes and also nucleic acids (RNA and DNA). Phospholipids are the primary structural components of cell membranes, while DNA serve as the instruction manuals for building proteins in cells.

Can too little or too much phosphorus be consumed?

Because most foods contain phosphorus, a deficiency is somewhat rare under normal circumstances. Toxicity is also rare perhaps with the exception of infants who receive a high phosphorus-containing formula. However, most commercially available infant formulas are not a threat in regard to their phosphorus content.

Sodium (Na)

As we discussed in Chapter 1, sodium is most comfortable when it gives up an electron. Thus, sodium in foods as well as in the body will have a positive charge (Na^+). In light of the involvement of sodium in the electrical events of the body, we often refer to sodium, along with chloride and potassium, as electrolytes. Again, an electrolyte is a substance that when dissolved into a body of water will increase the speed of the electrical conduction of the water.

What contributes to sodium intake?

The typical American diet includes about 3 to 7 g of sodium daily, which is a lot compared to other minerals. Oddly, the natural sodium content of most foods is very low. About 50 to 75 percent of the sodium consumed is added to foods by food manufacturers for taste or preservation purposes (see Table 10.4). Some of the foods having higher sodium content are snack foods (e.g., chips), luncheon meats, gravies, cheeses, and pickles. Another 15 percent is added in the kitchen during cooking and by "salting" foods at the table. Most people know that table salt is sodium chloride (NaCl). The sodium occurring naturally in foods such as eggs, milk, meats, and vegetables may supply only about 10 to 15 percent of total sodium intake. Finally, drinking water may contribute to sodium intake along with certain medicines. Foods that seem to make the greatest sodium contribution to the American diet include luncheon meats, snack chips, French fries, hot dogs, cheeses, soups, and gravies. In contrast to typical sodium intake of several grams per day, the adult dietary requirement for sodium may be as low as 100 to 500 mg of sodium daily.

TABLE 10.4. Sodium Content of Select Foods

Food	Sodium (mg)
Meat and alternatives	
Corned beef (3 oz)	808
Ham (3 oz)	800
Fish, canned (3 oz)	735
Sausage (3 oz)	483
Hot dog (1)	477
Bologna (1 oz)	370
Milk and milk products	
Cream soup (1 c)	1070
Cottage cheese (1/2 c)	455
Cheese, American (1 oz)	405
Cheese, parmesan (1 oz)	247
Milk, skim (1 c)	125
Milk, whole (1 c)	120
Grains	
Bran flakes (1 c)	363
Corn flakes (1 c)	325
English muffin (1)	203
Bread, white (1 slice)	130
Bread, whole wheat (1 slice)	130
Crackers, Saltines (4)	125
Other	
Salt (1 t)	2132
Pickle, dill (1)	1930
Broth, chicken (1 c)	1571
Ravioli, canned (1 c)	1065
Broth, beef (1 c)	782
Gravy (1/4 c)	720
Italian dressing (2 T)	720
Pretzels (salted), thin (5)	500
Olives, green (5)	465
Pizza, cheese (1 slice)	455
Soy sauce (1 t)	444
Bacon (3 slices)	303
French dressing (2 T)	220
Potato chips (10)	200
Catsup (1 T)	155
Bagel (1)	260

Within the past few decades many people have become concerned about how sodium in their diet might impact their health. This has applied some pressure upon food companies to reduce the sodium content of some of their products. In order for a product label to make certain sodium-related claims, it must meet the criteria listed in Table 10.5. We will take a closer look at the relationship between sodium and high blood pressure and cancers later on.

What does sodium do in the body?

Sodium is very well absorbed (about 95 percent) from the digestive tract. Therefore the primary means of regulating body sodium content is through urinary loss. Sodium is the predominant positively charged electrolyte dissolved in extracellular fluid. This, of course, includes the blood. Because of its abundance in the body, sodium is perfect for serving fundamental roles in the electrical activity of excitable cells such as muscle and neurons.

Sodium is also involved in regulating body water content as water is naturally attracted to sodium. Water will always move from one area to another in an effort to balance the total concentration of dissolved substances in both areas. This process is called *osmosis* and is a fundamental law of nature. Under certain circumstances the body will adjust the amount of sodium lost in the urine to decrease the amount of urinary water loss. This may occur as an adaptive measure during dehydration or a reduction in blood pressure such as after significant blood loss. Aldosterone is the principal hormone that governs the amount of sodium in urine.

TABLE 10.5. Labeling Guidelines for Sodium Content

Label Claim	Sodium Content (Per Serving)
Sodium free	Must contain < 5 mg per serving
Very low sodium	Must contain ≤ 35 mg sodium per serving
Low sodium	Must contain ≤ 145 mg sodium per serving
Reduced sodium	75 percent reduction in sodium content
Unsalted	No salt added to the recipe
No added salt	No salt added to the recipe

Can sodium deficiency develop?

Unlike most essential nutrients whereby aberrations resulting from a diet deficiency can take weeks, months, or even years to develop, electrolyte imbalances can lead to alterations much more rapidly. A reduced level of sodium in the body would result in alterations in the activity of excitable tissue, which certainly includes the brain, nerves, and muscle. This can occur within a day or two.

Because of the abundance of sodium in the human diet the potential for a deficiency is somewhat low. However, certain situations may place some people at a greater risk. These include eating a very low sodium diet in conjunction with excessive sweating and/or chronic diarrhea. Still, even under these conditions deficiency is very rare. Excessive sweating makes us thirsty and beverages would probably include some sodium. Furthermore, since the sodium concentration in our sweat is lower than in our blood it would take the loss of a couple of pounds of body weight in the form of sweat before any distress would occur.

Can sodium be toxic?

Provided that the kidneys are operating efficiently humans can rapidly remove excessive diet-derived sodium from the body without concern. However, individuals eating a very salty diet should include more water in their diet. Since water is attracted to sodium, more water will be urinated along with the excessive sodium. For people experiencing significantly decreased kidney performance, sodium becomes more of a concern. Dialysis may be necessary to remove excessive sodium and other substances from their body fluid.

Ingesting salt tablets on a hot day used to be a common practice, especially for athletes. However, this practice is no longer recommended for several reasons. First, it can cause intestinal discomfort and possibly diarrhea. Second, it would add more sodium to the body than is lost in sweat. To correct the elevated sodium concentration in the blood, more urine would have to be produced. This would lead to more water loss from the body, which during athletic performance could be a problem.

Potassium (K)

Similar to sodium, potassium atoms are most comfortable when they concede an electron and exist as a positively charged atom (K^+).

Potassium is one of the most important electrolytes in human body fluid; it is concentrated in the fluids inside of cells while sodium exists mainly outside of cells. The symbol for potassium is a K because of its Latin name *(kalium)*.

What foods contribute to potassium intake?

Unlike sodium, potassium is not routinely added to foods. Therefore, foods naturally containing potassium must be eaten to meet the body's needs. Luckily, potassium is found in most foods in the human diet (see Table 10.6). Many vegetables and fruits and their juices rank among the best sources of potassium. In fact, many athletes refer to bananas as "potassium sticks" with respect to their potassium content, although their potassium content really is not that outstanding compared to other fruits and vegetables. Along with fruits and vegetables, milk, meats, whole grains, coffee, and tea are among the most significant contributors to daily potassium intake. Adult requirements of potassium are approximately 2 g daily, a quantity that is easily obtained through a diet accommodating a variety of foods.

What does potassium do in the body?

About 90 percent of the dietary potassium eaten is absorbed by the digestive tract. Thus like sodium the amount of potassium in the body will need to be regulated by the kidneys. Unlike sodium and chloride though, about 98 percent of the potassium is located within the cells, making it the major positively charged electrolyte dissolved in the fluid within the cells. Therefore, potassium is extremely important in the electrical activity of excitable cells in the body.

Can too little or too much potassium be consumed?

Although dietary potassium intake is by and large adequate to meet human needs, situations can place the body at risk for potassium deficiency. Persistent use of laxatives can result in a lowered body potassium level by decreasing the amount of potassium absorbed from the digestive tract. Also, chronic use of certain diuretics used to control blood pressure may also result in increased urinary loss of potassium. Physicians will routinely monitor the potassium levels of patients following either of these prescribed protocols.

TABLE 10.6. Potassium Content of Select Foods

Food	Potassium (mg)
Vegetables	
Potato (1)	780
Squash, winter (1/2 c)	327
Tomato (1 medium)	300
Celery (1 stalk)	270
Carrots (1)	245
Broccoli (1/2 c)	205
Fruit	
Avocado (1/2)	680
Orange juice (1 c)	469
Banana (1)	440
Raisins (1/4 c)	370
Prunes (4)	300
Watermelon (1 c)	158
Meats	
Fish (3 oz)	500
Hamburger (3 oz)	480
Lamb (3 oz)	382
Pork (3 oz)	335
Chicken (3 oz)	208
Grains	
Bran buds (1 c)	1080
Bran flakes (1 c)	248
Raisin bran (1 c)	242
Wheat flakes (1 c)	96
Milk and milk products	
Yogurt (1 c)	531
Milk, skim (1 c)	400

Also, people who frequently vomit after a meal, either involuntarily or voluntarily, can reduce potassium absorption. Finally, people following a very low calorie diet (VLCD) for extended periods of time need to be concerned about their potassium consumption along with levels of other nutrients as well.

Potassium toxicity is not necessarily a concern provided that the kidneys are functioning appropriately. However, if the blood potassium level does become elevated (hyperkalemia) it would certainly affect the proper functioning of the excitable tissue, especially the heart and brain. The heart may actually fail to beat if hyperkalemia is severe and prolonged. Together with sodium, blood potassium levels are monitored closely in people diagnosed with diseases affecting their kidneys.

Chloride (Cl)

Chloride is the ion name for chlorine. Chlorine is an atom that is most comfortable when it removes an electron from another atom and as a result takes on a negative charge (Cl^-). Sodium and potassium as electrolytes often overshadow chloride, but chloride should not be underestimated in importance. Furthermore, chloride is involved in some interesting aspects of protein digestion as well as CO_2 elimination from the body.

What foods provide chloride in the diet?

Although some fruits and vegetables contain respectable amounts of chloride, the natural content of this mineral in most foods is naturally low. Chloride, as part of sodium chloride (table salt) added to foods, is the major contributor of chloride in our diet. Sodium chloride is 60 percent chloride by weight, thus 1 g of table salt is 600 mg chloride. The minimum requirement for chloride for an adult is about 700 mg per day, yet the average American diet contains about six times this amount.

What does chloride do in the body?

Similar to sodium and potassium, chloride functions as an electrolyte. In fact, chloride is the major negatively charged electrolyte in human extracellular fluid, which includes the blood. Chloride is important in the optimal functioning of excitable cells, which once again are nervous tissue and muscle. It is also part of hydrochloric acid (HCl), which is a key component of stomach juice. Furthermore, chloride is important in helping the body to remove CO_2. This process is very complex and involves changing CO_2 into a substance called *carbonate* that will dissolve more easily into the blood. Remember, gases such as O_2 and CO_2 do not dissolve very well in watery human blood. Therefore, the blood either carries them on hemoglobin (mostly O_2) or converts CO_2 to a more water-soluble substance. This allows for more and more CO_2 to be circulated to the lungs and breathed out of the body.

Chloride is almost entirely absorbed from the digestive tract. Therefore, the responsibility of body chloride regulation is placed upon the kidneys. Also similar to sodium and potassium, appropriate kidney function will be able to maintain optimal chloride levels in the body despite a high chloride diet. Human sweat should also be held accountable as a means for chloride loss from the body (along with sodium). However, sweat chloride and sodium losses are really only significant during heavy and prolonged sweating.

What happens if too little or too much chloride is consumed?

In light of Americans' heavy use of salt in food manufacturing, processing, and seasoning in the kitchen and at the table, chloride deficiencies are very rare. As mentioned, Western diets contain many times the estimated minimum requirement for chloride. Thus the potential for deficiency is believed to be rather low and is rarely seen. Provided that the kidneys are functioning properly, the risk of chloride toxicity is not necessarily a major concern either. However, if the kidneys are not functioning optimally this can result in elevations in the chloride in body fluid along with the other electrolytes. This then would most obviously affect the proper functioning of excitable cells in the body, although all cells would become compromised.

Magnesium (Mg)

Magnesium, like calcium, is most comfortable in nature when it gives up two electrons and takes on a double positive charge (Mg^{++}). Therefore, like calcium, you may be thinking that magnesium may provide at least some of its function by electrically interacting with other substances. This is certainly the case as is discussed next.

What foods provide magnesium?

Magnesium is found in a variety of foods; better sources include whole grain cereals, nuts, legumes, spices, seafood, coffee, tea, and cocoa (see Table 10.7). Certain processing techniques such as the milling of wheat and the polishing of rice may result in significant losses of magnesium from grains and other foods. Also, some magnesium can dissolve into cooking water during boiling, which results in some cooking loss as well. The RDA for adults ranges between 310 and 420 mg.

TABLE 10.7. Magnesium Content of Select Foods

Food	Magnesium (mg)
Legumes	
Lentils, cooked (1/2 c)	134
Split peas, cooked (1/2 c)	134
Tofu (1/2 c)	130
Nuts	
Peanuts (2 oz)	95
Cashews (2 oz)	140
Almonds (2 oz)	150
Grains	
Bran buds (1 c)	240
Rice, wild, cooked (1/2 c)	119
Wheat germ (2 T)	45
Vegetables	
Bean sprouts (1/2 c)	98
Black-eyed peas (1/2 c)	58
Spinach, cooked (1/2 c)	48
Lima beans (1/2 c)	32
Milk and milk products	
Milk (1 c)	30
Cheddar cheese (1 oz)	8
American cheese (1 oz)	6
Meats	
Chicken (3 oz)	25
Beef (3 oz)	20
Pork (3 oz)	20

What does magnesium do in the body?

Magnesium absorption from the digestive tract is fair (25 to 50 percent) with several factors being able to influence this efficiency. For example, a low body magnesium status results in a higher percentage of absorption. On the other hand, a high magnesium diet or excessive dietary calcium, phosphate, or phytate can decrease the efficiency of magnesium absorption.

Roughly 60 percent of the magnesium in the body is located in the bones. The remaining magnesium is found mostly in the intracellular fluid of cells throughout the body. Only a small percentage of magnesium is found in extracellular fluid. Magnesium in the bone can interact with calcium and phosphates to help increase the integrity of bones. The bones also serve as a reservoir or storage site for magnesium.

One thing that magnesium seems to do is to interact with the phosphates of ATP (see Figure 10.2). This adds stability to ATP and improves the ability of ATP to power cell operations. Many chemical reactions require the splitting of an ATP molecule to release the energy necessary to drive the reaction or cell activity. In fact, magnesium seems to be a vital factor in the proper functioning of more than 300 chemical reaction systems.

What happens if too little or too much magnesium is consumed?

Subtle alterations in blood magnesium content can affect the release of parathyroid hormone (PTH) and its activity. Further, a magnesium deficiency can negatively influence the ability of the cell membranes to maintain optimal sodium and potassium concentration differences across membranes. This is largely because magnesium is needed to stabilize ATP, which is the power source for pumping these ions across cell membranes. Thus, the proper function of excitable and other cells is jeopardized during magnesium deficiency.

Toxicity induced by a high dietary intake of magnesium can be thwarted by appropriately functioning kidneys.

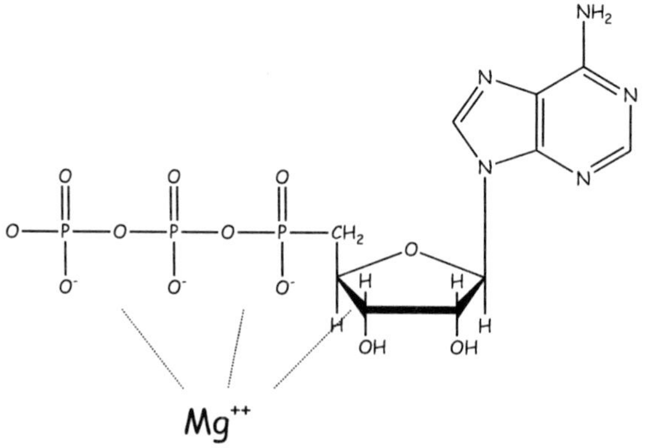

FIGURE 10.2. Because of its +2 charge, magnesium (Mg) has the ability to electrically interact with the phosphate tail of ATP (negative charge). This stabilizes ATP and allows it to be used more efficiently by cells.

Sulfur (S)

Sulfur is not really an essential nutrient but rather a vital component of essential nutrients. These nutrients include the amino acid methionine as well as biotin and thiamin. Therefore, the presence and actions of sulfur in the body is more of a reflection of what is going on with these substances rather than sulfur as an independent essential nutrient. Sulfur is also part of several food additives.

MINOR MINERALS FUNCTION AS COMPONENTS OF PROTEINS AND OTHER MOLECULES

Iron (Fe)

Iron is one of the most recognizable minerals in the body, although an adult may have a little less than a teaspoon's amount in his or her body. However, quantity should not be associated with importance as the effects of iron deficiency are tragic and severe. In animals, including humans, iron can be found as the central component of a very important molecule called *heme*. Heme is part of larger protein complexes that rank among the most important in the human body. One aspect that makes animals different from plants is the presence of heme. Plants do not have it.

What foods provide iron and what influences its absorption?

Iron is part of both animal and plant foods (see Table 10.8). The iron found in these foods exists in the form of either *heme* iron or *nonheme* iron. Animal foods (i.e., meats) contain both heme and nonheme iron. Meanwhile, plants and plant-derived foods contain only nonheme iron. The importance in the difference of these two forms of iron is largely in their efficiency of absorption. Nonheme iron is absorbed less efficiently (2 to 20 percent) in comparison to heme iron (25 to 35 percent). However, if the nonheme iron is part of a meal containing meat, fish, or poultry, its absorption can increase. Conversely, the presence of phytates and oxalates in some plant foods (vegetables) can interact with nonheme iron in the digestive tract and decrease its absorption (see Box 10.2). For this reason many nutritionists recommend that those people taking an iron-containing supplement should do so with a meal that has the least raw plant foods.

TABLE 10.8. Iron Content of Select Foods

Food	Iron (mg)
Meat and alternatives	
Liver (3 oz)	7.5
Round steak (3 oz)	3.0
Hamburger, lean (3 oz)	3.0
Baked beans (1/2 c)	3.0
Pork (3 oz)	2.7
White beans (1/2 c)	2.7
Soybeans (1/2 c)	2.5
Fish (3 oz)	1.0
Chicken (3 oz)	1.0
Fruits	
Prune juice (1/2 c)	4.5
Apricots, dried (1/2 c)	2.5
Prunes (5 medium)	2.0
Raisins (1/4 c)	1.3
Plums (3 medium)	1.1
Grains	
Breakfast cereal (1 c)*	4.0-18.0
Oatmeal (2 c)*	8.0
Bagel (1)	1.7
English muffin (1)	1.6
Bread, rye (1 slice)	1.0
Bread, whole wheat (1 slice)	0.8
Bread, white (1 slice)	0.6
Vegetables	
Spinach (1/2 c)	2.3
Lima beans (1/2 c)	2.2
Peas, black-eyed (1/2 c)	1.7
Peas (1/2 c)	1.6
Asparagus (1/2 c)	1.5

*Iron-fortified

For many people that meal is breakfast, which may also include citrus juice whose vitamin C may increase the absorption of nonheme iron.

Since the absorption efficiency of both forms of iron is low, it seems likely that the iron content of the body is primarily regulated at the point of absorption. This idea is reinforced by the fact that the efficiency of iron absorption increases during times of greater iron need, such as when iron stores are low. The efficiency of iron absorption also increases during periods of growth and pregnancy.

BOX 10.2. Factors Influencing the Efficiency of Iron Absorption

↑ **Absorption of Iron**
- Vitamin C at the same meal
- Normal stomach acid production
- Increased iron need (growth, pregnancy, poor status)
- Meat, fish, poultry at same meal

↓ **Absorption of Iron**
- Phytate, oxalates from plants
- Tannins such as from tea
- Decreased stomach acid production or the use of antacid medication

The RDA for adults ranges between 8 and 18 mg per day for men and women. Iron is the only essential nutrient for which the RDA is greater for adolescent and adult women than for their male counterparts. One of the most outstanding reasons for the higher RDA for females is iron loss during menstruation during childbearing years.

What does iron do in the body once it is absorbed?

As with other animals, iron is found in the cells as a part of heme and nonheme molecules. As mentioned, heme is an interesting molecule with iron situated at its core. In fact, iron seems to hold the whole molecule together (see Figure 10.3). Nonheme substances are mostly enzymes and iron storage molecules such as ferritin and hemosiderin.

Perhaps the most obvious function of iron is its involvement in the heme portion of hemoglobin. Of course, hemoglobin is a protein found in RBCs. The heme portion of hemoglobin binds O_2 so that it can be transported throughout the body in the blood. Since a healthy RBC may contain about 250 million hemoglobin molecules, each with the ability to bind four O_2, a single RBC could carry roughly one billion O_2 molecules. In the absence of iron, hemoglobin cannot be formed properly. This leads to less and less hemoglobin in the blood, which relates to decreased O_2 delivery to cells throughout the body.

A molecule similar to hemoglobin, called *myoglobin,* is found in muscle tissue. Similar to hemoglobin, myoglobin also binds O_2. This allows myoglobin to act as an O_2 reservoir in muscle fibers, which becomes readily available during exercise. When meat is eaten, which is just skeletal muscle of other mammals, much of the iron is derived from myoglobin. Also, because it is heme iron it will be better absorbed.

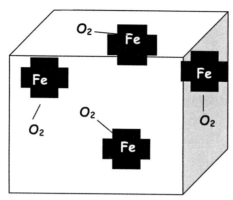

FIGURE 10.3. Red blood cells contain a lot of hemoglobin. There are four iron (Fe)-containing heme units found in hemoglobin. Iron holds the heme together as well as attaches it to the protein. In addition the Fe also binds O_2.

Iron is also a critical component of some of the molecules that form the electron-transport chain. Some of these molecules are called *cytochromes,* in which iron is again found as a component of heme. Therefore not only is iron important in delivering oxygen (hemoglobin) to cells for aerobic energy metabolism, it is also a key component of much of the aerobic ATP manufacturing machinery itself. Iron serves as part of an antioxidant enzyme called *catalase* and is part of many other metabolic enzymes as well. Iron is also fundamental in proper immune function.

What happens if too little iron is consumed?

A poor iron intake over time will result in a reduction of blood hemoglobin levels. *Anemia* is the medical term used to describe a condition whereby hemoglobin levels fall well below normal levels. Normal hemoglobin levels for men and women are less than 14 and 12 mg/100 mL of blood, respectively. In an anemic state (< 7-9 mg/100 mL) there is a decrease in the O_2 carrying capability of our blood. Less oxygen is able to reach cells and anemic people will often complain of lethargy as well as early fatigue when they exercise. Beyond oxygen transport in the blood, iron deficiency decreases the ability of cells to make ATP by aerobic means.

How can our body iron status be assessed?

Lower levels of iron in the body are indicated several ways. For the longest time we assessed hemoglobin levels and hematocrit (percent of blood that is RBCs) and used these as indicators of iron status. However, today we know that reductions in hemoglobin and hematocrit levels tend to occur later on as the body's iron status becomes more severely compromised. In the blood is an iron transport protein called transferrin. Transferrin has the capacity to pick up iron from tissues throughout the body. A good analogy would be a public transport system. A city can measure transportation capabilities based upon the number of buses driving around the city and the number of seats available on those buses. The amount of transferrin plus the potential (capacity) to bind iron are both used as indicators of iron status. Total iron binding capacity (TIBC) indicates the potential for iron transport above what is currently being transported on transferrin. For instance, if transferrin levels are somewhat normal yet the capacity to bind iron (TIBC) is relatively high, this suggests poor iron status. This is similar to having plenty of buses driving around but carrying fewer people than normal. The total people carrying capacity would be high.

Perhaps the most sensitive indicator of iron status is the level of ferritin in our blood. Ferritin is a large complex that stores iron in cells, such as in the liver. Therefore, the more iron in the tissues the more ferritin in the body. Now then, some of the ferritin seems to leak into the blood and can be used to gauge iron status in the body as it reflects tissue iron content. High levels of ferritin in the blood implies that more iron is in the body.

Can too much iron be consumed?

Recently, a fair amount of attention has been focused on what happens when there is too much iron in the body. For instance, researchers reported that men in Finland who have higher levels of ferritin in their blood were more likely to experience heart attacks in comparison to men with lower levels.

In support of the medical concern related to having too much iron in the body, people in certain sub-Saharan countries noted for drinking beer with a high iron content seem to develop cirrhosis of the liver beyond what would be expected from excessive alcohol consumption alone. Further evidence is genetic-based disorders in which iron absorption is dramatically enhanced. This can lead to an excessive body iron content in these people. The disorder is referred to as genetic-based *hemochromatosis* and is apparent in as many as 12 of every 1,000 people of European descent. This disorder is associated with severe liver disease and early death.

Zinc (Zn)

Zinc is one of the most active minerals in the body as it influences the functioning of hundreds of different enzymes. Although often overshadowed in the popular press by the likes of iron and chromium, lately zinc has been thrust into the limelight. Zinc supplements have been purported to reduce the length and severity of the common cold, which will be discussed.

What foods provide zinc?

In living things, zinc is more associated with amino acids and proteins. Therefore, it is logical to presume that animal foods, with their higher protein content, would be better zinc sources than plant foods. This is true. The best sources of zinc include organ meats, other red meats, and seafood (especially oysters and mollusks). Poultry, pork, milk and milk products, whole grains (especially germ and bran), and leafy and root vegetables are also respectable contributors of zinc (see Table 10.9). The RDA for adults is 8 to 11 mg of zinc.

Absorption of zinc from the digestive tract is not well understood. However, it does seem that many factors can influence how efficiently zinc is absorbed. For instance, zinc derived from meat boasts better absorption than zinc from plant sources. Zinc absorption from meat may actually be enhanced by certain amino acids, which would be present during simultaneous protein digestion. On the other hand, the efficiency of zinc absorption from plant foods seems to be lower which may in part be due to the presence of phytate, oxalates, and probably other substances (tannins) also found in many plants. The RDA for zinc takes into consideration the impact of various substances on zinc absorption.

What does zinc do in the body?

The distribution of zinc in the body may provide some indication as to its broad and extensive function. Zinc is found in all tissue of the

TABLE 10.9. Zinc Content of Select Foods

Foods	Zinc (mg)
Meats and alternatives	
Liver (3 oz)	4-5
Beef (3 oz)	4
Crab (1/2 c)	3-4
Lamb (3 oz)	3-4
Pork (3 oz)	2-3
Chicken (3 oz)	2
Grains	
Wheat germ (2 T)	2-3
Oatmeal, cooked (1 c)	1
Bran flakes (1 c)	1
Rice, brown, cooked (2 c)	~0.5
Rice, white (2 c)	~0.5
Legumes	
Dried beans, cooked (1/2 c)	1
Split peas, cooked (1/2 c)	1
Nuts and seeds	
Pecans (1/4 c)	2
Cashews (1/4 c)	1-2
Sunflower seeds (1/4 c)	1-2
Peanut butter (2 T)	~1
Milk and milk products	
Cheddar cheese (1 oz)	1
Milk, whole (1 c)	~1
American cheese (1 oz)	~1

body and is believed to be necessary for more than 200 different chemical reactions. Zinc largely functions as a necessary component of various enzymes, which would regulate all of those chemical reactions. In fact, the number of enzymes whose optimal function relies upon zinc is probably greater than the total number of enzymes that rely on all of the other trace elements combined. Zinc is involved with enzymes that affect body pH (carbonic anhydrase), alcohol metabolism (alcohol dehydrogenase), bone mineralization (alkaline phosphatase), protein digestion (carboxypeptidases), antioxidation (superoxide dismutase), and protein and nucleic acid metabolism (polymerases), not to forget heme production and immunity.

Can zinc supplements cure the common cold?

Although zinc supplements cannot cure the common cold, some evidence suggests that timely zinc supplements may reduce the severity and duration of a cold. The results of some clinical studies, but not all, have suggested that when people with a cold were provided zinc supplements their symptoms were less severe and they recovered more quickly than people not receiving the supplements. Most of the zinc tested was in the form of zinc gluconate lozenges; currently nasal sprays are also available.

Some scientists speculate that zinc might bind to the virus that causes the cold and decrease its ability to infiltrate cells. Because a virus is not a living thing in order for it to make new copies of itself, it must break into a living cell and use that cell's protein-making machinery to manufacture multiple copies of itself. This large-scale production of the virus allows it to spread. When the immune system catches up and the rate of destruction of the virus exceeds production, the virus is eliminated. This can take a week or so and the symptoms can be significant, as we all know.

It should be recognized that zinc supplements will not necessarily keep people from "catching a cold," and they should not be used preventively. Furthermore, not everyone will respond to zinc supplements so talking to a physician is recommended. Also, zinc supplements exceeding the RDA are not suggested as this can lead to a reduction in copper absorption.

What happens in zinc deficiency, and can zinc become toxic?

Zinc deficiency results in aberrations stemming from a decreased activity of zinc-dependent enzymes. These signs include stunted growth in children, abnormal bone growth and/or mineralization, delayed sexual maturation, decreased immune capacity, and poor wound healing.

Because of zinc's widespread function throughout cells, many people feel that zinc supplementation is a necessity. However, nutrition surveys have shown that most people consume adequate amounts of zinc. Complementing dietary zinc with a multivitamin/mineral supplement that contains zinc in an amount that does exceed the RDA probably does not pose a threat of toxicity. However, it should be recognized that copper absorption would decrease relative to an increase in zinc consumption. Furthermore, it is certainly possible to induce copper deficiency by consuming as little as three to ten times the RDA for zinc over several months. Because of the inverse relationship between dietary zinc and copper absorption, the utilization of zinc supplements is not recommended unless a physician has recognized a need. This is particularly true for people who use zinc supplements to treat the common cold. These supplements should not be continued beyond five to seven days.

One gram of zinc sulfate yields about 250 mg of zinc, which may induce nausea, vomiting, abdominal cramping, bloody diarrhea, and leave a persistent metallic taste in the mouth.

Copper (Cu)

Yes, copper is an essential nutrient. Although it brings to mind Abraham Lincoln's profile on the U. S. penny, copper is a very important mineral in many basic human functions. For instance, copper is needed to make collagen and it is a component of a powerful antioxidant enzyme.

What foods contain copper?

Like zinc, selenium, and other trace minerals, the amount of copper in foods is directly related to the conditions in which the plants were grown and/or animals raised. A soil rich in copper will increase the copper content of plants grown in that region. Thus, copper-rich soils produce copper-rich plants. This means then that when an animal grazes on those plants, they intake the copper. Also, copper-rich soils and rocks usually translate to copper-endowed water in streams and lakes.

The richest sources of copper include organ meats, shellfish, nuts, seeds, legumes, dried fruits, and certain vegetables such as spinach, peas, and potato varieties (see Table 10.10). Similar to the efficiency of absorption of several other minerals, copper absorption is also sensitive to the presence of other substances in the digestive tract. For instance, researchers have shown that substances such as vitamin C, fiber, and bile in excessive amounts can decrease the efficiency of copper absorption. Furthermore, increased consumption of zinc can decrease copper absorption, as mentioned previously.

TABLE 10.10. Copper Content of Select Foods

Food	Copper (mg)
Liver, beef (3 oz)	2-3
Cashews, dry roasted (1/4 c)	0.8
Black-eyed peas (1/2 c)	0.7
Molasses, blackstrap (2 T)	0.6
Sunflower seeds (1/4 c)	0.6
V8 drink (1 c)	0.5
Tofu, firm (1/2 c)	0.5
Beans, refried (1/2 c)	0.5
Cocoa powder (2 T)	0.4
Prunes, dried (10)	0.4
Salmon, baked (3 oz)	0.3
Pizza, cheese (1 slice)	0.1
Bread, whole wheat (1 slice)	0.1
Milk chocolate (1 oz)	0.1
Milk, 2% (1 c)	0.1

The current recommended intake for copper is 900 μg daily for adults. However, diet intake surveys have reported that the American population may not be meeting these recommendations.

What does copper do in the body?

Although a little bit of copper may be absorbed across the wall of the stomach, by and large most of the absorption takes place in the small intestine. The total amount of copper in an adult is only about .1 g. However, again we cannot confuse quantity with importance.

Copper is an essential component of many enzymes with various roles throughout the body. These enzymes are involved in iron metabolism (ceruloplasmin), antioxidation (superoxide dismutase), electron transport and ATP generation (cytochrome c oxidase) and the production of epinephrine, norepinephrine (dopamine β-hydrogenase), and the connective tissue protein collagen (lysyl oxidase).

The role of copper in iron metabolism is related to its transportation in the blood. A copper-containing enzyme is responsible for making sure iron is appropriate to hop aboard its primary transport protein in the blood. This transport protein is called transferrin. Without copper, iron is not efficiently transported to bones, which are responsible for making RBCs. At this time some research suggests that taking gram doses of vitamin C supplements for several months may reduce the activity of at least one copper-containing enzyme in our body.

What happens in copper deficiency, and can copper toxicity occur?

Because of copper's fundamental role in iron metabolism, copper deficiency can result in anemia. Scientists have also reported alterations in heart muscle tissue and function in animals fed diets low in copper. However, whether the same can be said for humans is not clear. Copper deficiency can alter white blood cell numbers in the blood as well as reduce immune functions.

A copper supplement containing copper sulfate (250 mg) yields about 64 mg of copper, which can result in nausea, vomiting, and diarrhea. Meanwhile, long-term use of large copper supplements may induce toxicity wherein the function of the liver, kidneys, and brain may become compromised. Wilson's disease is a rare genetic form of copper toxicity induced by increased copper storage.

Selenium (Se)

Although seemingly unknown by many for so long, selenium jumped into the spotlight a couple of decades ago when researchers identified that a mysterious type of heart disease in Asia was actually caused by selenium deficiency—another example of how a small amount of a mineral can have a huge impact on the normal functioning of the body.

What foods provide selenium?

Like many of the trace minerals, the quantity of selenium in foods is often a reflection of the soil content in which plants were grown and the animals grazed. Animal products, including seafood, seem to be better sources of dietary selenium than plants (see Table 10.11). The RDA for adults is 55 μg selenium.

What does selenium do in the body?

Selenium is absorbed well from our digestive tract. Therefore, absorption may not be the primary site of body selenium regulation. Se-

TABLE 10.11. Selenium Content of Select Foods

Food	Selenium (μg)
Snapper, baked (3 oz)	148
Halibut, baked (3 oz)	113
Salmon, baked (3 oz)	70
Scallops, steamed (3 oz)	70
Clams, steamed (20)	52
Oysters, raw (1/4 c)	35
Molasses, blackstrap (2 T)	25
Sunflower seeds (1/4 c)	25
Granola (1 c)	23
Ground beef (3 oz)	22
Chicken, baked (3 oz)	17
Bread, whole wheat (1 slice)	16
Egg (1)	12
Milk, 2% (1 c)	6

lenium contributes about 15 mg to the total weight of an adult. Although many functions have been suggested for selenium, only one or possibly two are clear at this time.

Selenium is a necessary component of an antioxidant enzyme called *glutathione peroxidase*. Glutathione peroxidase inactivates free-radical substances such as hydrogen peroxide and organic peroxides. Similar to other free radicals, these substances will lead either directly or indirectly to oxidative damage in cells. Since glutathione peroxidase is a water-soluble molecule, its antioxidant activities will usually take place in the watery portion of the cells rather than in and around cell membranes like vitamin E. However, the peroxides that glutathione peroxidase inactivate typically travel to and assault cell membranes. In fact, selenium and vitamin E seem to enjoy a co-protective function against oxidative damage to cell membranes. This means that having proper selenium status can moderately compensate for a reduced status of vitamin E and vice versa.

Selenium also appears to be incorporated into an enzyme (deiodinase) that is involved in iodide metabolism. This function of selenium is still unclear and scientists are currently engaged in trying to understand its function better. It appears that this selenium-containing enzyme helps convert the less potent form of thyroid hormone, thyroxine (T_4), to the more active form, triiodothyronine (T_3), in certain organs.

What happens in selenium deficiency, and can
too much be consumed?

Selenium deficiency has been determined to be the cause of Keshan disease. The major medical problem associated with Keshan disease is an enlargement and abnormal functioning of the heart and eventual heart failure. The disease was observed in discrete regions of Asia where the selenium content of the soil is extremely low. The people within this region relied exclusively on crops and livestock grown in that area for food yet both of these food sources had very low selenium contents. Keshan disease is preventable with selenium supplementation. On the other hand, selenium intakes greater than 750 µg/day over time can produce toxic alterations such as hair and nail loss, fatigue, nausea and vomiting, and a hindrance of proper protein manufacturing.

Manganese (Mn)

Similar to zinc, manganese is also involved in the proper functioning of numerous enzymes. However, manganese still struggles for recognition.

What foods provide manganese?

Whole-grain cereals, fruits and vegetables, legumes, nuts, tea, and leafy vegetables are good food sources of manganese. Animal foods are generally poor contributors of manganese. Additional substances in plants, such as fiber, phytate, and oxalate along with excessive calcium, phosphorus, and iron, can decrease manganese absorption. The RDA for manganese for adults ranges between 1.8 and 2.3 mg/day.

What does manganese do in the body?

Manganese is involved with several general functions in the cells. First, manganese can interact with specific enzymes to increase their activity. These manganese-activated enzymes are involved in many operations, including protein digestion and the making of glucose from certain amino acids and lactate (gluconeogenesis). Second, manganese is a component of many enzymes. These enzymes are engaged in many activities including urea formation, glucose formation, and antioxidation. Last, manganese may be involved in the activity of some hormones.

What happens if too little or too much manganese is consumed?

Manganese deficiency in humans is rare. However, nausea, vomiting, dermatitis, decreased growth of hair and nails, and changes in hair color can result from a deficiency. Manganese toxicity is also rare, although miners inhaling manganese-rich dust can experience Parkinson's-like symptoms.

Iodide (I)

Many people can recall iodine being applied to cuts and scrapes as children. Iodide is like chloride in that it is most comfortable in nature after it has acquired an extra electron and becomes negatively charged (I^-).

What foods contain iodide?

The iodide content of foods is mostly related to the soil content in which plants were grown and/or the iodide content of any fertilizers used to cultivate the soil. Furthermore, the iodide content in drinking water usually reflects the iodide content of the rocks and soils through which the water runs or is maintained. Seafood is typically a better source of iodide than freshwater fish (see Table 10.12). Dairy foods may be a fair source of iodide, but the iodide content of cows' milk reflects either the iodide content of the cows' feed and/or the soil content of their grazing region. Iodide deficiency for the most part has been eradicated from many regions of the world including the United States, where iodide is added to salt. Check your salt label for "iodized salt." The RDA for adults is 150 µg iodide daily.

What does iodide do in the body?

Iodide is one of the largest atoms found in the body, yet it appears to have only one function. Iodide is a key component of thyroid hormone, which is made in the thyroid gland located in the neck. Thyroid hormone is constructed from iodide and the amino acid tyrosine.

TABLE 10.12. Iodide Content of Select Foods

Food	Iodide (μg)
Salt, iodized (1 t)	400
Haddock (3 oz)	104-145
Cottage cheese (1/2 c)	26-71
Shrimp (3 oz)	21-37
Egg (1)	18-26
Cheddar cheese (1 oz)	5-23
Ground beef (3 oz)	8

Thus, by way of thyroid hormone, iodide has a significant impact upon body function.

Thyroid hormone is actually two substances: thyroxine (T_4) and triiodothyronine (T_3). Thyroid hormone affects most cells in the body, perhaps with the exception of the adult brain, testes, spleen, uterus, and the thyroid gland itself. Thyroid hormone promotes the activities associated with glucose breakdown and general energy metabolism and heat production. Since a higher blood thyroid hormone concentration increases metabolic rate, thyroid hormone was once prescribed to morbidly obese people. However, the effects of thyroid hormone are not only limited to increasing cell metabolism, and deleterious side effects limited its use for this purpose. Therapeutic thyroid hormone therapy also affects blood pressure and heart activity, as well as produces nausea, sweating, diarrhea, anxiety, headaches, and insomnia. Today, thyroid hormone is prescribed mostly to treat hypothyroidism, a condition in which the thyroid gland fails to produce adequate thyroid hormone. During the growing years thyroid hormone is very important because it promotes growth and maturation of the skeleton, the central nervous system, and the reproductive organs.

What happens in iodide deficiency?

A deficiency of iodide limits the ability of the thyroid gland to make adequate thyroid hormone. During childhood, an iodide deficiency can result in poor growth, poor maturing of organs, and mental deficits. A striking characteristic of iodide deficiency is an enlargement of the thyroid gland which is commonly referred to as *goiter.*

Treatment of goiter usually begins with iodide-rich foods including iodized salt, which will shrink the goiter with time but not necessarily correct any developmental problems (growth and mental aptitude) in children. Before the widespread use of iodized salt, various regions of the American Midwest were referred to as the "goiter belt" due to a low soil iodide content and decreased availability of iodide-rich fish.

Certain foods contain substances called *goitrogens* that appear to block iodide entry into the thyroid gland. Foods containing goitrogens include broccoli, kale, cauliflower, rutabaga, turnips, Brussels sprouts, and mustard greens. However, we probably do not eat enough of these vegetables to pose a threat. Routine blood tests include T_3 and T_4 concentrations thus providing a screening tool for thyroid deficiency or other thyroid hormone-impacting diseases.

Fluorine (F)

In nature, the element fluorine exists as a negatively charged atom or ion. Thus, similar to iodide (iodine) and chloride (chlorine), we commonly refer to fluorine as *fluoride* (F⁻). Fluoride salt (NaF) is routinely added to toothpaste.

What are fluoride sources in the human diet?

Most foods are poor sources of fluoride and probably should not be used exclusively to meet the human body's needs. However, the process of adding fluoride to drinking water (*fluoridation*) has greatly improved general fluoride consumption. However, the decision to use fluoride is not federal; it is regulated county by county in the United States. The RDA for fluoride for adults is 3 to 4 mg daily.

What does fluoride do in the body?

Earlier in this century it was recognized that people living in regions of the United States where the fluoride content in their water supply was relatively high had a much lower incidence of dental caries. From this it was realized that fluoride is important to protect the teeth against the development of cavities. This led to the widespread fluoridation of drinking water. Fluoride may function in part by associating with hydroxyapatite in teeth and, to a lesser degree, bone.

What happens if too much fluoride is consumed?

Although inadequate fluoride consumption is associated with greater dental caries, there is also reason for concern if too much fluoride is ingested. Fluoride seems to be very efficiently absorbed from the digestive tract regardless of the amount consumed. Even though excessive fluoride in the body is removed in the urine, humans can overwhelm this function by ingesting larger quantities of supplemental fluoride. Fluoride toxicity is called *fluorosis* and problems such as alterations in bones, teeth, and possibly excitable cells may result. Mottling of teeth is evidence of dental fluorosis in children.

Taking gram doses of fluoride, 5 to 10 g of sodium fluoride, can lead to subsequent nausea, vomiting, and a decrease in body pH (acidosis). Furthermore, irregular heart activity and death may also result.

Chromium (Cr)

Chromium has received a considerable amount of attention in recent years as supplemental chromium is purported to increase lean body mass and reduce body fat. Also, chromium supplementation has been suggested as a possible benefit for people diagnosed with diabetes mellitus.

What foods provide chromium?

Egg yolks, whole grains, and meats are good sources of chromium (see Table 10.13). Dairy products are not a particularly good source of chromium. Plants grown in chromium-rich soils may also make a significant contribution to the human diet. Many multivitamin/mineral supplements include chromium. The ESADDI for chromium is 20 to 35 µg per day.

What does chromium do in the body?

In the human body, chromium is involved in the regulation of blood glucose levels. Chromium seems to increase the activity of insulin, therefore reducing the amount of insulin required to maintain normal levels of glucose in the blood. Scientists believe that chromium is a key component of a molecule or complex of molecules called *glucose tolerance factor* (GTF). Although it is questionable

TABLE 10.13. Chromium Content of Select Foods

Food	Chromium (μg)
Meats	
Turkey ham (3 oz)	10.4
Ham (3 oz)	3.6
Beef cubes (3 oz)	2.0
Chicken (3 oz)	0.5
Grain products	
Waffle (1)	6.7
English muffin (1)	3.6
Bagel, egg (1)	2.5
Rice, white (1 c)	1.2
Bread, whole wheat (1 slice)	1.0
Fruits and vegetables	
Broccoli (1/2 c)	11.0
Grape juice (1/2 c)	7.5
Potatoes, mashed (1 c)	2.7
Orange juice (1 c)	2.2
Lettuce, shredded (1 c)	1.8
Apple, unpeeled (1 c)	1.4

whether chromium may have application to diabetes mellitus in people with good chromium status, scientists generally agree that poor chromium status may worsen type 2 diabetes mellitus. Therefore, those people diagnosed with type 2 diabetes mellitus should make sure that their diet provides adequate chromium either through foods or a supplement containing chromium.

What happens during chromium deficiency and toxicity?

Chromium deficiency can result in *glucose intolerance,* which is an inability to reduce blood glucose levels properly after a meal and throughout the day. Conversely, little is known about the toxic effects of chromium in larger doses. Some scientists have reported that supplements of as much as 800 μg daily are safe, while others question as to whether excessive chromium consumed chronically would build up in body tissues such as bone, and have milder long-term effects.

Vanadium (V)

What foods provide vanadium?

Although still only containing nanograms to micrograms of vanadium, breakfast cereals, canned fruit juices, fish sticks, shellfish, vegetables (especially mushrooms, parsley, and spinach), sweets, wine, and beer are good sources. A dietary requirement for vanadium has yet to be established, but 10 to 25 µg of vanadium per day may be appropriate.

What does vanadium do in the body?

Vanadium is present in trace concentrations in most organs and tissues throughout the body and has long been questioned in regard to essentiality. However, it is important to realize that the presence of a substance in the body does not necessarily indicate essentiality. Nevertheless, researchers have discerned that the absence of vanadium from animal diets reduces their growth rate, infancy survival, and levels of hematocrit, despite the inability of researchers to identify specific functions for vanadium.

On the other hand, vanadium administered in higher quantities exerts numerous effects upon metabolism. However, these activities cannot be considered vanadium dependent because they are observed only when vanadium is administered in excessive amounts. In this manner, vanadium acts as a pharmaceutical agent, not necessarily a nutrient. One such effect receiving much research attention is vanadium's ability to mimic the activity of insulin. Vanadium appears to be able to affect glucose metabolism in a manner similar to insulin. Promising research with diabetic animals has suggested that vanadium therapy may control high blood glucose levels (hyperglycemia). However, the application to hyperglycemia in humans is still questionable.

What do we know about vanadium deficiency and toxicity?

As mentioned, vanadium deficiency may result in reductions in growth rate, infancy survival, and hematocrit. Further, vanadium deficiency may alter the activity of the thyroid gland and its ability to utilize iodide properly.

Signs of vanadium toxicity such as a green tongue, diarrhea, abdominal cramping, and alterations in mental functions have been reported in people ingesting greater than 10 mg of vanadium daily for extended periods of time.

Boron (B)

What foods provide boron?

Fruits, leafy vegetables, nuts, and legumes are rich sources of boron, while meats are among the poorer sources. Beer and wine also make a respectable contribution to boron intake. Although not established to date, human requirement for boron is probably about 1 mg daily.

What does boron do in the body?

In the human body boron is found in relatively great concentration in bone. Although its exact involvement remains a mystery at this time, boron seems to affect certain factors that impact calcium metabolism. This is an area that has been receiving more and more attention as scientists attempt to better understand bone diseases.

What happens during boron deficiency and toxicity?

Boron deficiency results in an increased urinary loss of calcium and magnesium, assumedly derived from storage primarily in bone. Conversely, taking large amounts of boron may induce nausea, vomiting, lethargy, and an increased loss of riboflavin.

Molybdenum (Mo)

What foods provide molybdenum in the human diet?

Most of the foods humans eat contain a respectable amount of molybdenum, which ultimately reflects the soil content in which the plants were grown. Organ and other meats, legumes, cereals, and grains are among better sources of molybdenum. Diets high in molybdenum decrease copper absorption and also increase copper loss in the urine. The RDA for adults is 45 µg of molybdenum daily.

What does molybdenum do in the body?

Molybdenum seems to be active in the cells as part of a molecule that interacts with a few specific enzymes and makes them active.

These enzymes are involved in the metabolism of the sulfur-containing amino acids (methionine and cysteine) and the metabolism of pyrimidine and purines which are building blocks for nucleic acids (i.e., DNA and RNA).

What happens if too much or too little molybdenum is consumed?

Because of molybdenum's widespread availability in the human diet, a deficiency is somewhat unlikely. However, people receiving intravenous (IV) feedings for several months are at risk. In contrast, molybdenum is fairly nontoxic. Molybdenum is involved in the breakdown of purines to a waste product called uric acid. Uric acid is removed from the body in urine, and theoretically there is a greater risk for developing kidney stones formed by excessive uric acid. Excessive uric acid production may also increase the risk of developing *gout*, which is characterized by recurrent inflammation of joint regions and deposition of uric acid in those areas.

Cobalt (Co)

Cobalt is an essential part of vitamin B_{12}. Because vitamin B_{12} cannot be made in the body, independent cobalt is not an essential nutrient.

Nickel (Ni)

What foods contribute nickel to the diet?

In general, plants are more concentrated sources of nickel than are animal sources. Nuts are the most concentrated sources while grains, cured meats, and vegetables offer respectable amounts. Fish, milk, and eggs are recognized as poorer sources of nickel. The absorption of nickel from the digestive tract is probably affected by varying the amounts of copper, iron, and zinc, and perhaps vice versa. Adult requirements for nickel are most likely about 35 µg daily although the RDA has yet to be established.

What does nickel do in the body?

The possible essentiality of nickel was not seriously considered until about twenty years ago. Defining exact roles for nickel in the body remains somewhat elusive. However, nickel does seem to be involved in the breakdown of the amino acids leucine, valine, and isoleucine (branch-chain amino acids) and odd chain length fatty acids. Nickel research is relatively young and more clear-cut roles for nickel will probably emerge in the next decade.

Arsenic (Ar)

What foods are a source of arsenic?

As a natural constituent of the earth's crust, arsenic can be found in most soils and is taken up by plants grown in that area. However, the arsenic content of foods can also be affected by the arsenic in pesticides and airborne pollutants. Among the most concentrated sources of arsenic are sea animals (fish, shellfish). Dietary requirements for arsenic have not been established, although 12 to 15 µg daily is probably sufficient.

What does arsenic do in the body?

Although arsenic has long been regarded as an unwanted substance, it may be an essential component after all. Although its involvement has not been clearly identified, arsenic is most likely important in the metabolism of two amino acids, methionine and arginine.

What happens in arsenic deficiency and toxicity?

Arsenic deficiencies have resulted in a reduced growth rate in animals. Arsenic deficiency may also reduce conception rates and increase the likelihood of death in newborns. Perhaps no other constituent of the body conjures a stronger notion of toxicity than arsenic. It certainly is the only nutrient that can be fatal in milligram amounts. Arsenic, in the form of arsenic trioxide, can be fatal at doses greater than 0.76 to 1.95 mg.

Silicon (Si)

What foods provide silicon?

Not much is really known about the silicon content of various foods. Plant sources, including high-fiber cereal grains and root vegetables, seem to be better sources than animal sources. The RDA for silicon has yet to be established.

What does silicon do in the body?

Silicon, in the form of quartz, is one of the most abundant minerals on the planet. However, silicon makes only a minuscule contribution to human body weight. Silicon seems to be involved in the health of connective tissue. In bone, silicon seems to improve the rates of both bone mineralization and growth. The manufacturing of collagen, a predominant protein found in connective tissue, relies upon an adequate supply of the nonessential amino acid proline and a slightly modified form of proline called hydroxyproline. Silicon is probably required for the optimal production of both proline and hydroxyproline. Silicon is also important for the manufacturing of other proteins and substances vital to proper connective tissue.

What happens in silicon deficiency and toxicity?

Silicon deficiency can result in poor growth and development of bone, including decreased mineralization. Not much is known at this time regarding silicon toxicity.

Chapter 11

Exercise and Sports Nutrition

To move around is a fundamental part of human existence. Humans move to gather and prepare food, protect themselves, and reproduce. Scientists refer to this movement as physical activity or exercise. Meanwhile, exercise is viewed by the general public as the act of moving the body (as parts or as a whole) at various speeds and for various duration of time, and against a desired resistance. The exercise is planned, and there is a desired outcome in mind. To the public, the terms *exercise* and *workout* are synonymous.

Regular exercise can provide numerous benefits. Depending upon the type of exercise, these benefits can include

- improved cardiovascular health,
- a tool for weight management and changing body composition,
- a positive impact on bone density,
- a vehicle for relaxation and social interaction, and
- improved self-image.

THE INTENSITY AND DURATION OF EXERCISE DETERMINES THE ADAPTATION

What is exercise training?

When we exercise regularly the muscles that are involved can adapt to be more efficient in performing the exercise task. This is a "training effect" or "adaptation" that is visually obvious for weight trainers as the targeted muscles enlarge to provide more strength and power. Their exercises will involve near maximal or maximal intensity for very short durations. Meanwhile, in regular exercise, consisting of lower intensity tasks performed for longer durations, muscle will adapt to become more inclined to aerobic energy metabolism, as will be explained shortly.

The most important aspects of training are the *intensity* and *duration* of the exercise. The relationship between these factors is what determines the nature of the associated adaptation. Aspects of genetic predisposition also will influence the degree of adaptation as well as the inclination toward a certain type of training. More on the genetics of training and achievement in sports soon enough.

So then, it is intensity and duration that is planned for in training programs. Intensity refers to the level of exertion. For instance, lifting a weight that results in muscular fatigue after just a few repetitions or "reps" of an exercise is pretty high with respect to intensity. So too would be an all-out running or cycling sprint where fatigue occurs in a minute or so. Basically, the higher the intensity, the shorter the possible duration of the exercise. To reach such a high level of intensity, exercise often includes resistance against an otherwise simple movement of a muscle group or related groups. Examples of resistance training include weight training or running on an incline (e.g., running on hills or a graded treadmill) or cycling (e.g., cycling uphill or an exercise bike with variable resistance). It is the level of the resistance that dictates the necessary intensity. Higher intensity and muscular fatigue will be associated with muscle adaptations that will allow for greater strength and power. In this case, muscles should enlarge or "hypertrophy."

Conversely, running, cycling, or other exercises performed at a low or moderate intensity might exercise for a half to one hour or longer. Sustained lower intensity exercise is often called endurance training, as the exercise is endured over an extended period of time. It is also referred to as cardiovascular training as adaptations can include the development of a more powerful heart and more blood vessels in our heart and skeletal muscle.

Training Intensity Line

Mass, Strength, and Power Adaptation	← higher ——————— lower →	Aerobic and Cardiovascular Adaptation

In the "training intensity line" diagram, it is the intensity level that will be the primary determinant of the nature of adaptation. This means that although some sports are associated with a certain type of adaptation, it is not an absolute. For instance, weight training can be more aerobic and cardiovascular if the weights (resistance) are not heavy enough and the number of reps is very high. Running and biking are often associated with more aerobic and cardiovascular adaptations, but it is easy for runners or cyclists to train for greater strength and power by including more resistance in their training. Check out <www.athletefactory.net> for more on this subject.

MUSCLE IS FUELED BY CARBOHYDRATES, FATTY ACIDS, AND A SMALL AMOUNT OF PROTEIN

What fuels muscle activity?

Muscle contraction is fueled by ATP, which is generated by both anaerobic and aerobic energy metabolism. Because ATP is found in low concentrations in all cells of the body, these ATP-generating mechanisms must be increased with the onset of activity in an attempt to meet ATP demands of working muscle cells. This means that muscle cells need to stoke up those chemical reaction pathways that break down carbohydrate and fat for ATP generation (see Figure 2.8). Muscle cells have a little stored carbohydrate (glycogen) and fat and also receive glucose and fatty acids from the blood. So increased blood delivery to the exercising muscle delivers not only needed O_2 but also fuel.

Does creatine help power skeletal muscle efforts during exercise?

Another power source for working muscle is *creatine phosphate.* Creatine is a substance found mostly in skeletal muscle cells, but it is also found in heart muscle cells and brain. When ATP is abundant in these cells, such as during periods of rest for body muscle, a phosphate group is transferred to creatine. This forms creatine phosphate, which is a rapid ATP-regenerating source (see Figure 11.1). When ATP is used to power muscle contractions, the phosphate of creatine phosphate can be transferred to ADP to regenerate ATP. This involves only one chemical reaction and can happen very rapidly.

This regeneration of ATP from creatine phosphate is especially important for quick burst activities such as sprinting and weight train-

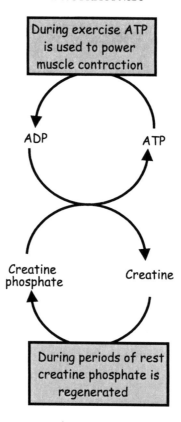

FIGURE 11.1. Muscle cell contraction is powered by ATP. The energy released by ATP allows myosin to pull actin filaments toward the center of the sarcomere. The net effect of all the sarcomere contraction results in the shortening of the whole muscle cell. Carbohydrate and fat are mostly used to regenerate ATP as it is being used.

ing. However, this system is extremely limited and will last only a few seconds. Yet this function helps muscle cells bridge the gap between the rapid depletion of ATP at the onset of exercise and the point when a muscle cell's other ATP-generating operations are appropriately stoked up. Then when the muscle cell is resting (in between sets or between sprints) creatine phosphate is regenerated to prepare for the next exercise effort. Later in this chapter supplementation practices involving creatine will be discussed.

MUSCLE CELLS ARE NOT ALL THE SAME

Are there different types of muscle fibers?

You will remember that scientists refer to skeletal muscle cells as fibers because they are thin and long. In fact, some muscle fibers can extend the entire length of a muscle group, such as in the biceps. That is several inches! In addition to their unique design, skeletal muscle cells are not all the same. In fact, humans are blessed with more than one type of skeletal muscle cell, which vary in performance and metabolic properties (see Table 11.1). This allows us to efficiently perform a broad range of activities or sports that vary in nature. This includes sports that are longer duration/lower intensity and short duration/higher intensity.

Scientists will often group muscle cells into two general categories or "types" (Type I and II). Type II muscle fibers are often sub-classified as IIa, IIb, and IIc. For this text, it is enough to distinguish between the two main types. Skeletal muscle is actually bundles of a mixture of Type I and II muscle fibers. In fact, the average person will tend to have about a 50/50 mixture of Types I and II muscle fibers. Meanwhile, highly successful athletes tend to have a significant imbalance one way or the other which, as will soon be dicussed, will allow them to excel at a particular sport (see Photos 11.1 through 11.3).

What is the nature of Type I muscle fibers?

Type I fibers (sometimes called "slow-twitch" [ST] or "slow-oxidative" [SO] fibers) are better designed for prolonged exercise performed at a lower intensity. In comparison to Type II fibers, Type I fibers will have more mitochondria and rely more heavily on the

TABLE 11.1. Performance and Metabolic Properties of Muscle Fibers

Type I Muscle Fibers	Type II Muscle Fibers
Develop force more slowly than Type II muscle fibers	Develop force more quickly (more powerful)
Have more mitochondria and capillaries and thus are more aerobic	Have fewer mitochondria and capillaries and thus are more anaerobic
Generate very little lactic acid (lactate)	Generate more lactate
Do not fatigue quickly	Fatigue quickly

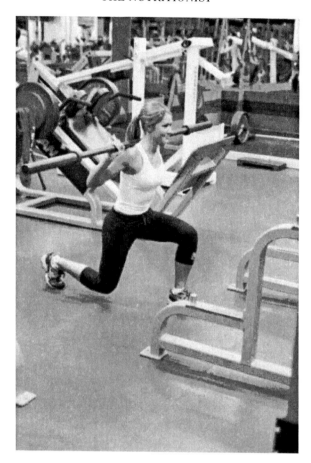

PHOTO 11.1. Lunges develop leg muscle.

aerobic generation of ATP. The primary energy molecules used to generate ATP in these muscle cells will be fatty acids and glucose. Since ATP production in mitochondria requires oxygen, proper function of these muscle fibers is very dependent upon O_2 supply via the blood. Luckily, Type I muscle cells always seem to have many capillaries around them to deliver O_2-endowed blood. In addition, Type I fibers contain a substance called myoglobin. As previously mentioned, myoglobin is an iron-containing protein that binds O_2 and serves as an O_2 reserve for these cells during exercise.

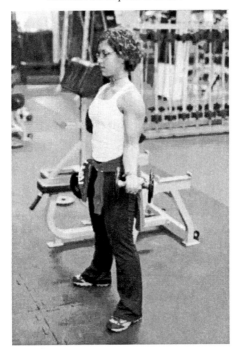

PHOTO 11.2(a)

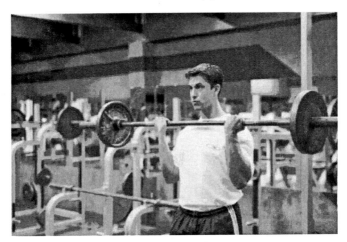

PHOTO 11.2(b)

PHOTO 11.2 (a) and (b). Curls performed with dumbbells (a) and barbells (b) can develop arm muscle.

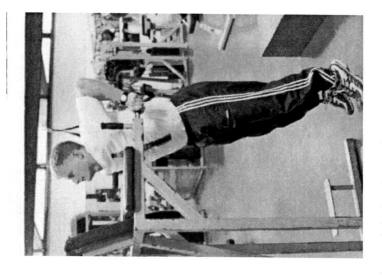

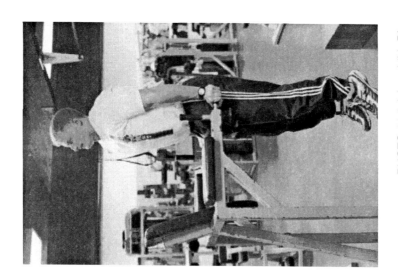

PHOTO 11.3 (a) and (b). Dips can work muscle in the chest and arms.

What about Type II muscle cells?

Type II muscle fibers (sometimes called fast twitch [FT] or fast-glycolytic [FG] fibers) can execute a much faster speed of contraction than Type I muscle fibers. This is to say that Type II muscle fibers are designed to generate force more rapidly, thereby allowing them to be more powerful as they will allow a job to be performed in a shorter amount of time. Work relates the amount of force necessary to move something (e.g., a weight) a certain distance—hence the term "work-out." Power is concerned with how long it took to perform the work. Mathematically:

$$\text{Work} = \text{Force} \times \text{Distance}$$
$$\text{Power} = \text{Work} \div \text{Time}$$

Type II muscle fibers are relatively limited in their ability to generate ATP by aerobic means. So, when these cells break down glucose to pyruvate and generate a couple ATP in the process, much of the pyruvate that is formed will then be converted to lactic acid (lactate). This is because these muscle cells have less mitochondria and receive less O_2 as they are served by fewer blood vessels (see Table 11.1 and Figure 8.3).

How does the brain know which type of muscle cells to use for different sports?

This is a no-brainer for the brain. This is because the brain will always call upon Type I muscle fibers first and then Type II. The major factor will be the required force to perform the exercise. For instance, when an exercise requires less force (e.g., jogging, fast walking, casual cycling) the brain will for the most part call upon Type I muscle fibers (see Figure 11.2). However, as the necessary force to perform an exercise increases (e.g., sprinting, weightlifting), the brain will also call upon Type II muscle fibers to generate force to support the force generated by Type I fibers.

Calling upon Type II fibers is sort of a win/lose situation for performance. It is a winner in that it will allow us to generate a lot more force to perform an exercise. However, it is a loser in that the exercise will become fatiguing as more lactic acid is generated in Type II fibers. This is why 5K runners cannot sprint the entire race. What they

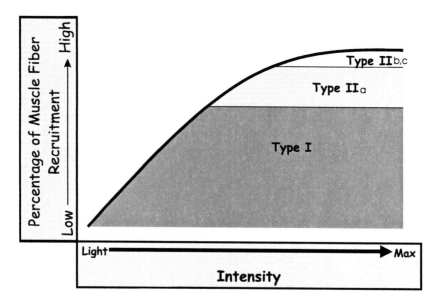

FIGURE 11.2. The order of recruitment of muscle fibers begins with our Type I fibers for lower intensity exercise (i.e., walking, casual cycling). Then as more force is needed, Type II fibers are also called upon (weight training, sprinting).

will do is run at the highest level they are able to, but that also keeps them from fatiguing before the end of the race. Their brains will call upon enough Type II muscle fibers to generate more force to allow them to run faster, however not enough Type II muscle fibers to generate critical levels of lactic acid that would cause fatigue before they cross the finish line.

Do successful athletes have an imbalance of muscle fiber type?

As mentioned, successful athletes seem to have an imbalance in muscle fiber types that favors excelling in a sport of a related nature. For instance, successful sprinters often have a higher percentage of Type II fibers, allowing them to generate more force in a very brief period of time. This then allows them to be more powerful, generate more speed, and complete a sprint distance more quickly. Conversely, successful endurance athletes tend to have a greater percentage of Type I muscle fibers. This allows them to generate more force through aerobic energy systems in muscle cells. They can perform at a higher intensity before they generate critical amounts of lactic acid.

Often the question is asked whether top athletes are born or bred. The answer is both, but probably more of the former than the latter. Most very successful athletes are born with the propensity to excel physically at a particular sport and training can then improve that potential. This is mostly true for sports that are endurance based or involve extreme power, as mentioned.

Can training allow muscle fibers to change type?

We do know that training results in changes in muscle metabolism which may make us think that it is possible for Type I fibers to change into Type II fibers and vice versa. However, this probably is not the case. For instance, endurance training can lead to changes associated with Type II muscle fibers that will make them more aerobic. The fibers will adapt to have an increased ability to generate ATP by using O_2. However, they will probably never really adapt to the point where we would classify them as Type I. Oppositely, we all know that resistance training (e.g., weight lifting) improves the strength and power of a muscle group. Although it would be logical to think that half of this effect might be related to adaptations in Type I muscle fibers—as though they are being transformed into Type II muscle fibers—surprisingly this is not the case either. In fact, as the muscle group grows in size, most of the growth is related to enlargement of Type II fibers.

RESISTANCE TRAINING IS HARD WORK BUT WELL WORTH THE EFFORT

Although weight lifting has long been associated with bodybuilding and power sports such as football and field events (shot put, discus, etc.), it is more popular with the general population than ever before. Clearly, resistance training can favorably influence bone density and increase the amount of muscle attached to the skeleton. Thus resistance training can reduce the risk of bone-related disorders such as osteoporosis and improve energy expenditure, reduce body fat content, and improve self-image.

Today there are numerous options for resistance training beyond free weights. Many people use pulley machines and resilient resistance materials such as bows (e.g., Bowflex) and elastic bands (e.g., Soloflex). Of course, in a pinch gravity alone may provide enough resistance. For instance, people accustomed to a regular workout will often do a few sets of push-ups on the floor if no gym equipment is available.

How does weight lifting increase muscle mass?

The goal of most weight lifters is to increase the size of the muscles that are targeted. Muscle mass development through weight training hinges on the "overload" principle. The use of weights places a greater than normal stress (load) upon the challenged muscle fibers. The overload stimulates the muscle to grow primarily by increasing the size (hypertrophy) of the overloaded muscle fibers. This means that the muscle cells get thicker. Therefore, as a biceps muscle enlarges from doing dumbbell curls it is really a reflection of an increase in size of the overloaded muscle fibers within that muscle. Although growth may occur in both Type I and Type II fibers, as mentioned, it is believed to be more significant in the challenged Type II fibers.

To overload a muscle, three sets of six to ten repetitions is probably adequate to stimulate growth. More sets will certainly provide a greater rate of hypertrophy, within reason. To begin, you need to estimate your "one-repetition maximum" (1-RM). This will be the maximum weight you can overcome to complete one repetition. Certainly it is not recommended that you try to determine your 1-RM by experimenting with heavy weights. You can experiment with light weights and determine the best weight for an exercise (e.g., shoulder press, bench press, curls) with which you are able to do about five to ten repetitions. This should be about 80 to 85 percent of your 1-RM.

As you continue to train that muscle, over time you will probably find it necessary to increase the weight. This is an indicator that your muscle is adapting and getting stronger. Initially, some of this adaptation is merely your muscle becoming more efficient in the exercise. However, overall most of the improvement in strength will be because the muscle is getting bigger.

How much rest do overloaded muscles need?

When you engage in resistance training you are making great demands upon your muscles. Therefore, the trained muscle should be given adequate time to rest and recover, both during the workout and after. Depending on the intensity of the set, muscle will need about 1 to 3 minutes to rest between sets. As muscle contracts it temporarily pinches blood vessels and hinders blood flow within that muscle. This not only decreases nutrient and O_2 delivery to working muscle fibers but also decreases the removal of waste such as lactate and CO_2. During a set the limited stores of ATP and creatine phosphate are rapidly depleted. Giving muscle a break between sets allows for the blood to bring more nutrients and oxygen and remove waste and at the same time also allows for regeneration of ATP and creatine phosphate.

If a muscle is trained hard it is generally recommended to rest a muscle for at least forty-eight hours before overloading it again. This allows muscle to recover and adapt. Often people will train the same muscles on Mondays, Wednesdays, and Fridays or Tuesdays, Thursdays, and Saturdays and rest the muscle in between. If a muscle is trained very hard in a given workout by doing extra sets, that individual may train that muscle only two times a week or every five days or even once a week.

Recovery and repair processes include those that prepare muscle to perform efficiently again. This includes: reducing the lactate level of the muscle fibers worked, which may not take that long; repleting of glycogen stores, which can take hours; and repairing cellular damage in the trained muscle fibers, which can also take hours or even a day or so. Adaptation, on the other hand, refers to those processes designed to allow the muscle to be better prepared to work again (see Box 11.1). This will include a net production of muscle proteins that will support contraction the next time around. As muscle cells accumulate more protein, they will also accumulate more water. Therefore, much of muscle hypertrophy is protein and water. In addition,

---

BOX 11.1. Processes Associated with Adaptation After Resistance Training

- Building of more protein for myofibrils
- An increase in number of mitochondria
- An increase in enzymes specific to the task
- Making more connective tissue for sheathing around muscle fibers and bundles
- A slight increase in glycogen stores

connective tissue providing integrity and support to the overloaded muscle will be enhanced as well.

Does our energy expenditure increase due to weight training?

The increased energy demand of weight training depends on the intensity level and duration of a workout coupled with the energy needed for recovery and adaptation. The energy needed for a workout may be along the order of 5 to 10 Cal per minute while recovery and adaptation may demand 100 to 300 Cal the next day. This additional energy expended should be calculated into your total energy expenditure (TEE). The predominant fuel powering weight training is carbohydrate, derived mostly from muscle glycogen stores and secondarily fat from fat tissue and within muscle tissue itself. One of the strongest influences will be epinephrine, which is released from the adrenal glands during intense training. Epinephrine will promote the breakdown of glycogen and fat stores, making those energy sources available to working muscle.

On the other hand, both fat and carbohydrate fuel adaptive processes over the next few hours up to the next day or so. The most important factors dictating fuel preference will be meals and corresponding fluctuations in insulin and glucagon levels.

How much energy should be eaten to make the body more lean and muscular?

To become more muscular and lean, people tend to complement weight training with dietary control. In addition, integrating aerobic training will certainly be beneficial. It is also important not to drastically restrict energy intake, if at all. Drastic energy restriction can place an extra demand upon skeletal muscle to provide amino acids for glucose production. Therefore, drastic energy restriction and weight training may place the body in sort of a futile cycle as muscle breakdown contradicts muscle hypertrophy.

Therefore, if you are at a fairly comfortable body size but you want to increase your muscularity and leanness, you will be best served by eating enough energy to meet your expenditure. That would include the energy expended due to exercise training while also choosing foods higher in carbohydrate and protein versus fat. The major thrust of your efforts should focus on the change in body composition, not necessarily body weight. In fact, as you add skeletal muscle, it is possible that you will gain weight.

For heavier people with a higher percentage of body fat who wish to become leaner, they can begin by estimating their TEE and then restrict energy intake by 10 percent. This is easily done by substituting foods with a greater percentage of energy from carbohydrate and protein versus fat. Also, engaging in regular aerobic activities will be of benefit, as discussed shortly.

How much protein is needed during weight training?

Protein is the major nonwater component of skeletal muscle. Logically, if you want to build more muscle, you need to eat more protein beyond the needs for normal maintenance. Scientists do not deny this logic, but they do tend to differ on how much more protein is necessary, and how much is too much.

Skeletal muscle is about 22 percent protein. Because 1 pound is equal to 454 g, there are about 100 g of protein per pound of skeletal muscle. Theoretically, then, to increase skeletal muscle mass by 1 pound per week, you would need an extra 14 g of protein a day (100 g/7 days) above your normal protein requirements. For example, the RDA for a 180 lb man is 65 g of protein. Adding 14 g to the RDA 65 g yields 79 g of protein, which is 1.2 times the RDA. But it really does not seem to be that simple. What we do know is that as we eat more protein, our liver becomes more efficient in breaking down amino acids. Therefore, we probably need to eat more protein than is mathematically predictable by a simple formula like this one. Many scientists contend that weight-training athletes may benefit most from a protein intake of 1.4 to 1.75 g per kilogram of their body weight or more. This translates to about 1.75 to 2.25 times the RDA for protein. Several research studies using protein intakes above this level have failed to show additional benefit (more muscle gain). Furthermore, the intensity and extent to which individuals train will dictate where they may fall with these ranges for protein recommendations.

How can protein intake be increased if need be?

If you assess your current diet and determine that you want to increase your protein intake, then items such as nonfat dry milk, cooked egg whites or egg substitutes (i.e., Egg Beaters), and lean cuts of meats and fish will offer protein with very little accompanying fat. Water-packed tuna is perhaps one of the most popular intact foods used by people to provide a significant source of protein. For instance, one can of Starkist Solid White Albacore Tuna (6 oz) contains roughly 45 g of protein. You can put the tuna on a salad or mix it with cut pickles, nonfat mayonnaise, or spicy mustard.

Most protein supplements are derived in laboratories from foods. For example, some popular protein supplements use casein and whey, which are derived from milk and/or albumin (ovalbumin) from eggs. Check the wrappers of protein bars or drinks for these names or terms such as "milk protein isolates." These protein sources are "complete" or "high biological value," as discussed in Chapter 6. One advantage that protein supplements have over many food protein sources is that many supplements provide the protein without much of the associated fat.

Whether there is an advantage to using supplements of different types of proteins is not clear at this time. By far the most popular is whey protein from milk. The amino acid composition is very similar to proteins in general. Soy protein is also quite popular. In addition, some researchers contend that soy protein supplements may actually increase thyroid hormone levels as well as lower blood cholesterol and triglyceride levels. These effects are probably not the result of the soy protein itself but associated molecules such as flavonoids.

There is no advantage to free amino acid-based protein supplements versus supplements containing intact protein. Intact protein is digested to amino acids and absorbed just as efficiently as free amino acids. Furthermore, protein supplements comprised of intact proteins tend to cost less. So unless there is a specific amino acid formulation you are looking for, you may want to save yourself a little money with intact proteins.

NUTRITION SUPPLEMENTS MARKETED TO ENHANCE MUSCLE MASS ABOUND

Sport supplements have evolved into a multibillion dollar industry, yet their evolutionary process really has not been that long. For instance, when I interviewed Red Lerille, Mr. America in 1960, he told me that in the 1960s bodybuilders mostly focused on higher protein diets. Sport supplements were not really in the picture until a few years later. Today there are numerous supplements available to people looking to improve their muscle mass or leanness. These include the following:

Arginine and lysine

Interest in possible athletic benefits from supplementing with individual amino acids was raised after researchers realized that when certain amino acids, such as arginine, are infused directly into the bloodstreams of hospital patients suffering from burns, there was a corresponding rise in growth hormone levels in their blood.

Some researchers have found that taking arginine and lysine supplements can increase growth hormone levels in healthy young men as well. Because it takes several grams of these amino acids to produce a growth hormone response, some participants of the studies complained of intestinal discomfort. Other researchers reported that supplementing these amino acids failed to raise growth hormone levels. Researchers at this time are not really convinced that this happens or would happen in everyone. In addition, even those research studies that found an increase in circulating growth hormone did not go further to determine if this resulted in increased muscle mass.

If gram doses of these amino acids truly do raise growth hormone levels, it would seem logical that these supplements should be taken either several hours prior to or after a training session. This is because researchers have reported that growth hormone levels already become elevated during a workout and that amino acid supplements prior to a high intensity workout fail to increase growth hormone levels beyond the training alone. Therefore, taking these supplements prior to or just after a workout would not have benefit, if indeed they were effective in the first place.

Ornithine alpha-ketoglutarate (OKG)

Ornithine and its derivative ornithine-α-ketoglutarate (OKG) have received considerable interest from weight-training athletes. Ornithine is an amino acid not found in our proteins. However, it does exist independently in our body and is fundamentally involved in the formation of urea. Like arginine, supplemental ornithine was popularized after scientists reported that when ornithine was infused into blood there was a corresponding increase in growth hormone. Some researchers have also reported that oral supplementation of ornithine also increases circulating growth hormone in a respectable percentage of participants. However, the needed dose translates to as much as 170 mg of ornithine per kilogram body weight, which amounts to 14 g of supplemental ornithine daily for a 180 lb male. Ornithine dosages of this size are usually associated with intestinal discomfort and diarrhea; again, it has not been determined whether the potentially induced increase in growth hormone leads to increased muscle gain. On the other hand, other researchers have not found that OKG raises growth hormone levels, and no one has found increases in muscle mass with supplementation.

Chromium and chromium picolinate

Chromium, especially in the form of chromium picolinate, has drawn the attention of some athletes. Because chromium appears to potentiate insulin activity, it has been theorized that supplemental chromium may increase amino acid uptake in skeletal muscle and promote muscle protein synthesis. This could lead to the building of more muscle. Picolinate is simply a molecule that, when bound to chromium, seems to enhance the efficiency of chromium absorption.

Earlier reports by some researchers stated that participants taking chromium picolinate for forty days in conjunction with weight-training programs increased their body weight. Furthermore, most of the increase in weight was attributed to lean body mass. Another research study described a slight weight reduction in chromium-picolinate supplemented football players. It was reported that these athletes became leaner as a result of a decrease in their body fat. However, other scientists challenged these studies because the methods used in these investigations suffered from flaws that easily cast doubt upon the credibility of the results. More recent and better designed studies, including those published in the highly reputable research journals, failed to show beneficial effects of chromium supplementation. Furthermore, studies exploring the potential toxic effects of long-term chromium supplementation have not been completed. Some scientists also speculate that picolinate itself may unfavorably alter brain neurotransmitter levels. So at this time chromium supplementation is not recommended for muscle mass development in otherwise healthy and well-nourished athletes.

Vanadium and vanadyl sulfate

Like chromium, vanadium as vanadyl sulfate has also received a fair amount of attention from weight-training individuals. However, contrary to the attention, there has been very little research performed regarding the possibility of vanadium as a mass-enhancing supplement. Like chromium, the potentially toxic effects of vanadium supplementation are not known, and many nutritionists caution against supplementation until more research is completed in this area.

Boron

When boron supplements led to elevated levels of testosterone, boron supplements became somewhat popular for weight trainers and bodybuilders, as it was believed that boron could increase testosterone levels. However, researchers have not been able to prove that boron supplementation increases testosterone levels, strength, and muscle mass in weight trainers. At this time, boron supplementation does not appear to be beneficial for weight-training athletes.

Creatine

Creatine is naturally made by the human body and has become one of the most studied sport supplements. Three amino acids (methionine, glycine, and arginine) and two organs (liver and kidneys) are involved in the production of creatine. As discussed, in muscle and other tissue, ATP is used to transfer energy and a phosphate group to creatine, forming creatine phosphate. This substance then becomes a readily available means of regenerating ATP when it is in demand. For muscle, this would be during the early stage of an exercise. In the brain, it can help to maintain ATP levels during brief periods of poor O_2 supply. The brain relies on aerobic ATP production so periods of decreased O_2 availability are extremely critical. ATP can be regenerated from creatine phosphate in a single chemical reaction, which does not require O_2.

As creatine is found in human muscle, it will also be found in the muscle of other animals. Therefore, meat eaters will already receive a gram or two of creatine in their diets. The practice of supplementing creatine became extremely popular in the 1990s as several scientific studies showed that muscle creatine levels could be increased with supplementation. This change was often (but not always) associated with increases in total body mass, lean body mass, strength, and power. Creatine is mostly supplemented as creatine monohydrate, but other forms do exist. It can be purchased as a powder to dissolve in a drink, or as a concentrated liquid to be administered orally via a dropper.

A few years ago it was more popular for individuals to begin creatine supplementation by way of a "loading" phase. In this phase, roughly 20 to 25 g of creatine may have been ingested for 5 to 7 days, followed by a longer "maintenance" phase involving about 3 to 5 g daily. What scientists found was that when young men were provided 20 g of creatine monohydrate daily for about a week they developed a 20 percent increase in muscle creatine levels. Furthermore, this increased muscle content of creatine could be maintained for thirty days when the loading phase was followed by a maintenance dose of only 2 g daily. Interestingly, the same researchers also found that you could get to the same level of muscle creatine after four weeks by starting off and maintaining a supplement dose of 3 g daily. This route is cheaper and safer, as it reduces the chances of toxicity.

At this time creatine supplementation is believed to be relatively safe when users follow the recommended levels. However, some scientists have speculated that more research must be performed on other tissue in which creatine is found. For instance, researchers have not yet properly studied the effects of creatine supplementation, especially "loading," on the heart and brain. Some of the effects of creatine are related to its spongelike properties. When it accumulates in skeletal muscle, it will pull water in with it. One interesting feature of skeletal muscle fibers is that when they swell they will increase protein production and grow bigger (hypertrophy). The neurons in the brain cannot do this as they are restricted in growth by the skull. Research is now under way to study the effects of creatine loading on neurological and cardiac tissue.

DHEA and androstenedione

DHEA and androstenedione are prohormone molecules. When the body makes sex hormones such as testosterone and estrogens, they are actually constructed during several chemical reactions beginning with cholesterol. In the gonads, which are the ovaries for females and testes for males, cholesterol can be completely converted to testosterone and estrogens and released into the blood. Two molecules along the way to the sex hormones are DHEA (dehydroepiandrosterone) and androstenedione, with the former coming just prior to the latter (see Figure 11.3). Androstenedione is just one chemical reaction shy of testosterone.

Testosterone is one of the most significant factors that evokes muscle protein production and promotes growth. However, it is a controlled substance, meaning that it is available only by physician's prescription. Androstenedione and DHEA are available as nutrition supplements at this time as they are naturally found in foods such as meats (muscle and organ). Many health professionals have questioned whether these two should be prohibited from the supplement scene until more is known about their effects. It should be mentioned that both of these substances are among the list of so-called sport doping agents banned by the International Olympic Committee (IOC) and the NCAA.

In order for androstenedione and DHEA to raise testosterone levels they must be absorbed from the digestive tract, circulate, and be converted to testosterone by enzymes in organs such as the liver and testes. Interestingly, skeletal muscle lacks the enzymes needed to convert DHEA and androstenedione to testosterone. It should also be

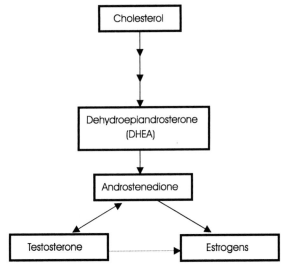

FIGURE 11.3. Potential reaction pathway for the production of popular steroid substances (DHEA and androstenedione) and derived hormones (testosterone and estrogens).

mentioned that both androstenedione and DHEA can be converted to estrogen molecules as well. To counter this, some supplement manufacturers recommend taking substances such as diadzein or chysin (flavonoids) in an attempt to block this undesirable conversion.

In general, researchers have failed to show that androstenedione and DHEA supplements do indeed increase testosterone levels in the blood when dosages mimicked manufacturer recommendations (100 mg of androstenedione and 25 to 50 mg of DHEA). However, when three times the recommended dosage was tested for androstenedione, testosterone levels did increase by 24 percent, which may seem encouraging. However, estrogen levels also increased by 128 percent, which was probably not what the males were hoping for.

At this time it seems that recommended levels for supplementation of androstenedione and DHEA may not be effective in increasing testosterone levels in the blood. Furthermore, while higher doses of androstenedione may raise testosterone levels, there may be an even greater increase in estrogen levels. This could lead to the development of feminizing features in men. Furthermore, one research study revealed that when men with more body fat were provided androstenedione supplements they were more efficient in converting androstenedione to estrogen than leaner men. This makes sense, as adipose tissue contains the enzymes necessary to convert androstenedione to estrogens.

Glutamine

Glutamine is a nonessential amino acid that is becoming a popular supplement for weight lifters and bodybuilders. It has been touted as a substance that results in a net gain of muscle protein and thus muscle mass. From the discussion of proteins, you will recall that body proteins are broken down and rebuilt on a daily basis. This is called *protein turnover* and it reflects the dynamic efforts of our cells to adapt to metabolic conditions that change minute by minute, hour by hour, and day by day. In muscle tissue, protein turnover reflects demands placed on muscle itself. During weight lifting there will be an increase in the breakdown of muscle proteins, which largely reflects recovery and repair processes. Also, in response to a workout, protein production is increased for several hours to a day or so afterward, which reflects repair and adaptive processes. When protein production exceeds breakdown, there will be a net growth of muscle tissue as seen in weight training. It is a matter of simple algebra. Glutamine is often purported to limit these breakdowns, which results in greater net gains of muscle protein.

Interestingly, there are several review articles related to glutamine and muscle protein turnover and the potential application to athletes. However, the review articles outnumber the research efforts actually testing glutamine. Therefore, at this time, there is limited information with regard to the efficacy of glutamine supplementation to enhance muscle development associated with resistance training.

HMB (β-hydroxy β-methylbutyrate)

HMB is the abbreviation for β-hydroxy β-methylbutyrate, which is a derivative of the essential amino acid leucine. HMB is a fairly popular supplement with weight trainers at this time and it also added to some sport bars, such as certain Met-Rx Protein Plus Bars. HMB may also be found in limited amounts in citrus and catfish.

At this time very few research articles are available describing the testing of HMB. The results of a couple of research studies suggest that supplementing 1.5 or 3 g of HMB daily for a couple weeks improved the strength and lean body mass of previously untrained men. However, other researchers have not found such an effect. Therefore, questions linger as to whether HMB supplementation can have a positive effect on muscle protein turnover and the development of greater lean body mass and strength.

AEROBIC OR CARDIOVASCULAR TRAINING IS GOOD FOR YOUR HEART AND METABOLISM

In the late 1970s and early 1980s, the aerobic boom took place and gyms and health clubs around the country began to include aerobic classes and early forms of cardiovascular equipment. Today, health clubs are often evaluated on the content and variety of their cardiovascular equipment, classes, and programs. Equipment now includes precision bikes, treadmills, steppers, gliders, and classes that are hybrids between classic aerobics and martial arts and weight training.

What adaptations occur from aerobic exercise?

Many of us engage in regular aerobic exercise such as running, cross country skiing, bicycling, rowing, fast walking, roller blading, distance swimming, and health club aerobic programs. During these activities the resistance against movement is not as great as weight training. Thus, muscle hypertrophy is much less pronounced, if at all. However, muscle will adapt in another amazing way. Here the adaptation allows the trained muscle to have greater endurance by increasing its aerobic ATP generative capacity. In doing so there is an increase in the number of mitochondria in the trained muscle cells. Furthermore, the trained muscle develops more capillaries to deliver blood. The increase in the number of capillaries provides more O_2 and energy nutrients during exercise. In addition, heart muscle thickens a bit (hypertrophy) to provide a more powerful stroke and greater cardiac output to working muscles. A greater heart stroke is often reflected by a slower heart rate when not exercising. Some top endurance athletes have resting heart rates as low as 40 to 45 beats per minute.

What nutrients fuel aerobic activity?

The primary fuel for aerobic and endurance activity depends on both the intensity and duration of the effort. The relative contribution of the different energy nutrients fueling the working muscle will vary depending upon whether exercise lasts for 15 minutes, 30 minutes, 1 hour, or 2 hours. Also, the mixture of fuel will be different at these time intervals when they are performed at different intensities.

During a fed state or a period of fasting, the most important factor determining what skeletal muscle will use for fuel is hormone levels. During exercise, epinephrine and insulin are the most important hormonal factors and the level of these hormones in the blood is controlled largely by the intensity of exercise. Scientists have come to realize that during cardiovascular exercise as the intensity of the effort increases the level of epinephrine will increase, while the level of insulin will decrease. The brain is mostly responsible for doing this by sending signals to the adrenal glands to release epinephrine and to the pancreas to limit the release of insulin. Insulin will promote the building of glycogen in muscle and fat in fat cells and to some degree in muscle cells. Conversely, epinephrine will promote the breakdown of these energy stores. Therefore, as exercise intensity increases, more glucose is available in muscle cells and more fatty acids are circulating to and available within muscle cells.

During sustained lower intensity efforts (e.g., brisk walking, slow swim) the brain will call upon mostly Type I muscle fibers. Here the intensity is low so epinephrine levels will only be slightly elevated. Working muscle cells will be primarily fueled by fatty acids, with the majority coming from the blood (see Figure 11.4 and Figure 5.4). However, as the intensity of the effort increases so too will epinephrine in the blood and as a result the breakdown of glycogen in working muscle. As this occurs, glucose from glycogen stores starts to become the largest single contributor to muscle energy expenditure. As the intensity level continues to increase, so too will the reliance on glucose. One reason for this is that as the intensity level is increased the brain will support Type I muscle fiber efforts with more and more Type II muscle fibers. Type II muscle fibers tend to use more glucose.

How do we burn more fat during cardiovascular exercise?

Figure 11.4 also reveals something very important: the amount of fat used as an energy source is greatest at a moderate intensity. So even though fat accounts for a lesser percentage of total energy expended, there is more total energy used at the moderate intensity, which leads to greater amounts of fat used. Think of it this way. Which would you rather have—60 percent of $100.00 or 40 percent of $200.00? This is one reason why cardiovascular exercise equip-

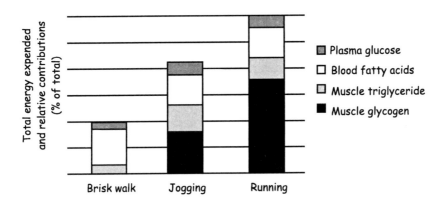

FIGURE 11.4. Approximate percentage contribution of carbohydrate and fat after 30 minutes of aerobic exercise (cycling) at either a lower (brisk walk), moderate (jogging), or higher (running) intensity. Although the lower intensity will allow for a greater percentage of fat (blood fatty acids and muscle triglycerides) utilization, the moderate intensity will allow for a greater quantity of fat to be burned.

ment often has a graphic on the display indicating the "target heart rate" or "fat burning zone." Here the target heart rate is associated with the moderate level of intensity in Figure 11.4, or the level of intensity in which you are burning the greatest amount of fat.

Another important consideration is duration. Cardiovascular exercise is always encouraged to last at least 20 minutes and preferably 30 to 45 minutes for most people. The reason for this is that it seems to take a little time for all the needed events for optimal fat utilization to come on line. This includes everything from mobilizing fatty acids from fat stores to increasing the delivery of O_2 to working muscle. There are a few other biochemical reasons for this as well, but they are beyond the scope of this text. The important thing is that it takes a while, often 12 to 20 minutes, to reach optimal fat burning efficiency. So be patient and include a period of lower intensity warm-up as well.

Do we use body protein for energy during endurance exercise?

The fuel used by our muscle fibers to make ATP during prolonged exercise is a mixture of carbohydrate, fat, and amino acid. Depending on the duration of exercise, amino acids may be counted on to generate as much as 6 to 10 percent of the ATP. The remainder of the energy burden will be split between fat and carbohydrate. A general rule is that for durations longer than 20 to 30 minutes the percentage of fat utilized climbs as the intensity level decreases. During lower intensity activities, such as brisk walking, bicycling (13 to 15 mph), jogging, and light roller blading, the muscle will make ATP mostly from fat (60 to 70 percent). However, at more moderate intensity activities, such as bicycling (16 to 20 mph) or running (8 to 9 mph), the reliance upon fat for ATP generation decreases to about 50 percent. Further, as even higher levels of intensity are performed, such as by professional marathon runners and endurance cyclists, carbohydrate is the primary fuel followed by fat and then amino acids.

The use of amino acids for energy is mostly a consideration for higher-level endurance athletes. This would include people who would train several times a week for extended periods and at higher intensities. This is one reason why marathoners often look lean but not as muscular as sprinters or milers, for example. One of the most significant reasons that more and more amino acids are used for energy is because cortisol levels in the blood are increased as the higher intensity activity is endured. Cortisol can cause the breakdown of muscle protein and the freed amino acids can be used for energy. Some amino acids will be used directly by muscle to make ATP, while others will circulate to the liver and be converted to glucose.

What causes muscle exhaustion in endurance activities?

A principal factor associated with exhaustion during endurance exercise is the availability of carbohydrates to working muscle. Quite simply, when muscle glycogen stores are depleted, muscle exhaustion ensues shortly thereafter. The depletion of muscle glycogen along with dehydration are the most significant contributors to exhaustion or what endurance athletes call "hitting the wall" or "bonking." From this it is easy to see why sport drinks such as POWERade and Gatorade are so popular. Electrolyte imbalances may also lead to fatigue, but this might occur only during very long efforts in which water is provided. Today, with the popularity of sport drinks and endurance foods the risk of an electrolyte imbalance is often reduced.

Can diet affect the onset of exhaustion?

Stored carbohydrate in the form of muscle and liver glycogen reflects dietary carbohydrate intake. During training or competition, researchers have shown that athletes can significantly increase their training time or time till exhaustion by eating a high carbohydrate diet. For instance, one athlete on a low carbohydrate diet will reach muscle exhaustion long before another athlete on a high carbohydrate diet (> 60 percent carbohydrate).

A high carbohydrate diet allows the body to replenish glycogen stores in between training sessions. Contrary to what many people think, it actually takes a while to rebuild muscle glycogen stores that have been used during exercise. In fact, if an endurance athlete reduces his or her muscle glycogen to nadir levels during training or competition, it can take nearly a day to rebuild them. This means that the athlete should eat carbohydrates immediately after completing the session and throughout that day to provide both the needed glucose and insulin to rebuild those stores.

What is carbo loading?

Some athletes preparing for a big event will attempt to *carbohydrate load* or *carbo load*. These events include marathons, triathlons, bicycle centuries or longer, and long-distance swimming. The desired outcome is achieving the highest possible level of muscle glycogen just prior to the onset of the competition by coordinating a high carbohydrate intake (> 60 percent) for at least one week prior to competition while at the same time tapering both the intensity and duration of training sessions.

Theoretically, if you start out with more glycogen you should be able to perform longer. A more common method of carbo loading is explained next and would be most beneficial when an event is to last more than one hour. Carbo loading would not be beneficial for shorter endurance efforts or sports involving only brief efforts (e.g., power lifting, velodrome cycling, or most track and field events). There may be benefit for intermittent effort yet longer duration sports such as soccer, football, and field and ice hockey, however, the practice and game schedule would make carbo loading unrealistic.

Carbo loading can be successfully performed with common high-carbohydrate foods such as pasta, grains, fruits, and vegetables; however, some athletes prefer purified carbohydrate supplements because they are free of fat and fiber. Dietary fiber will lead to more stool formation, which some athletes feel may be a slight performance hindrance. The preferred method of carbo loading involves maintaining a high carbohydrate diet (> 65 percent total Calories) during the week prior to the event. During the same period of time exercise is pretty much halved every two days in duration and intensity and halted one day prior to the event (see Table 11.2).

What are protein recommendations for endurance athletes?

Bodybuilders, power lifters, and football players recognize high protein intakes as an avenue to achieve and maintain enhanced muscle mass. Contrarily, endurance athletes recognize a relatively higher protein (total grams) intake as a means of replacing the body protein used for fuel during training, competition, and recovery and adaptation. Although individual protein requirements will vary with the level of intensity and duration of the activity, some sport nutritionists recognize that 1.4 to 1.75 g of protein per kilogram body weight will

TABLE 11.2. Protocol for Glycogen Loading

Prior to Competition	Training Protocol	Diet Protocol
6 days	90 minutes at intensity approximating 75% VO_2max	50% energy as carbohydrate and hydrate
5 days	40 minutes at intensity approximating 75% VO_2max	50% energy as carbohydrate and hydrate
4 days	40 minutes at intensity approximating 75% VO_2max	50% energy as carbohydrate and hydrate
3 days	20 minutes at intensity approximating 75% VO_2max; rest muscle	70% energy or 10 g carbohydrate/kg body weight and hydrate
2 days	20 minutes at intensity approximating 75% VO_2max; rest muscle	70% energy or 10 g carbohydrate/kg body weight and hydrate copiously
1 day (day before)	Rest muscle as much as possible	70% energy or 10 g carbohydrate/kg body weight and hydrate copiously
Competition	Rest prior to event	Eat carbohydrate-based meal > 2-3 hours before if possible; ingest carbohydrate 15-30 minutes prior. Hydrate appropriately

provide adequate protein along with a little margin of safety. This is pretty much the same recommendation discussed previously for weight trainers.

Many sport nutritionists feel that it may be more logical to approach protein needs for all athletes as a percentage of total energy instead of g/kg of body weight. This is to say that endurance athletes, as well as weight-training athletes, should plan for no more than 15 to 20 percent of the total energy to be derived from protein. Therefore, a 90 kg (200 lb) male bodybuilder eating 3,500 Cal daily and receiving 15 to 20 percent of his energy intake from protein will receive about 130 to 175 g of protein daily. This translates to 1.8 to 2.4 times his RDA or 1.4 to 1.9 g/kg body weight. Even a 68 kg (150 lb) endurance athlete eating 3,000 to 3,500 Cal daily but deriving only about 15 percent of that energy from protein is receiving about 110 to 130 g of protein daily, which is more than twice their RDA and 1.6 to 1.9 g of protein per kilogram body weight.

Do endurance athletes need a protein supplement?

Before traveling to the local nutritional supplement supplier for a protein supplement, first estimate current protein intake. Since many people, especially males, already eat 100 to 130 g of protein daily (about two times the RDA) only small if any dietary adjustments may be needed. Furthermore, endurance athletes tend to eat more energy than more sedentary people, so more protein is probably, but not definitely included. This is because many endurance athletes, especially runners, may eat more plant-based foods including pastas, breads, rice, etc. Thus, even though they may be eating more energy, more of it is coming from carbohydrate-rich sources. Endurance athletes should assess their diet prior to spending their money.

SPORT DRINKS ARE LIQUID PERFORMANCE

Sport drinks were pioneered in the 1960s when a scientist at the University of Florida (home of the Gators) developed a product designed to provide both fluid, energy, and electrolytes to athletes. The product became known as Gatorade, and a multimillion-dollar industry was born.

What are sport drinks and what is their composition?

Sweat is a combination of mostly water and electrolytes. It is needed to help remove the excessive heat generated from the body during exercise. One liter of sweat allows for the removal of about 600 Cal of heat. So, if an activity such as running for two hours generates about 900 Cal of heat, then theoretically about 1.5 L of sweat may have been lost. The primary electrolytes lost from the body in sweat are sodium and chloride. However, their concentration in sweat is lower than in the plasma of the blood. Thus, sweat is dilute compared to blood. Even when sweating profusely the sodium and chloride content of the sweat may be only about one-half of the concentration of human blood plasma. Many sport drinks provide the replacement of these electrolytes plus other nutrients, such as phosphorus, chromium, calcium, magnesium, iron, and certain water-soluble vitamins.

The energy in sport drinks is provided largely in the form of carbohydrates such as glucose, sucrose, fructose, corn syrup, maltodextrins, and glucose polymers. Maltodextrins and glucose polymers are mostly cornstarch that is partially broken down. Carbohydrates usually make up about 4 to 11 percent of the sport drink. Glucose and fructose are monosaccharides, whereas corn syrup is derived from cornstarch, which has been partially broken down to short, branching chains of glucose. Maltodextrin is just a few glucose molecules linked together with a branching point. Glucose polymers may just be short chains of glucose. Even Coca-Cola and other soft drinks can be regarded as sport drinks, and Coke is actually popular with many athletes, including the author of this book. Coke's carbohydrate source is a high-fructose corn syrup, which is corn syrup with added fructose.

As mentioned previously, one of the principal factors involved in the onset of exhaustion or fatigue is a depletion of muscle glycogen stores. The carbohydrate in these sport drinks becomes an available source of glucose to working muscle. It was once thought that the carbohydrate in a sport drink might slow the rate of glycogen breakdown and thus prolong endurance exercise. However, scientists now contest that the carbohydrate in a sport drink actually becomes a primary carbohydrate source for working muscle as glycogen stores wane. This contribution seems to be significant enough to push back fatigue by minutes or more. This could be the difference in finishing strong during a marathon or fatiguing at mile twenty-four.

Who would benefit from a sport drink?

For a well-nourished and hydrated weight-training athlete, there is probably not a need for a sport drink unless he or she is training for several hours and sweating profusely. The need for sport drinks for endurance athletes largely depends on the duration of exercise and the environmental conditions. Generally, for single shorter events such as 5K runs and half-hour aerobic sessions there is probably not a need. However, as an event or training session becomes longer, the need increases. For bouts lasting an hour or thereabouts, water replacement is certainly necessary. At this time, glycogen stores are not nearly depleted and therefore the need for the carbohydrate is not substantiated. However, many athletes will perform better in these moderate endurance efforts when they drink some sport drink just before and a little during the exercise. Because the electrolyte content of sweat is less than blood, electrolyte loss is not necessarily a concern at this point either. Eating after the event will replace these substances (glucose and electrolytes).

The bottom line on activities lasting up to one hour (e.g., 10 to 15 km run) is that it would be a good idea to drink some water prior to and during an event to help replace sweat water loss. Electrolytes and carbohydrates may not be necessary to prevent muscular fatigue. However, as mentioned, performance may be enhanced in some athletes by including some carbohydrate just prior to and during the endurance bout. This will require some experimentation by an athlete during training.

For longer endurance sessions, such as those lasting greater than two hours, a sport drink becomes more appropriate. The water helps replace the water lost in sweat while the carbohydrate provides a significant late energy source and delays the onset of exhaustion. At this point, electrolyte replacement begins to have some benefit. Even athletes competing in intermittent effort yet longer duration sports such as soccer, ice hockey, and football may benefit from a sport drink. If nothing else, the sweet taste will encourage greater fluid consumption and improve hydration status.

MANY PROGRAMS AND PRODUCTS ARE TOUTED TO IMPROVE ENDURANCE PERFORMANCE

Fat loading

Recently, attention has focused on a slightly different eating protocol called fat loading. The intention of this dietary protocol is to try to enhance fat utilization during exercise, thereby decreasing carbohydrate usage and thus slowing glycogen breakdown. One important consideration here is timing. For endurance athletes who eat more of their energy as fat, their cells will adapt to burn more fat over the course of the day as well as during exercise. However, it takes about a week or so for this adaptation to occur. So the athlete must follow a high fat diet during training, which may not be the healthiest and most tolerable diet.

Eating more fat and less carbohydrate may not build the same glycogen depth prior to competition. So even though they may use less carbohydrate during competition they might have less available to spend during exercise anyway. This may be okay for a marathoner running a slower pace (e.g., 8 minute/mile pace), however for a runner competing at a higher intensity (e.g., 5 or 6 minute/mile pace) this could be disastrous. This is something that an athlete would have to experiment with and become comfortable with prior to competition.

Medium-Chain Triglycerides (MCTs)

MCTs contain fatty acids, which are both saturated and are only six to twelve carbons in length. The shortness of these fatty acids gives them unique properties, including the ability to (1) be absorbed from the digestive tract into the blood (portal vein) and not generally incorporated in chylomicrons; (2) provide a rapid energy source for the liver and muscle; and (3) possibly increase fat mobilization from fat cells.

These properties make MCTs a possible candidate for supplementation during endurance events. Theoretically, MCTs can slow glycogen breakdown and decrease some muscle protein breakdown during endurance exercise by providing a readily available energy source for liver and muscle. However, researchers studying this have reported that MCTs do not enhance athletic performance.

Glycerol

Glycerol has also been considered a candidate for supplementation during endurance events. This notion is based upon glycerol's potential to be converted to glucose in the liver. The glucose could then circulate to muscle and support muscle operations during exercise. Theoretically, this could decrease the rate of breakdown of glycogen stores. However, it seems that the torpid rate of converting glycerol to glucose seriously decreases its candidacy.

Alternatively, glycerol supplementation in conjunction with water consumption may be of benefit to endurance athletes preparing to perform in warmer environments. It may be that glycerol can enhance water retention prior to an event and thus may allow more sweat to be lost prior to any reductions in performance due to dehydration. Scientists have also reported that glycerol supplementation prior to an event increases heat tolerance during competition in warmer environments—perhaps another potential aid for athletes competing in warmer environments without ample opportunity to drink fluids during training and competition. One example of this type of competition might be soccer. However, glycerol may lead to digestive tract discomfort so athletes will have to experiment here as well.

Vitamins

Since many of the water-soluble vitamins are involved in energy metabolism, they are a logical candidate for supplementation by athletes. Thiamin (vitamin B_1) supplementation of 900 mg per day for three days has been shown to provide some benefit in athletes riding a bike at high intensity until exhaustion. Whether this can be applied to other exercise situations, as well as the tolerance and development of adverse effects, is not known. Therefore, this practice is highly discouraged.

Niacin (vitamin B_3) supplementation seems to decrease fat mobilization from fat cell deposits. This effect is contradictory to what would be desirable for endurance events as athletes may succumb to fatigue earlier in the bout. Vitamin B_6 supplementation may increase the rate of breakdown of muscle glycogen stores, at least in theory. Although this effect may be beneficial in short-duration performances that rely more heavily on anaerobic metabolism, it may be detrimental to endurance athletes. Also, vitamin B_6 supplementation may decrease exercise-induced mobilization of fat from fat stores. This could lower the fuel available to competing athletes and cause a more rapid depletion of glycogen stores, leading to earlier fatigue. In addition, supplements containing larger amounts of vitamin B_6 are generally not advised for anyone due to toxicity concerns.

Iron

It seems that long distance runners, especially women, may be at increased risk for reductions in their blood hemoglobin concentration. This phenomenon is called *runner's anemia* and is believed to be the result of a few coinciding events. First, women average greater iron losses due to menstruation. Second, both men and women runners experience the destruction of RBCs due to the high repetition and force of foot impact. Furthermore, many long distance runners eat a diet in which their iron is derived mostly from plant sources, which is less efficiently absorbed. Last, and perhaps less important, small amounts of iron can be lost in sweat. Thus, distance runners should consider their iron status and possible need for a supplement.

Carnitine

Carnitine is necessary for the transport of longer chain length fatty acids into the mitochondria for ATP production. Once this function was established, carnitine was marketed to athletes to enhance performance and for anyone looking to reduce body fat content. However, once scientific investigation caught up with these claims, it became obvious that under most normal conditions carnitine supplements yield no benefit at all.

Carnitine is made in the liver from the amino acids methionine and lysine with a little help from vitamins B_6 and C. Beyond what is made in the liver, carnitine is found in foods, especially meats. At this time there does not seem to be a dieting or athletic benefit from carnitine supplementation under normal conditions.

Caffeine

Caffeine has been considered a stimulant and is used by many individuals in normal daily life as well as by athletes. Caffeine and related substances are found naturally in foods and beverages, such as coffee, teas, and chocolate; and as part of recipes, such as in various soft drinks. Coffee contains caffeine whereas tea contains theophylline and chocolate contains theobromine.

These substances indirectly act as stimulants by enhancing and prolonging the effects of certain hormones such as glucagon and epinephrine. Naturally, questions were raised as to whether caffeine could enhance athletic performance. Scientists have found conflicting results regarding caffeine supplementation both prior to and/or during activity. Several studies have reported that the beneficial effects of caffeine on performance are negated in people who use caffeine daily (coffee, soft drinks, etc). However, by going caffeine free for several days prior to an event, caffeine may enhance performance. Recent studies have shown that caffeine ingestion can indeed enhance endurance performance. Recently scientists have also come to agreement that 3-6 mg/kg of caffeine prior to training or competition can enhance endurance performance.

Caffeine seems to enhance mental alertness in smaller doses (200 mg), although many individuals complain of nervousness and anxiety when larger doses are used (> 400 mg). A cup of coffee contains 100 to 150 mg of caffeine while a cup of tea and cola contain 25 to 60 mg. The over-the-counter stimulant Vivarin contains 200 mg of caffeine per tablet. Caffeine is metabolized and removed from the body fairly slowly. It may take several hours for the caffeine in one cup of coffee to be completely removed in the urine.

Bee pollen

Bee pollen is not necessarily a single substance but rather a combination of several vitamins, minerals, amino acids, and other substances readily available in foods. Well-performed exercise studies have shown that supplemental bee pollen does not provide any benefits to exercise performance.

Coenzyme Q

Coenzyme Q, also known as Coenzyme Q_{10}, CoQ10, and *ubiquinone,* can be found in the cells as a key component of the electron-transport chain. It also seems to function as an antioxidant as it has been used as a supplement by individuals who recently experienced heart attacks. Some of the earlier studies regarding the effects of supplemental Coenzyme Q on athletic performance were positive; however, more recent and better designed studies have failed to show a significant athletic benefit of Coenzyme Q supplementation. Recently scientists have begun to focus on the possible benefits of Coenzyme Q supplements for people whose hearts have become compromised in performance. We will discuss this more in Chapter 13.

Bioflavonoids

Bioflavonoids, such as rutin and hesperidin, were at one time considered vitamins but have since been removed from the list of essential nutrients. However, bioflavonoids have been getting a second look in regard to potential antioxidant properties demonstrated in nonhuman studies. Studies involving bioflavonoids are now under way; and more will be known about these substances within the next few years, especially in the area of cancer prevention. In regard to enhancing athletic performance, at this time there appears to be no evidence to support supplemental bioflavonoids.

Para-amino-benzoic-acid (PABA)

A while back, scientists discovered that a substance called para-amino-benzoic-acid (PABA) was involved in building nucleic acids, such as adenosine (part of ATP). Therefore, it was theorized that supplemental PABA may enhance ATP content in cells and therefore enhance performance. However, it was later discovered that PABA is actually a component of the vitamin folate and does not have an independent role in the cells. Furthermore, since we lack the ability to make folate with supplemental PABA, there appears to be no logical reason to supplement the diet with PABA.

Lipoic acid

Lipoic acid seems to be needed in energy pathways, especially in those chemical reactions that generate CO_2. However, the body may make adequate quantities of this substance. At this time researchers have not found that lipoic acid supplements provide performance benefits to athletes.

Choline

Choline is a component of acetylcholine, which is a neurotransmitter of great importance to skeletal muscle activity. Nerve cells reaching skeletal muscle fibers release acetylcholine, which then "excites" skeletal muscle cells and evokes contraction. Naturally, choline became a candidate for supplementation to enhance athletic performance. Choline, along with *betaine (trimethylglycine [TMG]), dimethylglycine, sarcosine (N-methylglycine), methionine,* and *S-adenylsyl methionine,* is involved in some of the processes that build several molecules which may be important for muscle performance, such as creatine and nucleic acids. Choline supplementation and possible enhanced athletic performance (with and without other substances) requires further study.

Inosine

The molecule adenosine triphosphate (ATP) provides the energy that directly powers muscle contraction. Logic would have us believe that if we provide the building blocks of ATP in supplements, muscle cells would have more ATP available and exercise performance would be enhanced. Adenosine of ATP can be made from the molecule inosine. However, adenosine concentrations in the cells seem to be tightly controlled and it seems that humans make enough adenosine to suit their needs. Thus, excessive inosine (supplemented) is not efficiently converted to adenosine. Also, it has been suggested that the processes necessary to break down the excessive inosine may generate free radicals. In addition, inosine is broken down to uric acid, which may lead to the formation of certain types of kidney stones and gout if not proficiently removed from the blood.

Chapter 12

Nutrition Throughout Life

MAKING A BABY IS COMPLICATED

A female ovulates once a month during her reproductive years. Ovulation culminates in the liberation of an egg, which then settles in one of her fallopian tubes. There the egg sits and plays a waiting game, as it has but twenty-four hours or so to become fertilized by a sperm. Semen from a male counterpart is a compilation of sperm (produced by the testes) and nourishing and supporting fluids from various accessory reproductive glands, such as the prostate and Cowper's gland. Ejaculation produces about one-half teaspoon of semen, which will contain millions of sperm. This high number of sperm is very important because the task at hand is so great. Ultimately, however, only one sperm will fertilize the egg and initiate the genesis of human life.

What happens during pregnancy?

The fertilized egg now develops into a *zygote,* which is the very basis of human life. All humans begin their lives as a single cell. This single cell now has combined the genetic information (DNA) from the mother and father and has the potential to become human—to develop into a complex cell orchestration of metabolism, movement, and mentality. All the zygote needs is a nice warm and wet place to develop, such as the mother's uterus, and plenty of nourishment.

Within a brief time after conception, the zygote divides into two cells, which then divide into four cells, which then divide into eight cells, and so on. From conception to two weeks is referred to as the *preembryonic* period, while from week two to the closure of week eight marks the embryonic period. By the end of the embryonic period the embryo will show small but fairly developed organs and begin to take on a more recognizable human form. The commencement of week nine to the moment of birth marks the *fetal* period. During this time the fetus will show remarkable growth and maturation of organs and appendages. At approximately thirteen weeks, the heart begins to beat, even though the fetus still weighs but a few ounces.

Normal pregnancy lasts approximately forty weeks and is typically broken into three equal time periods called trimesters. It is desirable to deliver after at least thirty-seven weeks of pregnancy with the newborn weighing greater than 2.5 kg or about 5.5 lb. Infants born prior to the thirty-seventh week are referred to as premature, while infants born weighing less than 2.5 kg are called low birth weight (LBW) infants. Premature and low birth weight infants find life more challenging in the days, weeks, and months that follow as they are at greater risk for medical complications. Premature infants are often introduced into the real world before their organs, especially their lungs, are fully developed and capable of coping with the new environment. This is the price humans pay for having such a large head (full of brains). Humans must be born before the skull becomes too large to pass through the birth canal. From a developmental standpoint, humans probably should stay in the mother's womb for a few more weeks.

How much energy should a woman eat and how much weight should she gain during pregnancy?

During pregnancy the energy needs of a woman are increased to allow for a healthy gain in body weight. The mother's energy needs are slightly increased during the first trimester, while on the average an extra 300 Cal/day are needed during the second and third trimesters. A weight gain of roughly 1 pound per month during the first trimester is generally recommended. Then, during the second and third trimesters, a ¾ to 1 pound per week is considered healthy. This allows for a total pregnancy weight gain of 25 to 35 pounds.

If a woman is underweight at the onset of pregnancy, a 28 to 40 pound weight gain is often recommended. On the other hand, if a woman is overweight or obese at the onset of pregnancy, a weight gain of 15 to 25 pounds is considered safer. It is important to recognize that pregnancy is not the time to try to lose weight. A healthy weight gain for the mother translates into a healthy growth for the unborn infant. Weight loss is never encouraged during pregnancy.

If during early pregnancy a female experiences an excessive weight gain, she should not be encouraged to lose weight. However, she should be encouraged to be more careful and try not to exceed the 1 pound per week in the remaining weeks. In contrast, if a pregnant woman fails to gain the recommended weight during early pregnancy, she should be encouraged to gain at least 1 pound per week for the remaining weeks, while not dramatically overcompensating. She can divide her recommended weight gain by the number of remaining weeks and use that figure as a guide.

As a female gains weight during pregnancy, usually about 7 to 8 pounds is attributable to the weight of the infant at birth. The rest of the weight is distributed throughout the mother in various tissues developed during pregnancy. These tissue include the placenta, amniotic fluid, increased breast tissue, expanded blood volume, and fat storage and muscle. These all help support the mother and fetus during pregnancy and after birth. Even the mother's bones will become a little denser during pregnancy.

How much protein does a mother need during pregnancy?

Protein requirements are increased during pregnancy to allow for adequate protein production in the mother and developing baby. An increase of 10 g of protein per day above the RDA is recommended in pregnant women over twenty-four years of age. An increase of 15 g is recommended for pregnant women under twenty-four years of age. The use of a protein supplement is probably not necessary for most women as their typical protein intake is still greater than requirements during pregnancy or is accounted for through increased energy intake during pregnancy. Vegetarian females should be particularly careful of their protein intake, especially vegans or fruitarians.

Are vitamin needs increased during pregnancy?

Vitamin needs are generally increased during pregnancy with special consideration for folate and vitamin D. Since the manufacturing of DNA requires folate, and the unborn infant is comprised of rapidly reproducing cells, the need for extra folate is very important. The extra folate (55 percent above the nonpregnant RDA) also supports RBC formation in the mother's expanding blood volume. A woman can increase her folate intake by choosing folate-rich foods such as orange juice and many fruits and vegetables.

Vitamin D is also especially important during pregnancy. A pregnant woman's RDA is the same as a nonpregnant woman, but good status is crucial. Vitamin D is necessary to aid in calcium metabolism and fetal bone formation. Regular sunlight exposure as well as choosing vitamin D-fortified milk and dairy products can help meet additional vitamin D requirements. However, direct sunlight (or tanning beds) is not recommended during pregnancy because fetal tissue is very sensitive to damage by UV light.

It is important to realize that excessive vitamin A supplementation during pregnancy can result in birth defects. Furthermore, a vitamin A derivative is the active ingredient in Accutane, which is used to treat cystic acne. The use of this product should be discontinued during pregnancy, as well as when attempting to become pregnant. In fact, since this drug is metabolized slowly it can take several weeks to a couple of months before it is safe for a woman to become pregnant after discontinuing its use. If a female becomes pregnant while using Accutane, she should discuss this with her physician immediately, as the risk of birth defects is exceptionally high.

Are minerals needed in greater amounts during pregnancy?

As with vitamins, the need for many essential minerals increases during pregnancy. For instance, the RDA for iron increases from 8 to 27 mg daily. Iron is needed by the mother to form new hemoglobin for her expanding blood volume and by the fetus to meet new tissue needs. Calcium is especially important during fetal bone and teeth development. Fluoride also helps teeth and bone develop. Although the RDA for calcium for pregnant women is the same as nonpregnant women (1,000 to 1,300 mg), it is of the utmost importance to eat adequate quantities of this nutrient. Zinc requirements are increased by roughly 25 percent during pregnancy due to its general involvement in fetal growth and development.

Should pregnant women take prenatal vitamin/ mineral supplements?

Whether a pregnant woman needs prenatal vitamin/mineral supplements depends upon the ability of her current and expected diet to provide all essential nutrients in appropriate amounts during pregnancy. An argument for the use of prenatal vitamin and mineral supplements is supported by the occurrence of unusual eating patterns experienced by some women during pregnancy. Even the most nutrition-conscious women will admit to some unusual preferences, cravings, or eating patterns during pregnancy. Typically, prenatal vitamin and mineral supplements include folate, vitamin D, iron, zinc, and often calcium in an assortment of other essential nutrients.

What factors can affect the healthy growth of an unborn infant?

Other dietary and behavioral factors that may impact the proper growth and development of an unborn infant include caffeine, alcohol, smoking, and exercise. There may not be a greater common voluntary insult upon human health than cigarette smoke, which certainly holds true for unborn infants, although it is an involuntary insult to them. Pregnant mothers who smoke are at greater risk of delivering low birth weight and premature infants. Some research suggests that these infants are also more prone to childhood cancers and sudden infant death. A pregnant female's body should be a smoke-free environment.

The effects of abusive alcohol consumption during pregnancy are substantial. Fetal alcohol syndrome (FAS) is a group of abnormal characteristics common to children born to mothers who drank too much during pregnancy. These characteristics include low birth weight, physical deformities, and poor mental development. It is estimated that more than 7,500 infants are born in the United States each year with FAS, while another 30,000 to 40,000 show milder signs of FAS. Although many physicians believe that there may be a safe level of alcohol consumption during pregnancy (e.g., a glass of wine with dinner occasionally), it is not clear at this time where the threshold lies. It is therefore difficult to make general recommendations. Because of this difficulty it seems much more logical for most women to abstain completely from alcohol consumption during pregnancy.

Caffeine consumption during pregnancy and its potential effect upon the unborn infant has raised concern over the past couple of decades. Researchers have reported that there is probably a greater risk of spontaneous fetal abortion and low birth weight in pregnant women consuming the caffeine equivalent of greater than twelve cups of coffee per day. Many scientists believe that caffeine has a safety threshold, much like alcohol, and that daily caffeine intake below the threshold is not detrimental. However, many women choose to abstain completely from caffeine and caffeinelike substances (theophylline in tea and theobromine in chocolate) during pregnancy until more is known in this area.

Historically, many women have given up activity during pregnancy fearing adverse effects upon the growth and development of the fetus. However, times have changed, and regular exercise does not seem to affect growth or development of the unborn infant. In fact, newer research suggests that regular exercise may provide some benefits at delivery, such as a shorter delivery time and perceived discomfort and pain. Some caution should be applied, however, to the type of activity a pregnant woman chooses. Contact sports and movements involving rapid directional changes and jarring motions should be avoided. Exercise such as low impact aerobics, walking, and swimming is considered safe during pregnancy. However, a female must pay particular attention to her energy consumption and monitor her body weight and hydration status.

When is an unborn infant the most sensitive to harmful nutrition and other factors?

It should be understood that throughout pregnancy, the unborn infant is vulnerable to the effects of nutritional deficiency and toxicity as well as the impact of harmful substances. However, this is especially true during the embryonic period. Proper nutritional and environmental care should be taken throughout pregnancy to potentiate the possibility of a healthy offspring.

BABIES WORK THEIR WAY UP TO PEOPLE FOOD

What is lactation?

One of the changes that occurs in a female during pregnancy is an enhancement of breast tissue and the maturing of the enclosed mammary glands. This occurs due to hormonal changes during pregnancy. *Lactation* is a period of time when a woman is producing breast milk in her mammary glands. Increases in the level of the hormone *prolactin* in a female stimulates her mammary glands to produce milk. The suckling of an infant helps signal her pituitary gland to release more prolactin into her blood and is required for continued lactation.

What is breast milk?

Breast milk is not merely a single substance, as it changes in composition not only with time after birth but also during a single feeding. In the first few days after birth, mothers produce a very sophisticated form of breast milk called *colostrum.* Over the next two weeks or so of lactation, breast milk slowly loses many of the characteristics of colostrum and gains those of mature breast milk. Colostrum is a yellowish, viscous solution that contains more than nutrients; it also contains immune factors. These immune factors include antibodies and other factors that can help boost an infant's developing immune capabilities.

Since the infant's digestive tract is mostly unused during pregnancy, it is relatively immature at birth and will take the first few months after birth to develop. Many of the immune factors present in colostrum seem to pass through the infant's immature digestive tract wall intact and enter the blood. The immune factors in colostrum are believed to contribute to the fewer lung and intestinal infections observed in breast-fed infants versus formula-fed infants. Further, factors in breast milk seem to promote the formation of a healthy colon bacteria population, since an infant's digestive tract is also born sterile (without bacteria).

Mature breast milk is a thinner and almost translucent solution. It is not uncommon for it to present a slightly bluish tinge. Mature breast milk contains a greater ratio of whey to casein protein versus cow's milk. Infants digest whey protein more easily, whereas casein tends to form a curd during digestion. Mature breast milk also contains a protein called *lactoferrin,* which can bind iron and potentially reduce bacterial infections. This is because bacteria require iron to reproduce. In addition, the amino acid called taurine is also present in breast milk. Taurine is not used to make proteins, but it is necessary for proper bile formation and visual processes.

The fat content of mature breast milk increases during a single feeding. This is an excellent reason to encourage an infant to feed for longer periods of time (> 10 to 15 minutes). Infants need this energy-dense liquid available later in a feeding to help meet their needs for growth and development. Further, mature human breast milk contains linoleic acid and cholesterol, both of which are necessary for the proper growth of an infant's brain and other nervous tissue.

Lactose is the major carbohydrate in mature breast milk. You will remember that lactose is a disaccharide made up of the monosaccharides glucose and galactose. Beyond providing energy, galactose also seems to be important for the development of the insulating wrapping around nerve cells. Only small amounts of vitamin D are present in mature breast milk, so a supplement may be necessary, especially if an infant has minimal exposure to sunlight. Also, because the iron composition is also very low in breast milk, infants may benefit from a supplement by their second to third month.

The decision whether to breast-feed is up to the mother. Some women choose to breast-feed exclusively for the first couple of months, while others will also include infant formula. Some women choose not to breast-feed at all; they should be informed that breast-feeding is the healthier alternative and should consider the points listed in Box 12.1.

What are infant formulas?

Cow's milk-based infant formulas offer a nutritious complement to breast-feeding and can be used in place of it. These formulas, such as Similac, Enfamil, and Gerber, are different from breast milk in that they are taken from cow's milk and also do not contain the beneficial immune factors and several of the other substances noted previously. Cow's milk-based formulas generally contain casein as a protein source, which has been partially digested by heat treatment. This improves infant digestion of this protein and drastically decreases the likelihood of the formation of a discomforting curd in the digestive tract. In addition, many of these products are iron fortified and con-

---

BOX 12.1. Reasons to Breast-Feed

- Composition of breast milk more closely resembles an infant's nutritional needs for the first six months
- Breast milk contains immune factors that decrease an infant's risk of infection
- Breast milk-fed infants generally develop fewer allergies
- Breast milk is already at the right temperature
- Breast milk is a better economical value

tain a complement of vitamins and minerals to improve their composition. Soy protein-based infant formulas, such as ProSobee, Isomil, and Alsoy, are an option for formula-fed infants who do not tolerate the cow's milk-based formulas. Finally, the American Academy of Pediatrics advise mothers not to feed their infants plain cow's milk, especially skim milk, versus other options during the first year of the infants' lives. The composition is not compatible with an infant's needs and may be detrimental to the baby's health.

How much do humans grow during infancy?

Infancy is the time period between birth and a baby's first birthday. At no other time in life are nutritional needs higher per body weight. Infants will usually double their birth weight by the time they are halfway through their first year of life. Furthermore, they can easily triple their birth weight by their first birthday. At the same time, an infant will increase its length by roughly 50 percent by his or her first birthday. Also, the head is huge at birth, maybe accounting for one-third to one-quarter of the infant's length. As adults the head is about one-eighth of body height. No wonder an infant cannot support the weight of its head for a month or so after being born. Pediatricians and parents, checking indicators of normal growth patterns, follow changes in weight, length, and head circumference (see Appendix B). Generally, breast milk or formula meets an infant's nutritional needs during the first four to six months. Thereafter, the introduction of solid foods becomes a strong nutrient contributor.

How much energy and protein does an infant need?

An infant requires about 45 to 50 Cal per pound of body weight. This need is about twice as high as for adults when we look at it relative to body weight. Breast milk or most formulas will provide about 700 Cal per quart or liter. The addition of solid foods in the latter half of infancy makes a significant energy contribution.

Protein needs are also much higher for infants than for adults. Infants require about 1.5 to 2 g of protein/kg body weight (0.7 to 1.0 g of protein per pound). Furthermore, at least 40 percent of the protein should come from more complete protein sources. In general, protein should contribute 20 percent or a little less to an infant's energy intake, with fat (30 to 50 percent) and carbohydrate (30 to 50 percent) making up the remainder. The energy in mature breast milk is comprised of about 17 percent protein, 54 percent fat, and 40 percent carbohydrate. Cow's milk formulas approximate these percentages, although they are slightly higher in protein (18 percent) and lower in fat (43 percent). Fat recommendations are higher for infants than for adults due to their high energy need versus their relatively small food intake. Do not worry about their blood lipids yet as their growth and development are more important. In fact, recommendations by the American Heart Association for eating a lower fat diet do not begin until after they have reached two years of age.

Are vitamin and mineral needs greater during infancy?

Relative to body weight, vitamin and mineral needs are also higher during infancy versus adulthood. Because the vitamin K content of breast milk is low and an infant's digestive tract will not develop a healthy bacteria population for a few months, vitamin K is often administered to infants. A vitamin D supplement may be necessary for breast-fed infants who receive minimal exposure to sunlight or who have darker skin. Complementing breast-feeding with a vitamin D-fortified infant formula can assist in meeting an infant's needs. Because the iron content of breast milk is relatively low, the introduction to solid foods between ages four to six months becomes very important in supplying this nutrient. Iron-fortified cereals are very good choices. Many pediatricians will recommend an iron supplement for infants during their first few months of life. Again, complementing breast-feeding with an iron-fortified infant formula can assist in meeting an infant's needs. Also, infants fed a vegan or other meat-restrictive diets would need a vitamin B_{12} supplement.

When should an infant advance to solid foods?

The transition to solid foods (see Box 12.2) should begin when the infant is ready, not necessarily when the parent is ready. An infant will let you know through physical signs when they are prepared for solid foods. One of these signs is a relaxation of the gag reflex. The gag reflex propels undesirable items forward and out of the mouth. This reflex is strongest in infants and is still maintained to some degree throughout our life. This is the same reflex felt when adults put a finger in the back of the mouth. Relaxation of the gag reflex allows an infant to swallow foods of a more solid consistency, such as cereals

---

BOX 12.2. Recommended Progression of Feeding During Infancy

0-4 months	Breast milk or formula
4-6 months	Iron-fortified cereals when infant is ready while still breast-feeding or formula feeding
6-9 months	Strained vegetables, fruits, and meats are added to cereals while still breast-feeding or formula feeding
9-12 months	Gradual introduction to cut and mashed table foods; meats should be cooked well to minimize chewing; juice in a small cup becomes appropriate; breast-feeding or formula feeding continues

---

and purees. The ability of infants to form their mouths around spoons is another sign that solid foods are becoming more appropriate.

Early in the transition to solid foods infants will not have the hand dexterity and hand-to-mouth coordination to feed themselves. However, within the ensuing months they develop these capabilities. Also during this time, teeth begin to appear, and an infant may begin to take small sips from a cup. Usually by age nine months, infants are able to participate in a meal as they begin to play with plates, cups, and perhaps help support a cup when drinking. By ten months, infants may be feeding themselves finger foods and drinking from a cup; however, a thorough cleaning of the infant and the surrounding area usually is necessary following these feats.

How do food allergies develop?

The development of many food allergies or food intolerances is believed to originate in the earlier months of life. Scientists have estimated that about one-third of Americans are sensitive to one or more food components. Although the digestive tract is rapidly developing during the first few months of infancy, there remains the potential for complete or semicomplete food proteins to cross the wall of the digestive tract and enter the body. When this occurs, an infant's immune system recognizes this substance as foreign and destroys it. At the same time an infant develops "immune memory" of that substance for future reference. This immune memory includes a routine production of antibodies that specifically recognize that substance. These antibodies allow the body to develop a very rapid and full-blown immune response when exposed to that substance again in the future. This response causes the release of chemicals in the body (e.g., histamine and serotonin), which may cause any number of the following actions: itchiness, swelling, vomiting, asthma, diarrhea, headache, skin reactions, or a runny nose.

Even in the mature digestive tract of children and adults there still remains a slim chance that fragments of intact substances are absorbed. When this occurs, an allergic reaction ensues. Many factors in the diet may elicit the characteristics of a food allergy or intolerance. Some of the more common foods containing these substances include those food items listed in Box 12.3. Sometimes a food allergy is difficult to identify. Physicians who specialize in this area (allergists) may have the allergic patient eat a very plain diet and then introduce foods that are suspect one at a time until the culprit food is identified.

Food intolerance is often confused with allergies. However, the major difference is that the symptoms of food intolerance are mostly experienced in the digestive tract and include cramping, bloating, and diarrhea. The symptoms of a food allergy are said to be systemic, which means throughout the body and can include the digestive tract. The most common food intolerance is lactose intolerance, as described in Chapter 4.

KIDS GROW FAST

How are eating behaviors affected during childhood and adolescence?

The progression from infancy to childhood and then adolescence brings many new eating situations and experiences. During early

---

BOX 12.3. Food Items Suspect in Many Food Allergies

Fish and other seafood	Tomatoes
Oranges and citrus fruits	Wheat
Eggs	Cucumbers
Garlic	Nuts (especially peanuts)
Chocolate	Mustard
Various colorants and flavorants	Milk
Oats and oatmeal	Rye
Legumes	Corn

childhood if not well before, children are weaned from breast milk or formula completely and have also made the transition from infant foods to regular foods. Eating develops into a very social and impressionable time in our lives. The number of meals children eat in a day will decrease and many food likes/dislikes and eating behaviors are formed in childhood. Children watch others at the table and even respond to moods and changes in the environment at the table. During childhood, television, radio, and interaction with peers at day care, camps, and grade school impact the development of children's likes/dislikes and eating behaviors. Many of these characteristics remain throughout life, while others are phases.

How much growth can be expected during childhood and adolescence?

The rapid pace of growth of infancy slows during early childhood, and a typical weight gain for the second year is only five pounds. During this time, though, body composition is changing slightly as fat percentage decreases and lean tissue increases. Within the next few years the rate of gain in both height and weight further slows. Then, sometime around age seven, the rate of weight gain escalates and does not begin to taper off until the midteen years. The rate of height growth tapers until a growth spurt is recognized sometime around 10 to 12 for girls and 11 to 14 for boys (see Figure 12.1).

During infancy, the status of height, weight, and head circumference, relative to other infants of the same age and gender, can be used to gauge growth and ability to thrive. This assessment can be continued throughout childhood and adolescence as well, although only height and weight are used during this time. These measurements are used for placement at a certain percentile in reference to other children.

What if a child refuses to eat certain foods?

The number of meals and relative food intake decreases during childhood. Therefore, it is important to provide a variety of nutrient-dense foods, including meats (if applicable), fruits, and vegetables. Children should be encouraged but not necessarily forced to eat a variety of foods.

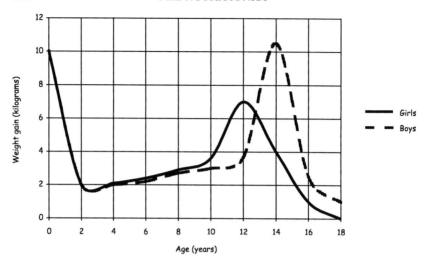

FIGURE 12.1. Average annual weight gain of boys and girls.

Since many children avoid or refuse to eat vegetables, what should a concerned parent do? First, be sure that you and others at the table set a positive example. Second, a policy of taking "one bite" of every item on the plate may help a child overcome an aversion to a food over time. Also, children may become more comfortable with a food if they participate in its preparation or serving. Perhaps even naming the dish after the child may increase interest. For example, Cindy's cool carrots, Gail's groovy peas, Mark's marvelous macaroni, David's delicious bread, Connie's crazy cauliflower, Lou's lovable lasagna, and Carol's wonderful broccoli.

Is childhood and adolescent obesity a concern?

Childhood and adolescent obesity is definitely a growing concern in the United States. It appears that the combination of reduced activity, more television and computer time, and the increased availability of foods (especially fat-laden foods), have rendered America's youth heavier than ever before. The incidence of Type 2 diabetes mellitus in adolescence continues to climb along with the diagnosis of hypercholesterolemia and hypertension.

Sadly, about 40 percent of obese children and 70 percent of obese adolescents maintain their obese status into adulthood. In addition, obese children who lose the excessive body fat before becoming adults are more prone to achieving obesity during adulthood than children who never were obese. This is a huge concern as we are all aware of the low success rates of weight reduction and maintenance in adults. It really seems that the key to lowering the number of obese adults is to decrease the inclination toward an obesity-prone lifestyle in children. This includes increasing the activity level in children and increasing nutrition and health awareness. Many nutritionists feel that focusing on adult obesity should be secondary to efforts to prevent obesity in children. Children are still forming many of their behaviors that will be with them throughout their lives. Meanwhile, adults who are inactive and who were not active as children have a more difficult time adhering to a lifestyle that is more active and includes exercise.

The television blitz of high-fat food commercials, such as cookies and snack chips, during child and teen programming seems to be very effective in boosting product sales along with the body fat of the targeted audience. Food and the money to buy food have never been so available to children and adolescents as they are today. On almost every child's walk to school or across town they encounter a convenience store, supermarket, cookie shop, pizza joint, or ice cream/yogurt parlor. One growing concern many parents have is the management of grade-school cafeterias and the installation of fast food chains in schools. This raises concern since children and adolescents are still developing eating patterns that may last a lifetime. It is not coincidence that every fast food chain seems to be found in every shopping mall. Malls are one of the primary locations where American kids spend their free time.

What are eating disorders?

Teens become a lot more involved in their self-image. A distorted body image for a teen, or an adult, may result in an eating disorder such as *anorexia nervosa* or *bulimia*. Anorexia nervosa is more common in teenage, white middle-class females who engage in chronic energy restriction to accommodate their fear of being "fat." Even when their body weight is below ideal standards, they still consider themselves "fat" and continue the energy restriction. Combined with reductions in body weight from fat stores are also reductions in body protein. As the ritual continues, the reduction in body protein ultimately affects heart muscle and other vital organs and tissue. Thus, these individuals jeopardize their very existence. Anorexics are obsessed with food and may play with their food when dining with family. They may also have memorized the energy and fat content of most foods.

Bulimia is the practice of bingeing on food only to purge it shortly thereafter. It is not uncommon for a bulimic to ingest several thousand Calories of food in one to two hours. Usually the choice of food during this time includes snack chips, cookies, ice cream, pizza, candy, and other fast food. Self-induced vomiting and an engrossment in guilt shortly follow the eating binge. Bulimia is a self-perpetuating behavioral disorder, as the next food binge becomes a coping vehicle for guilt from the previous binge/purge episode. Physical signs of bulimia may include a discoloration of teeth from frequent vomiting and also cuts to fingers and knuckles from frequent induction of vomiting. Often an individual will have disorder characteristics of both anorexia nervosa and bulimia, often called *bulimiarexia*.

Both anorexia nervosa and bulimia are psychological disorders, which makes them somewhat difficult to treat. Typically treatment will include the efforts of an eating disorders counselor and a dietitian who specializes in eating disorders. Usually there is a root psychological issue that needs to be addressed. Today, many professionals are characterizing some patterns of overeating, leading to obesity, as an eating disorder as well. Here, food is used as a coping or comforting tool. Again, there are probably pyschological issues at work here too.

ADULTS ARE FACED WITH A NEW SET OF NUTRITION CONCERNS

The threshold for adulthood is arbitrary and depends on whom you are asking. Some may define it based upon age, such as eighteen years of age and greater. Others may take a more physiological approach and define it as the point at which one's greatest stature is reached. However, this latter explanation becomes problematic as some humans may reach their maximal stature in their teen years while others may not obtain their peak stature until their early twenties. Since most of this book has discussed nutrition applicable to younger adults, most of the following discussion will focus upon older adults. However, alcohol consumption will first be addressed as the legal drinking age in the United States is twenty-one. Also addressed will be the importance of young adulthood when osteoporosis is discussed and in the next chapter on heart disease and cancer. Young to middle adulthood years are probably the most important years with regard to preventing the most significant diseases plaguing older adults, namely heart disease, cancer, and osteoporosis.

Is alcohol bad for us?

This may be one of the few books that even considers calling alcohol a nutrient. However, it does nourish our body by providing energy, and some research has suggested that ingesting small amounts of alcohol daily is associated with a lower occurrence of heart disease. However, in light of its widespread abuse in the United States and the numerous harmful effects to organs when it is abused, alcohol tends to be forsaken when making a list of human nutrients. Furthermore, it is more likely the other factors found in alcoholic beverages that are primarily responsible for preventing heart disease, not the alcohol itself.

What is alcohol and how does the body metabolize it?

Alcohol is a substance called ethanol or ethyl alcohol. Alcohol is not made in the body, thus alcohol circulating in the blood has been derived from drinking alcohol-containing beverages. Many tissues throughout the body can break down alcohol, but the liver handles the majority of the task by far. In liver cells, alcohol can be used to make a substance called *acetate* (a short chain fatty acid), which then leaves the liver and circulates to other tissue for ATP production. However, this seems to be about where the good news ends. When alcohol is present in the liver, it takes metabolic priority. It is broken down in the liver preferentially before other energy nutrients. When alcohol is consumed in higher amounts, its metabolism can disrupt normal liver cell operations, especially those that generate glucose when blood glucose levels begin to fall. Therefore, it is not uncommon for blood glucose levels to fall below normal several hours after heavy drinking without eating food. There probably is not much to be concerned about when enjoying a glass of wine or two with dinner occasionally or having a couple of beers during the ball game. However, when the quantity and frequency of alcohol consumption increases this can eventually lead to complications.

Other direct or indirect effects of alcohol abuse include impaired drug metabolism and elevated blood uric acid levels. The latter of these situations can lead to gout and kidney stones. Barbiturates, which are sedative drugs (i.e., pentothal, pentobarbital, seconal), are metabolized and inactivated by one of the same mechanisms that metabolizes alcohol. Since the metabolism of alcohol is given higher priority than the inactivation of barbiturates, these drugs stay active longer and build up in the body. Barbiturates depress the CNS, breathing, and heart activity. Therefore, combining barbiturates with alcohol can be a lethal combination.

Long-term alcohol abuse also results in excessive accumulation of lipids and disease in liver cells (fatty liver) as well as other cells throughout the body. Alcohol-related liver disease is the sixth leading killer in the United States. Luckily, the most important liver cells (hepatocytes) can regenerate themselves if the damage is not too severe and the alcohol abuse ceases.

How does nutrition change in later adulthood?

As humans progress through life, many changes occur in nutrition and body function. One such change is a decrease in basal metabolic rate (BMR). Therefore, energy expenditure will generally not be as high as during younger years. Regular exercise can help minimize this reduction by slowing the loss of muscle tissue. In fact, when researchers studied the effects of weight training in older adults they found that their muscularity increased, as did their metabolic rate. So keep up the resistance training!

Scientists have also realized that levels of certain hormones may also decrease with age. We are all familiar with estrogen and menopause for women. Men too seem to experience reductions in testosterone as they age. In fact, physician prescription testosterone for aging men has been called the hormone replacement therapy of the twenty-first century. Not every man's testosterone level decreases over their lifetime, so the best thing to do is monitor the levels regularly.

Adults of an even more advanced age also tend to experience reduced digestive capabilities and decreased senses of taste, smell, and thirst—all of which can certainly impact their nutritional status.

How does the need for vitamins and minerals change with age?

Recent scientific studies have reported that people fifty-one years of age and older can maintain adequate vitamin A status on intakes below their RDA. Contrarily, the requirement for vitamin D in this population may actually be greater than RDA recommendations. It seems as though there is a reduced ability to make vitamin D in the skin as we get older. Furthermore, there may be reductions in the ability to properly metabolize vitamin D in the organs, especially in the liver and kidneys. Some scientists have reported that a dietary intake of vitamin D at about two times the current RDA may be necessary to maintain optimal vitamin D status in older people who receive limited sunlight exposure. Many scientists also feel that the RDAs for other vitamins such as vitamin B_6 and B_{12} and riboflavin are also too low for older people. Increased vitamin E consumption may also be helpful in the prevention of heart disease. Furthermore, the reports of many scientific studies suggest that the 800 mg recommendation for calcium may be inadequate for people fifty-one years of age or older. For these reasons, a multivitamin and mineral supplement would probably benefit most adults over the age of fifty.

OSTEOPOROSIS IS BONES WITH HOLES

Osteoporosis is a reduction in the density of bone. The remaining bone is then compromised in strength and resistance against fracture. It is perhaps the most common medical problem for older women and occurs six to eight times more frequently in women than in men. It is estimated to afflict 25 million Americans. A primary problem resulting from osteoporosis is the greater occurrence of fractures. In fact as many as 1.5 million new fractures are attributable to osteoporosis in the United States each year. Sadly, many of these fractures result in permanent immobility.

The World Health Organization (WHO) has set guidelines for characterizing the degree of bone loss. In order to do so, bone density must be compared to what is typically seen in younger people. *Osteopenia* is a level of bone density reduction that places a person at greater risk of fracture. It is said to be a measured bone density that is 1 to 2.5 standard deviations (SD) below an average (or statistical mean) for a younger person of the same gender. Osteoporosis is more severe, whereby the reduction of bone density is greater than 2.5 SD below the average. Individuals should talk to their physicians about where they are relative to others.

What is the composition of bone?

Bone represents about 12 percent and 15 percent of young adult women's and men's body weight, respectively. That is roughly 5.5 kg (15 lb) for a woman and 11 kg (23 lb) for a man. Typically, when we think of bone, we think of minerals such as calcium and phosphorus, but minerals make up only 30 to 40 percent of bone weight. Beyond minerals, bone is also comprised of bone cells, nerves, blood vessels, collagen, and some other proteins.

Is bone dead or inactive tissue?

Bone is often considered dead or at least inactive tissue. Maybe this comes from images of skeletons at Halloween or the bone fossils of animals that lived long ago. Whatever the case, bone is actually fairly active. It is constantly engaged in remodeling processes by bone cells called osteoblasts and osteoclasts. The osteoblasts are responsible for making and laying down new collagen protein and other substances. The collagen provides the network for the deposition of calcium and phosphorus mineral complexes such as hydroxyapatite to cling to. This is an important and often overlooked point, because without collagen you cannot mineralize bone. For this reason the osteoblasts are said to be active in making new bone tissue and are often called "bone makers."

Osteoclasts, on the other hand, are primarily responsible for initiating the events leading to the breakdown of bone substances. For this reason they are often called "bone destroyers." Osteoclasts ooze acids that will dissolve the mineral complexes as well as enzymes (collagenase) that will dissolve collagen. The actions of osteoclasts may seem destructive, but their role in bone remodeling is pivotal. Also, when osteoclasts break down bone mineral complexes, the minerals can become available to the blood. This could be important in maintaining blood calcium levels.

The activities of osteoblasts and osteoclasts are indeed antagonistic and occur simultaneously. Therefore the body is building new bone at the same time as it is breaking down older bone. This is referred to as "bone turnover" and is similar to tearing up and pouring new concrete for a street or tearing down and constructing a new wall in a building. This reconstruction allows for that street or wall to be most appropriate in its functions.

Throughout life there are periods when the activities of these cells are out of balance. This can be purposeful or pathological. The imbalance in turnover results in either a net gain or loss of bone. For example, in childhood, as bones are lengthening and growing thicker, the activities of osteoblasts will exceed those of the osteoclasts, and new bone is built. On the contrary, in later adulthood, osteoclast cell activity seems to be greater than osteoblast activity. This results in a slow loss of bone matrix. During periods when there is neither a net loss nor gain of bone, the activities of osteoblasts and osteoclasts are in balance and coordinated to properly remodel bone.

Even though a finalized bone length and therefore adult height is realized in the late teens to early twenties, bone is constantly being remodeled. The turnover process is governed by factors such as hormones (growth hormone, PTH, estrogen, testosterone, and calcitonin) and vitamin D. Mechanical forces, such as pressure exerted upon bone during resistance exercise, also play a big role in bone turnover. These factors affect bone remodeling primarily by increasing or decreasing the activity of osteoclasts and osteoblasts.

When are bones the densest, and how much mineral is lost from that point?

Throughout the first few decades of human life, and providing that adequate minerals are provided by diet, the body deposits these minerals into bone in order to strengthen it and also to serve as a future mineral reservoir. Humans typically reach peak bone mass (PBM) or maximal bone density (MBD) by their late twenties to very early thirties. After this time, bone density seems to decrease slowly.

The decrease in bone density appears to be more substantial in women versus men. It has been estimated that a woman may lose 27 percent or more of her bone mineral from peak bone mass to her seventies. Bone mineral losses of up to 50 percent have been reported in women diagnosed with osteoporosis. Generally, osteoporosis develops without symptoms. It is usually not until a person fractures a bone or complains of severe back pain that an X-ray diagnosis is made. The point should again be made that while the focus has largely been on minerals, osteoporosis is a disease resulting from loss of bone material in general. This means that protein as well as minerals are lost, and as mentioned above, some scientists believe that the key to preventing osteoporosis may actually be founded in preserving the collagen foundation. Without collagen, the minerals could not stick in bone. Perhaps the analogy of hanging drywall on the wooden frame of a house will help. Here the wooden frame is collagen and the drywall is hydroxyapatite. In fact, hydroxyapatite crystals resemble sheets of drywall (see Figure 10.1).

What factors are involved in the loss of bone mineral?

A reduction in blood estrogen levels, as typical after menopause (postmenopausal), is directly associated with a decrease in bone density. Thus, estrogen is a principal factor in the development of osteoporosis. Researchers have reported that osteoblasts (bone makers) have receptors for the hormone estrogen, and estrogen also appears to decrease the activity of osteoclasts (bone destroyers). Despite these findings, the exact mechanisms for how estrogen protects women against excessive bone material losses is not clear. Postmenopausal estrogen replacement therapy (ERT) has proven effective in slowing the rate of postmenopausal bone mineral loss in women. Beyond reductions in circulating estrogen in postmenopausal women, other factors can increase the loss of bone mineral. These factors include poor calcium and/or vitamin D intake as well as abnormalities in metabolism.

Beyond hormonal and nutritional influences, other factors directly affect bone mineral content. Physical activity increases the mechanical stress placed on bone and stimulates a reinforcement of bone strength. Perhaps this effect is most obvious in the absence of any weight-bearing demands upon bone. For instance, astronauts subjected to extended periods of time in space at zero gravity (weightlessness) experience decreases in bone density. On the other hand, regular weight-bearing exercise seems to help strengthen bone and also to slow the gradual loss of bone material as the body ages.

Smoking seems to exert a negative influence upon bone mineral content and the rate of bone mineral loss, especially in postmenopausal years. Smokers tend to have lower bone densities than nonsmokers. One reason for this occurrence is that smoking reduces blood estrogen levels. Smokers also seem to reach menopause at a younger age.

Can osteoporosis occur earlier in life?

Although osteoporosis is most often diagnosed in postmenopausal women, it should be noted that signs of osteoporosis have been observed in younger women as well. Younger female athletes who are excessively lean can reduce or halt their estrogen production and establish the opportunity for bone loss. In addition, the positive effects of weight-bearing exercise are not apparent in excessive lean women. The positive effects of resistance training will not balance out the negative impact of reduced estrogen levels.

Anorexia nervosa, which is most common in teenage and younger adult women, is characterized by abnormally low body weight. This state can also reduce estrogen production and invoke bone demineralization.

What are the most conventional ways to prevent osteoporosis?

The best defense against osteoporosis is a good offense. Some weight-bearing exercise and a diet providing adequate protein, vitamin D, calcium, manganese, boron, zinc, vitamin C, copper, and iron in the years prior to peak bone mass will optimize bone density. The latter minerals and vitamin C are important for making proper collagen. An early start and a continuation of these practices throughout adulthood in conjunction with regular medical checkups and a periodic X ray will provide the most benefit. In fact, it seems that one of the most important times for the positive effects of activity on bone density is during the prepuberty years. Children should be encouraged to be involved in physical activities. Also, discuss menopausal/postmenopausal hormone replacement therapy with a physician; and do not smoke and encourage others to quit as well.

Are there nutraceuticals that can help prevent osteoporosis?

Recently the limelight has been upon some interesting factors in foods that may have an impact on bone health. Perhaps the most promising nutraceutical (see Chapter 3) substances in the prevention of osteoporosis are isoflavones found mostly in soybeans and soy foods (tofu, tempeh, and miso). There are about twelve forms of isoflavones in soy, including genestein and daidzein. Scientists believe that these factors may have the ability to bind to estrogen receptors and that would include those in bone tissue. At this time scientists are optimistic that a positive link exists between soy or isoflavone consumption and bone health. However, it will probably take time and a few well-performed human studies to draw more specific conclusions. So at this time it would seem wise to include some soy in the diet (see Box 12.4).

Can caffeine or coffee cause osteoporosis?

The results of a couple of studies revealed a correlation between excessive coffee consumption and a higher hip-fracture rate. However, even if there is a true effect many researchers believe that there is a safe level of consumption. It does seem that one to three cups of coffee a day is probably not at all a factor in osteoporosis.

BOX 12.4. Ways to Improve Your Soy Intake

Soy nuts

• Eat soy nuts out of hand as you would roasted peanuts; use in party mix; chop up and use to replace other nuts in baking; scatter on chef's salad.

Soybeans

• Cook fresh green soybeans (also called edamame) as you would lima beans and serve as a fresh vegetable. The fresh soybeans have a sweet taste, like peas.
• Use dry soybeans as you would use other dried beans. Soak overnight, cook slowly one to two hours, then use where the recipe calls for kidney, pinto, black, or navy beans.

Soy milk

• Use soy milk in place of regular milk when cooking (puddings, soups, cream sauces) and baking (cakes, cookies, yeast, and quick breads).

Soy flour

• Replace up to one-fourth of the total flour in a baked recipe with soy flour.

Tofu

• Blend softer tofu with tomato sauce or a can of cream soup.
• Use tofu in place of mayonnaise or sour cream in salad dressings or dips.
• Substitute for all or part of the cream cheese in a cheesecake.
• Use in place of cottage, ricotta, and mozzarella cheese in stuffed pasta shells, manicotti, or lasagna.
• Use firm tofu in salads, stir-frys, and soups.
• Make "egg" salad: cut tofu into small pieces, add celery, onion, salt, pepper, low-fat mayonnaise, and mustard.

- Marinate tofu cubes in teriyaki sauce. Grill on skewers with sweet peppers, cherry tomatoes, mushrooms, and zucchini.
- Use in place of beef, pork, or chicken in a stir fry, fajita, or create-a-meal dish.

Tempeh

- Barbecue tempeh, crumble it in chili, stews, and soups, or make it into sloppy joes.
- Cube for kabobs after marinated in teriyaki and broil or grill.
- Crumble it and use in recipes where you would use ground beef or small chunks of meat, like taco meat, burrito meat, or spaghetti sauce.

Soy cheese

- Top a pizza with tempeh crumbles.
- Add a couple of slices of soy cheese as you prepare macaroni and cheese.
- Use in all recipes calling for cheese, baked and unbaked.

Chapter 13

Nutrition and the Major Killers of Humans

A little more than a century ago, infectious diseases including smallpox, tuberculosis, cholera, typhoid, and yellow fever were among the major killers of Americans. Today, advancements in medicine have controlled or nearly eliminated these diseases. However, we are left to deal with seemingly more complicated killers, namely heart disease and cancer. When combined, these two diseases account for roughly 75 percent of the deaths of Americans and are also very prominent medical problems in other developed countries as well. Stroke is the number three killer of Americans and people of many developed countries. The mechanisms that lead to a stroke are often the same as those that contribute to heart disease.

Yet as prominent as heart disease and cancer are, many health professionals are convinced that these diseases are largely preventable or their critical points can be pushed back years to decades for most people. In addition, nutritional intake has proven to be one of the most important factors with regard to the development and treatment of these diseases. The influence of nutrition can be both a matter of what is eaten that supports the development of these diseases as well as what is not eaten that could potentially prevent or slow the progression of these diseases.

Information on these diseases is certainly abundant. However, the Web sites developed by the American Heart Association <www.americanheart.org> and the American Cancer Society <www.cancer.org> are very informative and credible. In addition, look for information and breaking news on *The Nutritionist's* Web page <www.DrNutrition.com>.

HEART DISEASE IS A MATTER OF BAD PLUMBING

Diseases of the heart are many, but heart disease is the term most often used to address a condition in which atherosclerotic development in the arteries of the heart (coronary arteries) impedes blood flow to a region of the heart. When blood flow through a coronary artery is inhibited, the region of the heart that it supplies will suffer—in fact, that tissue suffocates! This type of heart disease is also referred to as coronary heart disease (CHD) or coronary artery disease (CAD) or atherosclerotic heart disease (ASHD). Like many medical terms, atherosclerosis has its roots in the Greek language. *Athero* means gruel or paste and *sclerosis* means hardness.

From the standpoint of energy metabolism, heart muscle cells rely almost exclusively upon aerobic energy metabolism. Heart muscle cells will die in a short period of time (minutes) if they are deprived of O_2. When cells in a region of the heart die, it is medically known as an infarction and is realized in the form of a *heart attack*. The medical term *myocardial infarction* (MI) means death of heart muscle cells.

What are the major components involved in atherosclerosis?

Atherosclerosis is a complex process with many players. The major players of atherosclerosis include macrophages, lipoproteins, platelets, and smooth muscle cells. Other factors involved include calcium and connective tissue proteins. Macrophages are derived from circulating monocytes, which are a type of white blood cell. Remember that many white blood cells function by recognizing substances that are either foreign or no longer of use to the body and then facilitate its destruction. They are the protectors of the body, sort of "biological bouncers," if you will.

Circulating monocytes normally leave the blood by squeezing through the wall of the capillaries, then they patrol the spaces in between the cells. This occurs in tissue throughout the body and can be viewed as a purification operation. When patrolling monocytes come in contact with something that does not belong, they swell and become very mean and aggressive. As these cells will then engulf the undesirable matter and break it down, they are called macrophages. As you know *macro* means large, while *phage* is derived from a Greek word that means to eat. Macrophage literally means big eater!

As discussed several times, lipoproteins are a normal component of the blood. They function to shuttle water-insoluble fat and cholesterol throughout the body. They are basically lipid-laden submarines. Since the cholesterol in the blood is found aboard lipoproteins, total blood cholesterol must then be the sum of the cholesterol being carried in the different types of lipoproteins. A clinical laboratory is able to determine the quantity of cholesterol in each lipoprotein class (e.g., HDL-cholesterol or LDL-cholesterol).

You will also recall that the liver packages up cholesterol and triglyceride (fat) into very low density lipoproteins (VLDLs), which are then released into the blood. As VLDLs circulate, they unload their fat cargo with most of it going to fat (adipose) tissue and other tissue such as skeletal muscle and the heart. As they lose their fat, VLDLs become LDLs, which are left with mostly a cargo of cholesterol. LDLs then can continue to circulate and drop off cholesterol in tissue throughout the body. Also, as LDLs circulate and unload their cholesterol, they are subject to removal from the blood by the liver and other tissue.

HDLs are made by the liver and intestines. As HDLs circulate they pick up excessive cholesterol from tissue throughout the body. HDLs then transfer this cholesterol back to LDLs, which are subject to removal from the blood, or HDLs themselves are removed from the blood by the liver. In either case, much of the cholesterol that HDLs accumulate on the journey through the body is returned to the liver. So in essence LDLs are cholesterol delivery vehicles, while HDLs go out and pick up the excess.

Where does atherosclerosis occur?

Our arteries can be thought of as blood-filled tubes, the walls of which contain distinct layers. The innermost layer, or the layer closest to the blood, is called the *intima* (see Figure 13.1). The middle layer is referred to as the *media,* as it sits in the middle of the wall and serves as the median of the layers. In between the intima and the surging blood is a fine layer of cells, which is covered with a thin layer of connective tissue proteins (e.g., collagen). It is within the intima that atherosclerosis develops. This means that the fine layer of cells functions as the doorway for blood components to participate in atherosclerosis. As there is not a true doorway by design, one must be cre-

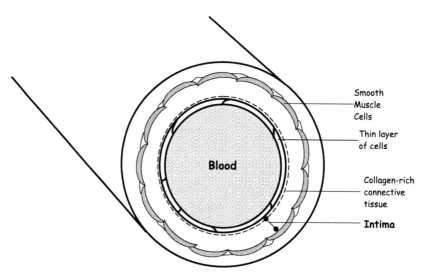

FIGURE 13.1. Basic structure of an artery. The intima is the site of the development of atherosclerosis.

ated to allow atherosclerosis to develop. The damage to the cell lining and connective tissue is often referred to as "injury."

Interestingly, atherosclerosis is much more common at branching points in arteries. Although atherosclerosis can occur in arteries throughout the body, the most common sites are in those arteries supplying the brain and heart. Hindrance of blood flow within the brain and heart can result in a stroke or heart attack, respectively.

How does atherosclerosis occur?

Quite simply, atherosclerosis is a buildup of substances within the intima of arteries. This buildup or *plaque* consists mostly of lipid, protein, and calcium in conjunction with an excessive presence of macrophages and smooth muscle cells. The lipid is mostly cholesterol derived from LDLs while the protein is largely connective tissue proteins, such as collagen. As the atherosclerotic plaque grows in size, it causes the wall of that artery to protrude further and further into the blood vessel. This in turn decreases the area for blood to flow through (see Figure 13.2). If the narrowing becomes severe enough, it becomes an occlusion and blood flow is reduced to a critical level. Furthermore, if a blood clot develops in this location or it circulates to

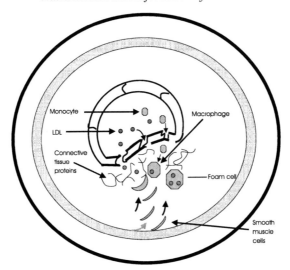

FIGURE 13.2. Injury to the wall of an artery allows LDLs and monocytes access to the intima. Monocytes become macrophages and smooth muscle cells also migrate to the intima. Both macrophages and smooth muscle cells engulf LDLs, especially after they are oxidized. Smooth muscle cells produce connective tissue proteins and calcium becomes deposited in the intima as well.

and gets lodged in this narrowed area, it will dam up blood flow. This is often how heart attacks occur, making them seem so sudden. Basically heart tissue "downstream" does not receive the oxygen that it needs to survive.

As mentioned, scientists believe that an initial injury must occur to the cell wall lining an artery to kick things off. Then a continual insult must occur to allow for atherosclerosis to progress. The injury allows for a lot of monocytes to leave the blood and enter into the intima area. The injured cells lining the artery probably release chemicals that signal monocytes to come in. Platelets arriving on the scene to repair the artery wall also release chemicals. Furthermore, some of the chemicals also encourage the relocation of smooth muscle cells from the media to the intima. LDLs start to move through the injury opening. What we now have is a mixed bag of a lot of stuff arriving in the intima.

The monocytes, which are soon transformed into insatiably hungry macrophages, begin to ingest the LDLs in the intima. It seems that these LDLs are slightly modified from the typical LDLs in the blood.

These modified LDLs are called "oxidized" LDLs, a meal that macrophages find most delicious. Some scientists believe that smooth muscle cells may also begin to engulf the oxidized LDLs. The ingestion of oxidized LDLs by macrophages gives them a foamy appearance (foam cells) when seen with a microscope. Furthermore, smooth muscle cells begin to release fibrous proteins into the area, and calcium-rich complexes also begin to accumulate. While all this is happening, new monocytes and LDLs continuously enter the intima from the blood and smooth muscle cells migrate from the media.

When does atherosclerosis begin?

Although the medical complications of atherosclerosis (i.e., blood vessel occlusion and heart attack) can occur suddenly, the disease really develops over a very long stretch of time (see Box 13.1). Atherosclerosis is a chronic degenerative disease, which means that the inception of atherosclerosis may be established very early in life and merely progresses from there to a critical point. In fact, cadavers of children have shown evidence that the foundations of atherosclerosis may be noticeable as early as ten to twelve years of age. Therefore, it should be realized that atherosclerosis is not a disease of old age but is more likely a disease that builds throughout a lifetime. It is mostly associated with older people because later life is usually the time at which the blockage reaches a critical point, and blood flow becomes insufficient and invokes clinical signs and symptoms such as angina (chest pain).

BOX 13.1. What Is Sudden Cardiac Death?

For many people, atherosclerosis may be undetected as early warning signs of a heart attack have not been experienced. Therefore, when the heart attack does occur it seems unexpected and happens suddenly and without warning. In fact, about half of the people in the United States who die of heart disease experienced sudden cardiac death. This means that early detection is very important.

Warning Signs:
- Chest pain (angina)
- Shortness of breath
- Lightheadedness
- Unexplainable nausea
- Mild anxiety

What influences the development of atherosclerosis?

The origin of atherosclerosis, as well as its progression, probably has an underlying genetic nature. However, various aspects of human lifestyle, such as diet, stress, exercise, smoking, and drinking can indeed modify the rate of progression. Since atherosclerosis is believed to exist to some degree in most people, perhaps disease management should be practiced throughout life. This management would include a low-fat, low-cholesterol diet, no smoking, no chronic heavy drinking or stress, and lots of fruits, vegetables, and exercise. Those of us with better management practices would be at lower risk for experiencing the medical problems associated with advanced atherosclerosis.

What are the risk factors associated with heart disease?

Because various factors seem to promote the development of atherosclerosis, these are referred to as "risk factors" for heart disease. Among the significant controllable risk factors for heart disease are tobacco smoking, high blood pressure (hypertension), obesity, and diabetes mellitus. Also as LDLs are a major player in the development of atherosclerosis, blood lipid profile can help to assess risk as well. Table 5.6 presented a typical lipid profile for a young man. Among the several telling indicators are elevated total and LDL-choleterol levels, reduced HDL-cholesterol levels, and elevated ratios of total cholesterol to HDL-cholesterol and LDL-cholesterol to HDL-cholesterol levels. Furthermore, several ratios have determined to be indicators of risk as well. Because elevations in LDL-cholesterol are associated with increased risk of heart disease, it is often deemed the "bad cholesterol" in our blood. Although it may not be this simple, higher LDL-cholesterol levels would mean that more LDL would be needed to carry the extra cholesterol. This in turn means that there is more LDL in the blood that can participate in atherosclerosis.

On the other hand, as having a higher level of HDL-cholesterol decreases the risk of heart disease, it is often referred to as the "good cholesterol" in the blood. It is believed that some of the virtuous nature of HDLs is due to their ability to gather some of the cholesterol associated with atherosclerotic plaque. This could slow the progression of atherosclerosis. Others believe that HDLs carry an antioxidant.

Having a total blood cholesterol greater than 200 mg/100 mL, LDL-cholesterol > 140 mg, and a ratio of LDL to HDL-cholesterol greater than 4:1 places an individual at an increased risk of heart disease. Other aspects of human lifestyle that also increase the risk of heart disease include obesity; eating a high fat and high cholesterol diet with a high percentage of saturated fat; inactivity; smoking; stress; poor fruit, vegetable, and whole grain consumption; and chronic overconsumption of alcohol. These latter factors may express an independent risk as well as contribute to the development of major risk factors.

The above factors are deemed risks because of their statistical relationship to atherosclerotic disease. For people diagnosed with heart disease, usually one or several of these risk factors is present. However, the presence of one or more of these risks does not guarantee the development of heart disease—again, reemphasizing the probable underlying genetic component. Further support for an underlying genetic component is the incidence of heart disease within a given family even when individuals attempt to minimize their risk factors by doing all the "right things." Therefore, family history or genetic predisposition is often regarded as one of the strongest risk factors.

What is the relationship between LDL-cholesterol and HDL-cholesterol?

Because cholesterol is transported in more than one form of lipoprotein, and different lipoproteins seem to carry a different risk for heart disease, it is important to determine lipoprotein-cholesterol fractions. In general, higher levels of HDL-cholesterol are associated with a lower risk of heart disease. Many medical professionals believe that a HDL-cholesterol less than 35 mg/100 mL of blood and/or 15 percent of total cholesterol may be a better predictor of heart disease than total cholesterol itself. In addition, recent research efforts suggest that this threshold may be too low for women. These research findings suggest that HDL-cholesterol less than 50 mg/100 mL of blood may be a more sensitive risk factor for women. Aerobic exercise, moderate continuing alcohol consumption, estrogen replacement therapy, and loss of excessive body weight appear to increase HDL-cholesterol levels in the blood. Smoking seems to decrease HDL-cholesterol levels. Normal levels of HDL-cholesterol are about 30 to 90 mg per 100 mL of blood.

LDL is called bad cholesterol because as its level increases in the blood, so does the risk of heart disease. As mentioned above, the more LDL in the blood, the more LDL can move into the artery walls and participate in atherosclerosis. As discussed shortly, high fat diets with a greater amount saturated fat increase LDL-cholesterol levels. Smoking may also increase LDL-cholesterol levels in some people. Normal levels of LDL-cholesterol are about 50 to 140 mg per 100 mL of blood. As HDL- and LDL-cholesterol are considered "good" and "bad" cholesterol respectively, their ratio can also be used to predict the risk of heart disease. Here the risk of heart disease increases as the LDL-cholesterol to HDL-cholesterol ratio exceeds 4:1. Similarly, total cholesterol to HDL-cholesterol ratio can be used to assess risk as well. A ratio of total cholesterol to HDL-cholesterol of 3.5:1 is considered healthy and risk increases as the ratio climbs above 5:1. This is because most of the cholesterol in the blood is found in LDL, so total cholesterol would reflect LDL-cholesterol. This is especially true in inactive people.

How does diet cholesterol impact the development of heart disease?

One of the earliest recommendations for reducing blood cholesterol levels was to follow a low cholesterol diet. This was evident on food labels: following guidelines established by the federal government, food manufacturers may have used claims such as *low* or *reduced cholesterol* or *cholesterol free* (see Table 3.3). However, it soon became apparent to researchers that blood cholesterol levels are influenced more by how much saturated fat is eaten rather than cholesterol. Cholesterol is derived from animal foods; as a general rule, animal foods that are higher in saturated fat usually contain a significant cholesterol content. Thus, focusing on reducing the level of saturated fat in the diet usually results in a reduction in cholesterol as well.

To go into more detail about the influence of saturated fat and cholesterol upon blood cholesterol levels, first, about 500 to 1000 mg of cholesterol is made in the body daily, with the liver producing the most. This production of cholesterol can be much greater than the amount of cholesterol humans eat, depending on diet. On average, American men and women tend to eat about 337 and 217 mg of cholesterol per day, respectively. Cholesterol is found in meats, poultry, seafood, dairy foods, egg yolks, and organ meats. Some lean foods, such as shrimp and crayfish, are somewhat high in cholesterol. Furthermore, although turkey, chicken, and fish are considered healthier animal foods, their cholesterol content is about the same as lean beef, lamb, and pork.

Interestingly, as more and more cholesterol is ingested, less and less is made in the body. On the other hand, as less cholesterol is ingested and body cholesterol levels decrease, more cholesterol is made. It seems, then, that the body can measure its content of cholesterol and attempts to regulate the amount of cholesterol it makes with respect to the amount of cholesterol in the diet and body cholesterol status. For instance, the impact of eating a diet containing 400 mg of cholesterol versus 300 mg of cholesterol a day results in an increase of only a couple of milligrams of total blood cholesterol. Thus, the negative impact of eating more cholesterol may not be as significant as we think.

The American Heart Association recommends that dietary cholesterol be less than 300 mg daily, a feat easily accomplished when total fat and saturated fat are reduced to less than 30 percent and 10 percent of total daily Calories, respectively. Although some home blood cholesterol testing kits are available, one huge drawback at this time is that they do not assess HDL-cholesterol levels. A total cholesterol level of 210 mg/100 mL of blood may sound alarming, but what may not be known is that perhaps 65 mg may be attributable to HDL-cholesterol. If this were the case, concern would not be as great. However, for those people who use the home test kits to monitor total cholesterol levels in between visits to their physician, the information can be useful.

Can blood cholesterol levels be too low?

Lower levels of HDL-cholesterol can increase the risk of heart disease, but what about low total cholesterol levels? Scientists spend so much time dealing with the opposite situation that often this question is overlooked. But we should probably know more about this as almost 5 percent of American men have a total cholesterol less than 140 mg/100 mL of blood. Although the risk of heart disease is certainly not a concern, there seems to be a trend toward increased mortality as blood cholesterol levels decrease further and further below 140 mg/100 mL of blood. This condition should be addressed with a physician if it is indeed the case.

How might a diet higher in saturated fat influence risk factors for heart disease?

Eating a diet higher in saturated fat seems to increase total and LDL-cholesterol levels. This is especially true for saturated fat sources endowed with more lauric acid (12:0), myristic acid (14:0), and palmitic acid (16:0). These saturated fatty acids may impact blood cholesterol levels by slowing the mechanisms that remove circulating LDL from the blood. As a result, there is a general increase in total cholesterol complemented by an increase in LDL cholesterol and LDL:HDL-cholesterol ratio. Palmitic acid is the primary saturated fatty acid found in the American diet. Palmitic acid is most concentrated in the fatty tissue of animals (meats). So animal fats and higher fat dairy products (e.g., butter, cream) can raise blood cholesterol levels. Other fat sources to avoid are coconut and palm kernel oil, which contain higher amounts of these "bad" fatty acids.

Today, food labels include the amount of both total cholesterol and saturated fat. However, it is worth mentioning that other saturated fatty acids, such as the stearic, butyric, caproic, caprylic, and capric acids do not seem to have the same blood cholesterol-elevating effect as those saturated fatty acids mentioned previously. It is likely that we may see a more descriptive listing of fatty acids on food labels in the near future.

Do unsaturated fatty acids affect blood cholesterol levels?

Regarding unsaturated fatty acids, neither monounsaturated fatty acids (MUFAs) nor polyunsaturated fatty acids (PUFAs) have a cholesterol-elevating impact. In fact, if they are used to replace saturated fatty acids in the diet, total cholesterol will probably be lowered. This is especially true for people whose blood cholesterol levels were elevated well above recommended levels.

Much interest in MUFAs was generated when studies of heart disease in various populations around the world revealed that certain Mediterranean countries enjoyed a relatively lower incidence of heart disease despite eating a diet that would be considered rich in fat. Further evaluation revealed that these people ingested much of their fat in the form of olive oil, which has a high percentage (77 percent) of the MUFA oleic acid. This spawned several investigations which determined that when oleic acid replaced palmitic acid in a diet, blood cholesterol levels were lowered by decreasing the amount of LDL-cholesterol in the blood.

How do omega-3 and omega-6 PUFAs impact heart disease?

Two PUFA families, omega-3 and omega-6, have received much more attention than others. Linoleic acid, an omega-6 PUFA, has been shown to reduce total blood cholesterol in people. However, some concern followed when it was also revealed in certain studies that a portion of the lowered total cholesterol may be attributable to reductions in HDL-cholesterol as well as LDL-cholesterol. However, many scientists feel that the positive effects of reduced total cholesterol and LDL-cholesterol outweigh the potentially negative impact of reduced HDL-cholesterol levels. Furthermore, as lifestyle recommendations for heart disease prevention include regular HDL-raising aerobic exercise, the effect of omega-6 PUFAs on HDL-cholesterol levels may be counterbalanced.

Omega-3 PUFAs, such as linolenic acid and DHA (docosahexaenoic acid) and EPA (eicosapentaenoic acid) can have a favorable impact on the human blood lipid profile, especially if cholesterol and triglyceride levels are higher to begin with. Substituting saturated fatty acids (the bad ones) with these fatty acids can lower LDL-cholesterol levels and thus total cholesterol levels. However, if the ω-3 PUFA is added to a diet that also maintains a higher amount of saturated fatty acids, then the lowering of LDL-cholesterol may not occur. This reinforces an important point. The most potent way to lower total and LDL-cholesterol is to without question start with a reduction in the saturated fat content of the diet.

At this time, linoleic (18:2 ω-6 PUFA) and linolenic acid (18:3 ω-3 PUFA) are dietary essentials. They are needed by the body to make a family of hormonelike substances called eicosanoids (thromboxanes, prostaglandins, and leukotrienes). EPA (eicosapentaenoic acid) and DHA (docosahexaenoic acid) are ω-3 PUFAs in fish and other sea animals and can substitute for linolenic acid. One of the eicosanoid substances derived from the ω-3 PUFAs is a prostaglandin called prostacyclin or PGI_2. This eicosanoid is very potent in inhibiting blood clotting. This seems to be very significant as many heart attacks occur because a blood clot forms or becomes lodged in a narrowed coronary artery. In fact, individuals who eat diets higher in omega-3 PUFAs, such as certain Eskimo populations, show a lower incidence of heart disease. Omega-3 PUFAs such as EPA and DHA are found in Atlantic and Pacific herring, Atlantic halibut and salmon, coho, albacore tuna, bluefish, lake trout, and pink and king salmons. It is probably a good idea to include these fish in a regular diet a couple of times a week. Linolenic acid can also be found in small quantities in canola oil and soybean oil, and in even smaller amounts in corn oil, beef fat, and lard.

The ω-6 PUFA linoleic acid can be found in safflower, sunflower, corn, soybean, and canola oils. This PUFA is used by certain cells to make a particular thromboxane, namely thromboxane A_2, which enhances blood platelet aggregation. This is a key event involved in blood clot formation. With respect to heart disease, humans may benefit by not exceeding a diet ratio of omega-6:omega-3 PUFA of about 2 to 4:1.

Should fish oil supplements be used to lower cholesterol?

Although some evidence suggests that fish oil supplements may lower cholesterol levels, this may only be the case in people with very high cholesterol levels. Several questions about the safety and appropriate therapeutic doses for people to take remain unanswered. For these reasons it is difficult to generally recommend fish oil supplements. Perhaps people with very high blood cholesterol and triglyceride levels who have not responded to more conventional nutrition practices may consider their use. However, these individuals should make their physicians aware of the supplementation.

Fish oil supplementation has also been suggested to lower blood pressure in people with high blood pressure as well as improving glucose tolerance in Type 2 diabetes mellitus. While at times research with high blood pressure has shown promise, in many of the studies that did reveal a positive effect, the reduction was small and often did not last. With regard to glucose intolerance and Type 2 diabetes mellitus, which often occurs with hypercholesterolemia, there just is not enough convincing scientific evidence at this point in time to recommend general supplementation.

If an individual decides to try fish oil supplements, he or she should also keep in mind that it may be harder for the blood to clot. As mentioned, the eicosanoids made from omega-3 PUFAs generally make it harder for the blood to clot by decreasing the activities of platelets at the site of a hemorrhage. However, for those people at extreme risk of a heart attack, meaning that coronary arteries are significantly occluded and heart pains (angina) have been experienced, fish oil supplements may decrease the likelihood of sudden cardiac death. This activity is related to a reduction in the clotting capability of the blood, thus reducing the potential for a sudden blockage and heart attack. Fish oil supplementation is often no bed of roses; it's more like a barrel of fish, as an individual can develop a fishy odor. Furthermore, he or she may experience nausea and possibly nosebleeds and a greater sensitivity toward bruising.

Do trans *fatty acids increase the risk of heart disease?*

Trans fatty acids are naturally found in low percentages in most animal fats, including milk and dairy products. These fatty acids are made by bacteria in the stomachs of cows and other grazing animals, by converting *cis* unsaturated fatty acids in grass and leaves to *trans* (see Chapter 5). Also, when vegetable oils are hydrogenated, some of the points of unsaturation are converted from a *cis* to a *trans* design.

It does appear that *trans* fatty acids impact blood lipids in many people by raising total and LDL-cholesterol when compared to oils containing *cis* fatty acids. In addition, HDL-cholesterol levels may also be reduced. Also, when *trans* fatty acids are substituted for saturated fatty acids, blood cholesterol levels are not reduced in a manner similar to *cis* fatty acids. This effect, or lack of an effect, may be partly explained by the influence of fatty acids on LDL receptor cycling. The types of fatty acids eaten will be reflected by the fatty acid composition in the plasma membranes (phospholipid fatty acids). When more of the fatty acids are unsaturated with *cis* double bonds, the plasma membrane will be a little less crowded and more fluid. When LDL receptors surface on the plasma membrane, they actually must migrate to anchoring sites (see Figure 13.3). Once they are anchored they can then bind circulating LDLs and bring it into that cell. The LDL is then broken down and the cholesterol is available to that cell. Meanwhile the receptor is then able to resurface on the plasma membrane and migrate to the anchoring site. This process is often called LDL receptor cycling and the rate-limiting step is the LDL receptor migration from its surfacing site to its anchoring site. Therefore if the migration takes longer, the whole cycle takes longer and less LDL is removed from the blood throughout the day. The kinking of *cis* double bonds of plasma membrane allows neighboring mole-

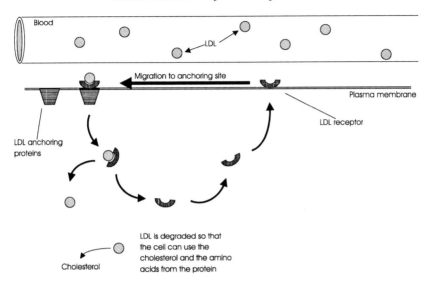

FIGURE 13.3. LDL receptors surface at one point in the plasma membrane and then must migrate to anchoring proteins. Once anchored, LDL can interact with the LDL receptor and the LDL/LDL receptor complex enters the cell. The LDL receptor then dumps the LDL and resurfaces on the plasma membrane. Meanwhile, the LDL is degraded so that the cholesterol can be used by that cell.

cules to push away from one another and render the membrane less crowded. It is like a packed subway station. It is more difficult to get to the correct train when it is packed with people.

The important point is that *trans* fatty acids can have an unhealthy effect similar to saturated fatty acids, only not as potently. Therefore margarine is still better than butter, but, reducing or eliminating both would be healthier still! Furthermore, since hydrogenated fat sources are very integrated into many manufactured foods (e.g., snack foods), the best recommendation for reducing *trans* fatty acids is to reduce total fat intake while also looking for those recipe foods that use vegetable oils or unhydrogenated vegetable oil, not hydrogenated vegetable oils.

What other dietary factors influence the development of heart disease?

Beyond fat and cholesterol, other dietary factors appear to impact the development of atherosclerosis. Studies investigating different diets and the incidence of heart disease have shown that diets richer in fruits and vegetables, fiber, and possibly other diet-derived factors, such as garlic, are associated with a lower incidence of the disease. Fruits and vegetables probably exert a beneficial effect in several ways. First, they can replace fat- or cholesterol-rich foods and also provide more essential nutrients compared to less nutrient-dense foods. Second, fruits, vegetables, and whole grains are sources of health-promoting factors called nutraceuticals (nutrients with pharmaceutical properties), as was discussed in an earlier chapter. Those nutraceutical chemicals derived from plant sources are often referred to as phytochemicals. Among the many nutraceuticals important to heart disease are fibers, antioxidant nutrients, and those that can limit the changes in the heart as it becomes diseased. These factors include vitamins C and E, folate, vitamins B_{12} and B_6, sulfur compounds in garlic and onions, flavonoids in soy, and carotenoids in fruits and vegetables.

Does supplemental vitamin C help deter atherosclerotic development?

Whether supplemental vitamin C at greater than ten times the RDA helps to deter the onset of heart disease is still questionable. Research studies on animals suggest that larger intakes of vitamin C may decrease total blood cholesterol and blood pressure, as well as key events in blood clotting. It is also speculated that vitamin C may reduce the production of LDLs. Whether many of these beneficial effects can be applied to people has been debated by scientists. However, some evidence looks promising. Also, one of the roles of vitamin C in helping prevent heart disease may be to recycle vitamin E, as discussed next.

How about vitamin E?

Vitamin E probably provides some protection against heart disease. Vitamin E circulates throughout the body aboard lipoproteins. As discussed, one of the primary factors associated with atherosclerotic development is the oxidation of fatty acids and proteins in LDL to form oxidized LDL. Vitamin E may provide some antioxidant protection for these molecules. Also, as more and more people try to replace saturated fatty acid sources (i.e., animals fats) with unsaturated fatty acid sources (i.e., vegetable oils), it is feasible that more vitamin E is warranted. Unsaturated fatty acids are much more vulnerable to free-radical attack than are saturated fatty acids. Interestingly, ω-3 PUFAs, such as from fish, may not be a prime target of free radicals as once thought.

In order for vitamin E to provide antioxidant protection it yields one of its electrons to free radicals, thereby inactivating the free radical. When this occurs, vitamin E no longer has antioxidant activity and, in order to become active again, it must acquire another electron. Vitamin C and another substance called glutathione may be key in reloading vitamin E with an electron and thus recycling it.

Does β-carotene decrease the risk of heart disease?

The carotenoids, especially β-carotene, appear to be effective antioxidants. Several large population studies have reported that the incidence of heart disease is lower in people who eat a diet rich in these substances. Whether there is additional benefit of supplementation for individuals eating a diet already rich in carotenoids has not been resolved. Most scientists believe that eating a diet rich in fruits and vegetables and whole grain products will have a greater positive impact than supplements.

Can garlic help prevent heart disease?

Garlic contains three sulfur-containing substances (diallyldisulfide, allicin, and alliin) which are purported to have medicinal properties. Several researchers have reported beneficial effects in reducing risk factors of heart disease with garlic supplementation. These benefits included a lowering of blood cholesterol, reduced blood pressure, and less blood coagulation. However, it should be mentioned that many other researchers have reported that garlic does not provide these benefits. Therefore, the efficacy of garlic supplementation is debatable but does seem promising. All people are encouraged to include more garlic, onions, and leeks in their diet. Garlic supplements may also provide benefit to some people as well. A physician would know if an individual would be a good candidate for experimentation. Also, keep in mind that greater exposure to garlic may be a problem for some people with food allergies.

What role do folate and vitamins B_6 and B_{12} play in relation to heart disease?

Recently it was determined that higher levels of homocytsteine can increase heart disease risk, maybe because homocysteine is involved in oxidizing LDL. Homocysteine is naturally produced in the cells as they go about their molecule-making business. As displayed in Figure 9.3, homocysteine can be converted to the amino acid methionine via the assistance of folate and vitamins B_6 and B_{12}.

How does fiber impact heart disease prevention?

Dietary fiber, especially soluble fiber, which is found in oatmeal, oat bran, beans, some vegetables, and some fruits, may also slow the development of heart disease. These fibers influence blood cholesterol levels by interacting with cholesterol in the digestive tract, and decrease its absorption. Some of this cholesterol is actually in the form of bile, which was made by the liver. Because bile would otherwise be reabsorbed and reused, this forces the liver to use some of the cholesterol it makes daily and/or is present in the blood to make new bile. This ultimately allows small decreases in LDL-cholesterol and total blood cholesterol.

Fiber may impact blood cholesterol in a second manner. When bacteria in the colon metabolizes certain fibers, a small amount of short-chain fatty acids are produced (namely acetic acid [2:0], propionic acid [3:0], and butyric acid [4:0]). Some researchers believe that these fatty acids can be absorbed through the colon and possibly decrease the manufacturing of cholesterol by the liver.

If animal sterols (e.g., cholesterol) are bad, what about plant sterols?

Sterols are a large family of molecules made by plants and animals. While animals are very good at making the sterol called cholesterol, plants make other sterols. In fact, many of us might have a hard time telling the difference between these plant sterols and animal cholesterol (see Figure 13.4).

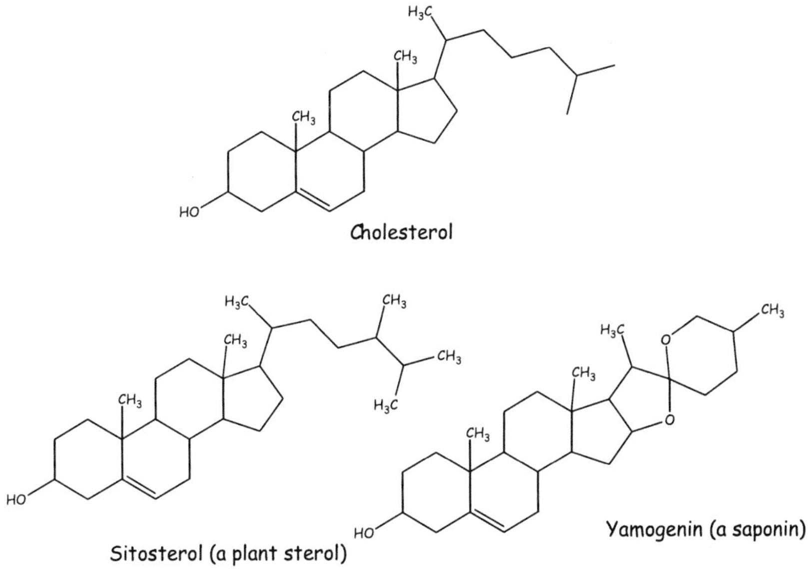

FIGURE 13.4. Cholesterol (animal sterol) and the structure of two plant sterols.

Depending on the quantity of natural plant foods eaten, the diet may contain a couple hundred milligrams of sterols, which interestingly approximates the level of cholesterol in the diet. Research by scientists in the United States and around the globe (such as in Finland) has suggested that sterols such as sitosterol, stigmasterol, campesterol, and sitostanol can lower blood cholesterol levels in some people. As these sterols are found in plant oils, this may help explain some of the cholesterol-reducing properties of those oils. In addition, other related molecules, such as squalene, which is not quite a sterol, and cafestol (in coffee) may help lower blood cholesterol levels. Rice bran oils contain significant amounts of these factors.

Can eating more flavonoids lower the risk of heart disease?

In short, probably. However, the details and recommendations are still a little out of reach at this point. Flavonoids (isoflavones or isoflavonoids, flavones, flavonols, catechins, and anthocyanins) are a class of chemicals produced by plants and are often called polyphenolic compounds with respect to their molecular structure. Onions, citrus, some teas, and red grapes (red wine) contain a flavonoid called quercetin. Researchers in the United States, Finland, and around the world have determined that people who eat or drink less of these chemicals seem to have a higher death rate from heart disease. Some of these flavonoids may act to decrease the level of total and LDL-cholesterol in the blood, while others may decrease free-radical activities, thereby protecting LDL from oxidation as well as helping to protect the walls of the arteries. So again, eat more fruits, vegetables, and whole grains and, if you like, enjoy a glass of red wine daily or a few a week.

Is obesity related to heart disease?

Heart disease is certainly among the list of disease states for which obese people are at a greater risk. The risk appears to increase as the body-fat content increases. Furthermore, obesity is associated with many other risk factors of heart disease such as diabetes, high blood pressure, elevated total cholesterol and LDL-cholesterol, and decreased activity.

As discussed in a previous chapter, scientific understanding of fat (adipose) tissue is evolving. It now seems that as fat cells swell during body fat gain, these cells release substances into the blood (hormones) that may promote some of the risk factors for heart disease listed previously.

Why is smoking related to heart disease?

Cigarette smoke is concentrated with free-radical substances, and some of the effects of these free radicals impact atherosclerosis. Smokers experience more free-radical-generated oxidation of LDL components. This leads to more oxidized LDL and a greater risk of heart disease. Researchers have also reported that smokers may more readily form blood clots as their platelets become more sticky and adhere to blood vessel walls and to each other.

Can drinking wine decrease the risk of heart disease?

A few years back it was recognized that there was a decreased incidence of heart disease in France despite the consumption of a high-fat diet, a phenomenon referred to as the "French paradox." Since it was well known that this population also drinks a lot of red wine, scientists began to investigate the potential benefits of red wine.

The consumption of wine in France, as well as in other countries such as Denmark where similar observations have been reported, is chronic yet only moderate. This is to say that these populations tend to drink wine regularly but in smaller quantities (one to four glasses daily) than in America. Alcohol consumed daily but in small quantities has long been known to reduce the incidence of heart disease in people by perhaps reducing high blood pressure and blood clot formation. Furthermore, it is also likely that certain substances found within the red wine, such as flavonoids and similar molecules, may provide the benefit. These substances may act as antioxidants or have other beneficial effects in regard to heart disease.

The prophylactic effects of alcohol are not limited only to wine. Researchers have determined that alcohol in a variety of forms (i.e., liquor, wine, and beer) consumed chronically but in smaller quantities is associated with reduced risk of heart disease.

What general changes in diet and behavior help reduce the risk of heart disease?

It would seem at this time that many nutritional and behavioral factors are related to heart disease. It is probably best not to focus upon any one or two of these factors but to try to embrace all of them as part of the human lifestyle, at least to some degree.

- Reduce total fat, saturated fatty acid, and cholesterol intake
- Exercise regularly, especially aerobic activities
- Reduce body fat percentage if necessary
- Increase fiber intake to 20 to 35 g/day
- Eat fish at least one to two times weekly
- Do not smoke; and reduce excessive drinking and stress factors

What drugs are prescribed to reduce blood cholesterol?

The drugs commonly prescribed to treat hypercholesterolemia include those that either decrease cholesterol synthesis in the liver, decrease VLDL production, or decrease dietary cholesterol absorption. Drugs such as lovostatin are known to reduce the manufacturing of cholesterol by the liver, although the benefits of this medication may also include increased LDL removal from the blood. Cholestyramine or colestipol will bind cholesterol in the digestive tract and render it unavailable for absorption. Gram doses of nicotinic acid, a form of niacin, seem to decrease the production of VLDL in the liver. It is believed that nicotinic acid impedes fat mobilization from the fat cells, which ultimately decreases fatty acids returning to the liver. If fewer fatty acids are in the liver, then less VLDL will be made.

Does estrogen replacement therapy during and after menopause decrease heart disease risk?

In a word, yes! Time and time again researchers have determined that while estrogen replacement therapy (ERT) can help protect women from osteoporosis-related bone fractures, it can also help protect them against heart disease. However, while ERT is generally recommended, it should not be taken lightly. Some studies have found that while the risk of osteoporosis-related fractures and heart attacks can decrease, the risk of breast cancer may increase. This issue will be addressed later in this chapter.

Is iron status in the body related to heart disease?

A few years ago research reported that a relationship may exist between heart attacks and higher levels of an iron-storing protein that may be found in our blood. The protein, ferritin, is typically found in tissue such as the liver and is a storage container for iron atoms. However, some ferritin can leak out of cells and circulate. As the level of ferritin in the blood increases, it is assumed that there is more iron in the body. The researchers noted that the risk of a heart attack was highest in those individuals with higher ferritin levels in conjunction with a higher LDL-cholesterol level (> 193 mg/100 mL of blood).

Since then other researchers have reported that while total dietary iron intake was not associated with a greater risk of a heart attack, higher intake of heme iron was indeed associated with a greater risk. Heme iron comes from animal sources, largely red meat. Those men with a higher heme iron intake who took a vitamin E supplement were at a slightly lower risk for heart attack than those men without a vitamin E supplement. In addition, factors such as smoking and diabetes also placed those men with a higher heme iron intake at an even higher risk of heart attack.

Can ubiquinone be helpful in preventing heart attacks?

Ubiquinone (coenzyme Q) is found in a variety of plants and animals, and better food sources include meats (especially organ meats such as heart and liver), sardines, mackerel, soybean oil, and peanuts. The research involving ubiquinone is difficult to assess for several reasons. Often the studies are short, not long term, or the ubiquinone is provided in addition to other drugs. Some researchers believe that ubiquinone, acting as an antioxidant, can be yet another protective factor against free-radical activity and thus heart disease development. Furthermore, some researchers believe that ubiquinone may decrease damage to heart muscle after it has been deprived of O_2 for a brief period of time. In this situation, when O_2 floods back into the deprived cells, there is an increased opportunity for free-radical production. Ubiquinone may be helpful in dealing with this situation.

HYPERTENSION HURTS THE HEART AND BLOOD VESSELS

As many as one in five Americans (one in four adults) have high blood pressure. This means that as many as 50 million Americans ages six and older have high blood pressure. Of these people, roughly 30 percent do not even realize their blood pressure is elevated. This is because they have not really experienced significant symptoms or have not had a physical examination in a long time.

What is hypertension?

Hypertension is a disorder of circulation in which elevated blood pressure results in increased tension in the walls of the blood vessels. Since it is impossible to routinely measure blood vessel wall tension, hypertension is assessed indirectly by measuring blood pressure. Thus, high blood pressure and hypertension are used to describe the same condition.

Typically, a resting blood pressure greater than 140/90 (read as "140 over 90") is regarded as hypertension. Here, 140 is the *systolic* blood pressure (measured in millimeters of mercury) or the pressure in large arteries when the heart contracts. In contrast, the 90 refers to *diastolic* blood pressure or the pressure in large arteries when the heart relaxes. Many physicians consider blood pressure measures around 120/80 to be healthier.

Why is hypertension deleterious?

Chronic hypertension is a medical problem for at least two reasons: The first problem results from the founding principle of blood flow. Blood always moves down a pressure gradient—from an area of greater pressure to lesser pressure. When the heart contracts (beats), it develops a blood pressure of about 120 millimeters of mercury. This pressure is normally satisfactory to move blood throughout the blood vessels. This is analogous to turning on a garden hose and seeing the water move down a pressure gradient out of the end of the hose. However, if the end of the garden hose is attached to a tank of water which has a certain pressure, the water from the hose cannot move into the tank unless the water pressure in the hose is greater than the water pressure in the tank. The same principle holds true for the heart and circulation. The heart must generate sufficient pressure to overcome the blood pressure in the arteries, otherwise blood will not flow. If the pressure in the arteries is elevated, as occurs in hypertension, the heart has to work harder to generate more pressure to keep the blood flowing. This extra work causes the heart muscle to enlarge or hypertrophy.

Enlargement of the heart as a result of hypertension is called *pathological hypertrophy*. Pathological hypertrophy of the heart is not necessary healthy and is somewhat different from the healthier hypertrophy typically developed with exercise. So the first complication associated with chronic hypertension is an increased workload on the heart. Furthermore, a larger, overworked heart will require much more O_2 and nutrients to perform. This certainly becomes a problem if coronary arteries are partially or significantly occluded due to atherosclerosis.

The second complication associated with chronic hypertension is that the elevated pressure can traumatize blood vessel walls, which leaves them more susceptible to atherosclerotic development, as explained previously. Hypertension can result in other medical complications such as damage to nephrons, the tiny blood processing units of the kidneys.

What factors are associated with hypertension?

Obesity is associated with the development of hypertension. In many obese people, reductions in blood pressure go hand in hand with reductions in body fat. In addition, if exercise is incorporated into the weight-reduction program, blood pressure is reduced beyond that which can be accounted for by weight loss alone. Stress reduction has also been shown to lower elevated blood pressure significantly. Also, individual diet components such as high fat and high saturated fat foods as well as high sodium foods have been associated with the development of hypertension.

The relationship between diets high in sodium and hypertension does not seem to exist in everyone and will be realized in only about 10 percent of people with high blood pressure. These people are sometimes labeled "salt sensitive." This means that their blood pressure can be reduced by following a low-sodium diet (2 g of sodium/day or less). Finally, smoking and/or chronic and excessive alcohol consumption are also associated with hypertension.

How is hypertension treated?

Ideally, the treatment of hypertension begins with nonpharmaceutical intervention, meaning no drugs. If a person is overweight, weight reduction is encouraged; heavy drinkers are encouraged to cut down their intake. Also, regular cardiovascular exercise and stress management is strongly encouraged. If these practices are not successful in reducing the hypertension then the next step usually includes medication in conjunction with dietary and behavior modifications.

Drugs collectively known as *antihypertensives* are used to treat high blood pressure (see Table 13.1). Antihypertensives focus on relaxing blood vessels to lower blood pressure, reducing the production of an enzyme (ACE) in the blood, and maybe even decreasing the performance of the heart. Other drugs include diuretics and central nervous system agents. These drugs generally hinge on modifying the determining factors of blood pressure, which are cardiac output and resistance to blood flow through vessels. Cardiac output, which is how much blood is pumped out of the heart in a minute's time, is the product of stroke volume and heart rate. Resistance to flow is largely influenced by the diameter of blood vessels. The more narrow

TABLE 13.1. Common Drugs Used to Treat Hypertension

Beta-Blockers	Propanolol (Inderal), Nadolo (Corgard), Timolol (Blocadren), Atenolol (Tenormin), Metoprolol (Betaloc, Lopressor), Acebutolol (Sectral), Oxprenolol (Trasicor), Pindolol (Visken), Labetalol (Trandate)
Calcium Antagonists	Verapamil (Calan, Isoptin, Verelan), Felodipine (Plendil, Renedil), Diltiazem (Cardzem), Nimodipine (Nimptop), and Nifedipine (Adalat)
ACE Inhibitors	Captopril (Capoten), Enalapril (Vasotec), Lisinopril (Prinivil, Zestril), Ramipril (Altace), Qunapril (Accupril), Fosinopril (Monopril), Amlodipine (Norvasc), and Nicardipine (Cardene)

the vessels (constriction) the more resistance there will be to blood flowing through them.

$$\text{Blood Pressure} = \text{Cardiac Output} \times \text{Vascular Resistance}$$

The calcium antagonists (Ca channel blockers) slow heart rate and relax blood vessels. Therefore they may decrease blood pressure by addressing both cardiac output and circulation resistance. The ACE inhibitors act by decreasing the activity of an enzyme in the blood called angiotensin converting enzyme (ACE). Angiotensin loosely translates to vascular tension. This enzyme is responsible for activating a hormone called angiotensin to its active form. Active angiotensin (Angiotensin II) is a potent constrictor of blood vessels and also increases aldosterone levels in the blood. Aldosterone in turn can increase the volume of the blood by decreasing the loss of sodium in the urine. The extra sodium in the blood attracts water, which thus swells blood volume. This in turn may increase blood pressure by increasing the resistance of blood flow through blood vessels. Other drugs act to decrease the potency of angiotensin by interfering with its ability to interact with its receptors.

Beta-blockers can decrease heart rate and stroke volume by decreasing the potency of norepinephrine (noradrenaline). To do so the beta-blockers "block" the ability of norepinephrine to interact with receptors called beta-adrenergic receptors. Diuretics work by increasing water loss in urine, which in turn can decrease blood volume, which then may decrease blood pressure.

CANCER IS WHEN GOOD CELLS GO BAD

Cancer is by no means a new disease. Scientists have found evidence of cancer in dinosaur fossils and mummified remains of ancient civilizations. All animals can and do develop cancer (even sharks). Yet because cancer is granted so much attention today it is easy to think of cancer as a modern biological phenomenon. However, it is more likely that cancer is merely a consequence of life, one that perhaps humans have significantly potentiated. Each year more than 550,000 Americans will die as a result of cancer—more than 1,500 Americans lives a day are cut short.

What is the basis of cancer?

Like many diseases, cancer is merely an alteration of normal biological processes. The basis of the cancer is the very foundation of life itself, cell reproduction. As a rule of nature, all cells must come from existing cells. In order to make a new cell, an existing cell grows in size, makes an exact copy of its DNA, and then divides into two identical cells, each with a complete copy of DNA. These two cells can then grow in size, copy their DNA, and divide, creating four cells total. These four cells grow, copy their DNA, and divide to make eight cells. Therefore, in just a few more generations of cell division, thousands of cells can be created (see Figure 13.5).

Throughout life, all tissue in the body grows in this manner until its genetically predetermined size is realized. Thus the brain and other organs will get only so big under normal conditions. At this point there are two possible scenarios. One scenario is that the current cells will exist for extremely long periods. For example, once tissue such as the brain, pancreas, and adrenals reach their intended size, their cells may exist for several decades or even throughout life. These cells simply are arrested in their ability to grow and divide.

The second scenario is that cells of a particular organ or tissue will continuously undergo turnover. The term *turnover* describes the balance between cells being broken down and those being made. New cells are constantly being made to replace cells of the same type that have a limited life span. The replaced cells are either broken down in the body, such as blood cells, or are removed from body surfaces, such as cells lining the digestive tract and skin cells. Cells that line the

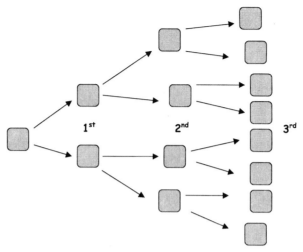

FIGURE 13.5. All cells come from existing cells.

stomach and small intestine may have a life span of only a few days, while a red blood cell will live about four months.

It is important to realize that almost all of the cells in the body inherently possess the ability to grow and divide and that these functions are tightly regulated by certain proteins within these cells. These cell proteins are ultimately produced from DNA genes. Quite simply, cancer is a disruption in this fine regulation. Cells that are arrested in their ability to reproduce can begin to reproduce. Or cells that are already reproducing at a specific rate, such as in the colon, uterus, or prostate, can reproduce at a rate greater than normal, thus resulting in more cells being produced than broken down.

What is the difference between a tumor and cancer?

Not all forms of rapid uncontrolled cell growth are cancerous. Therefore, the term *tumor* is more appropriately applied to any unregulated cell growth. Once the presence of a tumor is recognized, the next step is to discern whether it is benign or malignant. The characteristics of benign compared to malignant are listed in Table 13.2.

Cancer is a disease that is in essence unregulated cell growth of a malignant nature. Thus, cancer is a malignant tumor. Because a benign tumor grows within a fibrous sack of connective tissue with uniform expansion boundaries, it can often be treated by surgical re-

TABLE 13.2. Tumor Characteristics

Benign	Malignant (Cancer)
Usually encapsulated in a fibrous sack which may be surgically removed	Not encapsulated in a fibrous sack therefore making it more difficult to remove surgically
Tumor growth is uniform in expansion boundaries	Cell growth is not uniform in boundaries, again making accurate surgical removal difficult
Has not spread to other regions of the body	Utilizes the blood or lymphatic circulation to spread to other regions of the body
Limited blood supply (arteries and capillaries)	Development of blood vessels to support rapid growth and spread

moval. However, malignant cell growth is not contained and does not show even and somewhat organized expansion. This certainly makes it more difficult to remove completely by surgery.

One deplorable characteristic of malignant cell growth is the ability of some of the cancerous cells to break away from the original tumor site. They then travel in the blood or through lymphatic circulation to find new residency and reproduce in a different region in the body. Thus the cancer is able to spread throughout the body (see Figure 13.6).

What causes a normal cell to go awry?

One way a normal cell can be converted to a tumor-producing cell is by inflicted alterations in the associated genes in DNA. These genes are very special because they contain the instructions for a cell to make the proteins involved in the reproduction of that cell. The process of altering DNA is called a *mutation*.

The factors that can cause mutations to genes include a variety of chemicals and ultraviolet (UV) light. Collectively, substances that can cause DNA mutations relevant to tumor production are referred to as *carcinogenic* agents. Carcinogenic means to potentially give rise to cancer. Fortunately, most mutations in DNA are not harmful. Scientists have estimated that the human body's cells collectively face millions of these assaults on DNA every day. In many cases the mutation does not involve the cell reproduction genes and/or DNA-repair mechanisms quickly repair the damage. DNA repair involves

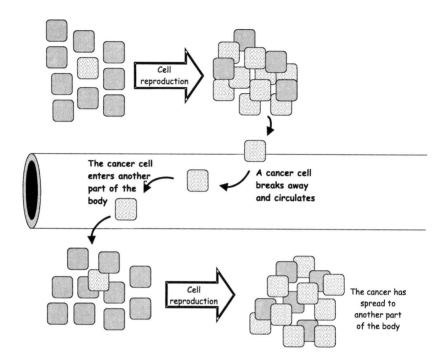

FIGURE 13.6. A single tumor cell will reproduce new tumor cells. If the tumor cells are cancerous, they can break away and circulate elsewhere in the body and spread the cancer.

"proofreading enzymes," so called because they endeavor to check over the DNA, looking for abnormalities, and when found they fix them if they can. Certainly, however, by exposing ourselves to more and more carcinogenic agents we increase the likelihood of developing tumors and cancer.

How is cancer treated?

The treatment of cancer typically involves one of three medical options or a combination of them: surgical removal, radiation therapy, and chemotherapy. These are the proven or conventional modes of treatment. In addition, several other options (see Box 13.2) are available that can be used in conjunction with the conventional modes. These are often called complementary therapies.

BOX 13.2. Complementary Cancer Therapies

Music Therapy	Prayer, spiritual practices
Aromatherapy	Biofeedback
Meditation	Art therapy
Tai Chi	Yoga

Surgical removal of cancerous tissue is somewhat tricky. If the tumor is benign, then cutting out the tumor is somewhat like removing seeds from an apple. However, when the tumor is cancerous, it may be spreading out in an organ unpredictably, which makes it difficult to remove entirely. Theoretically speaking, if even one cancerous cell remains in the body, the tumor can regrow.

How bad is smoking to human health, and is it associated with cancer?

Smoking is the most preventable cause of premature death for people. In fact, one of five deaths of Americans can be directly attributed to tobacco smoking. Almost 90 percent of all lung cancers are due to smoking, and smoking is also highly associated with cancers of the mouth, pharynx, larynx, esophagus, pancreas, uterus, cervix, kidney, and bladder. Clearly, the best thing a smoker can do for himself or herself is to stop smoking as soon as possible.

How is nutrition involved in cancer prevention?

There are many components of the food supply or human lifestyle that have either been shown to or are at least speculated to impact cancer either by increasing or decreasing its occurrence. Those that may provide benefit include vitamins A, E, C, and folate, calcium and selenium, dietary fibers, omega-3 fatty acids, carotenoids, organosulfur compounds, and polyphenolic substances. Those that possibly increase the risk of cancer include fat, alcohol, smoking, nitrites, aflatoxin, and pesticides.

Many chemical carcinogens can be rendered powerless by optimizing normal cell defense mechanisms such as antioxidants and detoxifying enzyme systems. Optimal nutrition helps assure us of maximal defensive mechanisms. Furthermore, once cancer has established itself, optimal nutrition has been reported to slow and in some situations reverse the spread of cancerous cell growth.

Does obesity place us at a higher risk for cancer?

Large studies of populations have indicated that obesity is a significant risk factor for almost all types of human cancer including endometrial, colon, breast, and prostate. Quite simply, individuals who eat less energy and maintain body weights closer to their ideal body weight tend to be at a lower risk for most cancers. Whether increased body fat directly causes cancer is doubtful, but many scientists feel that some of the chemicals that swollen fat cells release can increase the rate of developing cancer. This is because some of these chemicals are associated with the growth of cells and tissue.

Is dietary fat related to cancer?

Eating a diet with a higher percentage of the Calories derived from fat appears to place people at greater risk of many cancers. This may partly be explained by the association between a high fat diet and the development of obesity. However, some researchers believe that a high fat diet exerts an independent effect as well. In addition, diets containing higher amounts of linoleic acid, an essential omega-6 PUFA, have been reported to place people at a greater risk of various cancers.

Why are antioxidants important in cancer prevention?

Vitamin C, carotenoids, vitamin E, selenium, copper, zinc, iron, and manganese are very important factors in normal antioxidant activities. These factors then become very important in cancer prevention as many cancers begin with free-radical damage to key cell components, such as DNA. All of these factors can be found to some degree in fruits and vegetables, which probably is a primary reason why people eating a diet rich in fruits and vegetables are at a lower risk of most cancers. Also, people eating a diet rich in fruits and vegetables tend to eat less fat and exercise more frequently. Whether there is a need for antioxidant supplementation is the subject of much debate.

Can vitamin C decrease the incidence of cancer?

Among all of the vitamins, perhaps vitamin C has received the most attention as an anticancer agent. In many cancer studies involving animals, higher doses of vitamin C have been reported to reduce the incidence of induced cancer. These studies are indeed suggestive of potential benefits for people. However, before making this quantum leap, it is important to realize that many of vitamin C's beneficial effects were shown under conditions which do not necessarily apply to people.

Much of the research involving vitamin C and cancer in people has been correlation studies, which are used to determine an association between the two or more entities. In regard to cancer of the mouth, larynx, or esophagus, as the vitamin C content of the diet increases, the risk for these cancers decreases two to three times. Furthermore, individuals not consuming adequate vitamin C had a two to three times greater risk of stomach cancer. However, several studies failed to show that vitamin C intake was beneficial in reducing the risk of breast, pancreas, or colon cancers.

Although it appears that the benefits of vitamin C are most likely in prevention and not in the treatment of cancer, the dietary amount required to produce benefits is still subject to debate among cancer researchers. There is little doubt that a diet providing less than the RDA for vitamin C places us at greater risk for many cancers; however, the question of debate is whether a vitamin C intake at 5, 10, or 100 times the RDA provides an additional benefit. It is likely that vitamin C intake is not a panacea but instead a very important piece to the puzzle of living a healthier life. An adequate vitamin C intake may not be any more important than abstinence from smoking and heavy drinking, maintaining a lower body fat percentage, engaging in frequent exercise, and eating a lower fat/saturated fat diet rich in fruits and vegetables. A higher vitamin C intake will not necessarily negate other risk factors of cancer.

One important consideration for vitamin C consumption is recognized in smokers. Researchers have reported that it may take as much as a four to six times greater vitamin C intake for smokers to achieve the same blood level of vitamin C as nonsmokers. This is especially important as cigarette smoke contains an abundant supply of free radicals and free-radical-creating substances, and appears to increase the risk for many cancers, especially lung cancer.

Is β-carotene important in cancer prevention?

β-carotene has long been speculated as reducing the risk of cancer. In accordance, several studies of populations have suggested that when people ate more β-carotene the presence of cancer was lower. Recent research has also presented that women with a higher intake of carotenoids have a lower incidence of breast cancer and for a while it became one of the more popular supplements. It has been speculated that the protective properties of β-carotene are related to its antioxidant capabilities. However, when researchers provided β-carotene supplements to smokers, the incidence of lung cancer failed to decrease; it actually increased. Many scientists believe that this was not a direct effect of β-carotene but an indirect effect. Quite simply, as the level of β-carotene increased in their blood, the level of other nutraceuticals decreased. The reason is because many of these substances are lipids and circulate aboard lipoproteins. In order to climb aboard, say, VLDL in the liver, lipids actually must compete with one another for space. Thus when there is an excess of one of these chemicals it can inhibit others from circulating. So perhaps the negative effects of decreased presence of other protective factors overshadowed the potentially positive effects of β-carotene. This further emphasizes the virtues of eating a diet rich in fruits, vegetables, and whole grains rather than looking for "magic bullet" supplements.

Is fiber related to cancer prevention?

Research suggests that as fiber increases in the diet, the risk of colon cancer and certain other cancers decreases. Dietary fiber, by increasing the rate of feces movement through the colon, decreases the time that carcinogenic agents in the digestive tract interact with cells lining the colon. Fiber may also bind carcinogenic substances in the digestive tract and decrease their absorption or interaction with colon cells. On a related note, scientists have suggested that the risk of colon cancer decreases with a healthy calcium intake.

What other substances in food may be important in cancer prevention?

As mentioned several times, people who eat more fruits and vegetables are at a lower risk for various cancers. It now appears that many other factors in these foods, beyond the established nutrients, impact the development of cancer. These substances include phenols, indole, aromatic isothiocyanates, terpenes, and organosulphur compounds. Many of these substances have been studied in cell cultures and also in animals and appear to be very promising. Together with naturally occurring antioxidants such as vitamin C and β-carotene, these products may account for much of the cancer risk-reducing effects associated with diets high in fruits and vegetables.

So, the best things to do nutritionally are

- eat five or more servings of fruits and vegetables a day,
- eat more whole grain products,
- choose foods lower in fat and saturated fat,
- maintain a body weight closer to your ideal body weight,
- engage in regular exercise (especially aerobic) to assist in maintaining a lower body weight and reducing stress,
- limit consumption of fatty red meat, and
- do not use alcohol excessively.

APPENDIX A:
PERIODIC TABLE OF ELEMENTS

1 H Hydrogen								
3 Li Lithium	4 Be Beryllium							
11 Na Sodium	12 Mg Magnesium							
19 K Potassium	20 Ca Calcium	21 Sc Scandium	22 Ti Titanium	23 V Vanadium	24 Cr Chromium	25 Mn Manganese	26 Fe Iron	27 Co Cobalt
37 Rb Rubidium	38 Sr Strontium	39 Y Yttrium	40 Zr Zirconium	41 Nb Niobium	42 Mo Molybdenum	43 Tc Technetium	44 Ru Ruthenium	45 Rh Rhodium
55 Cs Cesium	56 Ba Barium	57 La Lanthanum	72 Hf Hafnium	73 Ta Tantalum	74 W Tungsten	75 Re Rhenium	76 Os Osmium	77 Ir Iridium
87 Fr Francium	88 Ra Radium	89 Ac Actinium	104 Unq Unnilquadium	105 Unp Unnilpentium	106 Unh Unnilhexium			

☐ Component of Human Body

58 Ce Cerium	59 Pr Praseodymium	60 Nd Neodymium	61 Pm Promethium	62 Sm Samarium	63 Eu Europium
90 Th Thorium	91 Pa Protactinium	92 U Uranium	93 Np Neptunium	94 Pu Plutonium	95 Am Americium

								2 **He** Helium
		5 **B** Boron	6 **C** Carbon	7 **N** Nitrogen	8 **O** Oxygen	9 **F** Fluorine	10 **Ne** Neon
		13 **Al** Aluminum	14 **Si** Silicon	15 **P** Phosphorus	16 **S** Sulfur	17 **Cl** Chlorine	18 **Ar** Argon

28 **Ni** Nickel	29 **Cu** Copper	30 **Zn** Zinc	31 **Ga** Gallium	32 **Ge** Germanium	33 **As** Arsenic	34 **Se** Selenium	35 **Br** Bromine	36 **Kr** Krypton
46 **Pd** Palladium	47 **Ag** Silver	48 **Cd** Cadmium	49 **In** Indium	50 **Sn** Tin	51 **Sb** Antimony	52 **Te** Tellurium	53 **I** Iodine	54 **Xe** Xenon
78 **Pt** Platinum	79 **Au** Gold	80 **Hg** Mercury	81 **Tl** Thallium	82 **Pb** Lead	83 **Bi** Bismuth	84 **Po** Polonium	85 **At** Astatine	86 **Rn** Radon

64 **Gd** Gadolinium	65 **Tb** Terbium	66 **Dy** Dysprosium	67 **Ho** Holmium	68 **Er** Erbium	69 **Tm** Thulium	70 **Yb** Ytterbium	71 **Lu** Lutetium
96 **Cm** Curium	97 **Bk** Berkelium	98 **Cf** Californium	99 **Es** Einsteinium	100 **Fm** Fermium	101 **Md** Mendelevium	102 **No** Nobelium	103 **Lr** Lawrencium

APPENDIX B:
CDC GROWTH CHARTS,
UNITED STATES

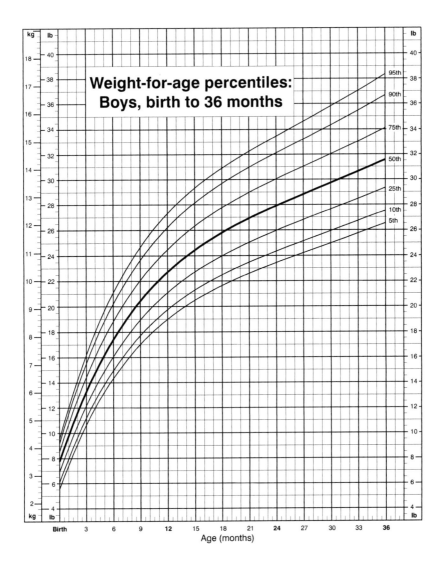

Source: Developed by the National Center for Health Statistics in collaboration with the National Center for Chronic Disease Prevention and Health Promotion (2000).

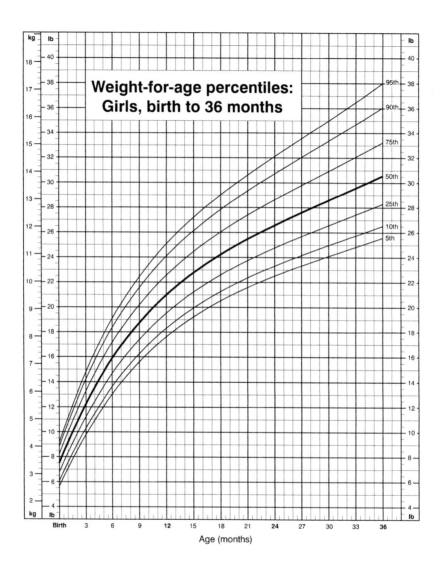

Source: Developed by the National Center for Health Statistics in collaboration with the National Center for Chronic Disease Prevention and Health Promotion (2000).

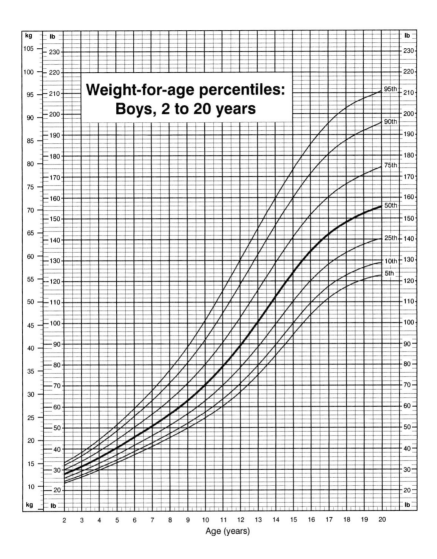

Weight-for-age percentiles: Boys, 2 to 20 years

Source: Developed by the National Center for Health Statistics in collaboration with the National Center for Chronic Disease Prevention and Health Promotion (2000).

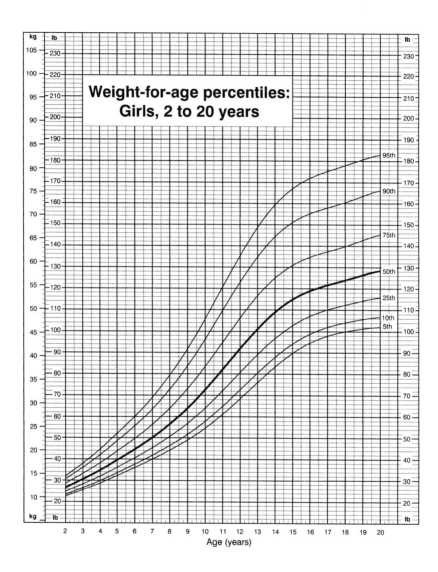

Source: Developed by the National Center for Health Statistics in collaboration with the National Center for Chronic Disease Prevention and Health Promotion (2000).

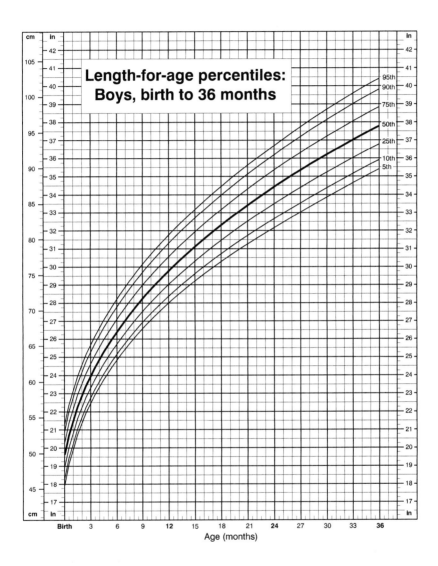

**Length-for-age percentiles:
Boys, birth to 36 months**

Age (months)

Source: Developed by the National Center for Health Statistics in collaboration with the National Center for Chronic Disease Prevention and Health Promotion (2000).

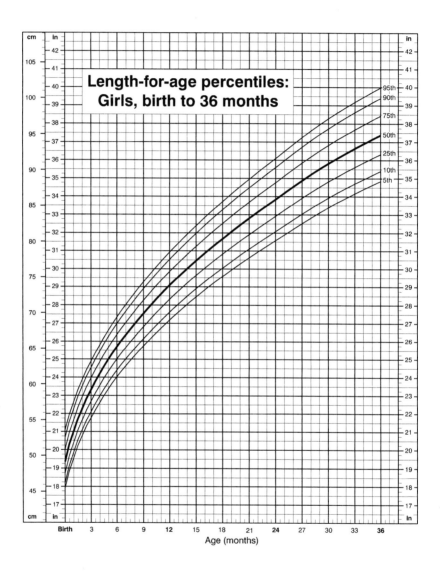

Source: Developed by the National Center for Health Statistics in collaboration with the National Center for Chronic Disease Prevention and Health Promotion (2000).

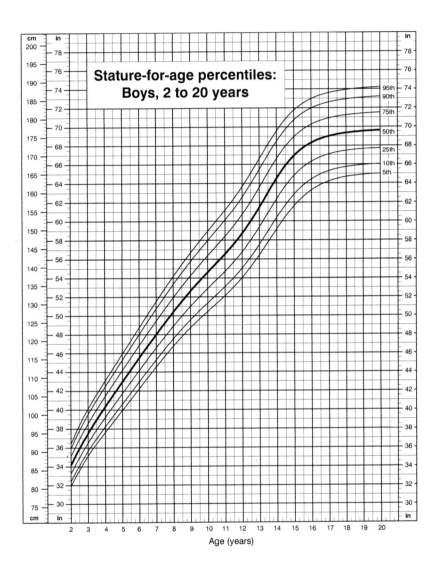

Stature-for-age percentiles:
Boys, 2 to 20 years

Age (years)

Source: Developed by the National Center for Health Statistics in collaboration with the National Center for Chronic Disease Prevention and Health Promotion (2000).

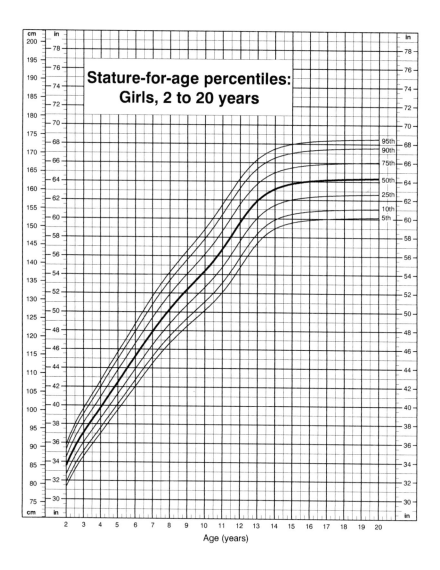

Source: Developed by the National Center for Health Statistics in collaboration with the National Center for Chronic Disease Prevention and Health Promotion (2000).

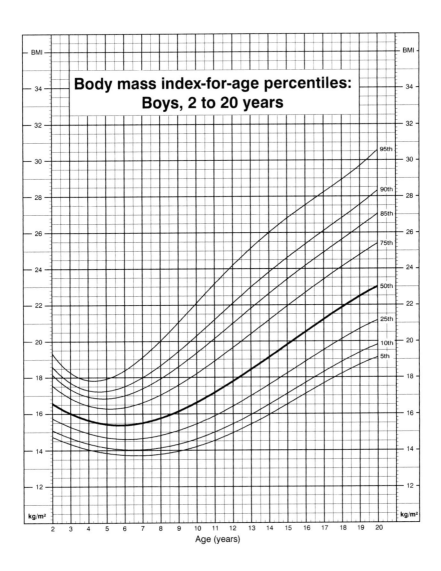

Source: Developed by the National Center for Health Statistics in collaboration with the National Center for Chronic Disease Prevention and Health Promotion (2000).

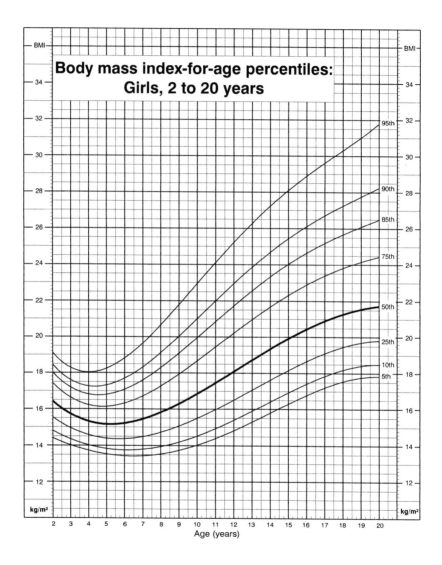

Source: Developed by the National Center for Health Statistics in collaboration with the National Center for Chronic Disease Prevention and Health Promotion (2000).

Suggested Readings

General Reading

American Heart Association (1998). *American Heart Association Low-Fat, Low Cholesterol Cookbook: Heart-Healthy, Easy-to-Make Recipes That Taste Great.* New York: Times Books.

Bernedot, D. (1999). *Nutrition for the Serious Athlete.* Champaign, IL: Human Kinetics.

Foster, S. and Tyler, V.E. (1999). *Tyler's Honest Herbal,* Fourth Edition. Binghamton, NY: The Haworth Herbal Press.

Gershoff, S. and Whitney, C. (1996). *The Tufts University Guide to Total Nutrition.* New York: HarperCollins.

Peirce, A. (1999). *The American Pharmaceutical Association Practical Guide to Natural Medicines.* New York: William Morrow and Co.

Willett, W.C. (2001). *Eat, Drink, and Be Healthy: The Harvard Medical School Guide to Healthy Eating.* New York: Simon and Schuster.

Winawer, S.J. and Shike, M. (1996). *Cancer Free—The Comprehensive Prevention Program.* New York: Simon and Schuster.

Advanced Reading (Academic Texts)

Brown, A. (2000). *Understanding Food—Principles and Preparation.* Belmont, CA: Wadsworth Publishing.

Insel, P., Turner, R.E., and Ross, D. (2001). *Nutrition.* Sudbury, MA: Jones and Bartlett Publishers.

Wardlaw, G.M. (2000). *Perspectives in Nutrition,* Fourth Edition. Burr Ridge, IL: McGraw Hill College Division.

Wildman, R.E.C. (2001). *The Handbook of Nutraceuticals and Functional Foods.* Boca Raton, FL: CRC Press.

Wildman, R.E.C. and Medeiros, D.M. (2000). *Advanced Human Nutrition.* Boca Raton, FL: CRC Press.

Wildman, R.E.C. and Miller, B.S. (2002). *Sport and Fitness Nutrition.* Belmont, CA: Wadsworth Publishing.

Internet Resources

American Academy of Pediatrics. Available online: <www.aap.org>.

American Cancer Society. Available online: <www.cancer.org>.

American College of Sports Medicine. Available online: <www.acsm.org>.
American Diabetes Association. Available online: <www.diabetes.org>.
American Dietetics Association. Available online: <www.eatright.org>.
American Heart Association. Available online: <www.americanheart.org>.
Discovery Health Channel. Available online: <www.discoveryhealth.com>.
National Association of Anorexia Nervosa and Associated Disorders. Available online: <www.anad.org>.
National Osteoporosis Foundation. Available online: <www.nof.org>.
Robert Wildman. Available online: <www.dr.wildman.com>.
Supplement Watch. Available online: <www.supplementwatch.com>.
WebMD. Available online: <www.webmd.com>.

Index

Page numbers followed by the letter "b" indicate boxed material; those followed by the letter "i" indicate illustrations; and those followed by the letter "t" indicate tables.

Order a copy of this book with this form or online at:
http://www.haworthpressinc.com/store/product.asp?sku=4593

THE NUTRITIONIST
Food, Nutrition, and Optimal Health

_____in hardbound at $49.95 (ISBN: 0-7890-1478-5)
_____in softbound at $24.95 (ISBN: 0-7890-1479-3)

COST OF BOOKS_____

OUTSIDE USA/CANADA/
MEXICO: ADD 20%____

POSTAGE & HANDLING_____
(US: $4.00 for first book & $1.50
for each additional book)
Outside US: $5.00 for first book
& $2.00 for each additional book)

SUBTOTAL_____

in Canada: add 7% GST____

STATE TAX____
(NY, OH & MIN residents, please
add appropriate local sales tax)

FINAL TOTAL____
(If paying in Canadian funds,
convert using the current
exchange rate, UNESCO
coupons welcome.)

❑　　**BILL ME LATER:** ($5 service charge will be added)
(Bill-me option is good on US/Canada/Mexico orders only;
not good to jobbers, wholesalers, or subscription agencies.)

❑ Check here if billing address is different from
shipping address and attach purchase order and
billing address information.

Signature_____

❑　**PAYMENT ENCLOSED: $**_____

❑　**PLEASE CHARGE TO MY CREDIT CARD.**

❑ Visa ❑ MasterCard ❑ AmEx ❑ Discover
❑ Diner's Club ❑ Eurocard ❑ JCB

Account # _____

Exp. Date_____

Signature_____

Prices in US dollars and subject to change without notice.

NAME_____

INSTITUTION_____

ADDRESS_____

CITY_____

STATE/ZIP_____

COUNTRY_____ COUNTY (NY residents only)_____

TEL_____ FAX_____

E-MAIL_____

May we use your e-mail address for confirmations and other types of information? ❑ Yes ❑ No
We appreciate receiving your e-mail address and fax number. Haworth would like to e-mail or fax special
discount offers to you, as a preferred customer. **We will never share, rent, or exchange your e-mail address
or fax number.** We regard such actions as an invasion of your privacy.

Order From Your Local Bookstore or Directly From
The Haworth Press, Inc.
10 Alice Street, Binghamton, New York 13904-1580 • USA
TELEPHONE: 1-800-HAWORTH (1-800-429-6784) / Outside US/Canada: (607) 722-5857
FAX: 1-800-895-0582 / Outside US/Canada: (607) 722-6362
E-mail: getinfo@haworthpressinc.com
PLEASE PHOTOCOPY THIS FORM FOR YOUR PERSONAL USE.
www.HaworthPress.com

BOF02